Gestational Diabetes Mellitus

Gestational Diabetes Mellitus

Edited by Eden Kerr

AMERICAN
MEDICAL PUBLISHERS
www.americanmedicalpublishers.com

American Medical Publishers,
41 Flatbush Avenue,
1st Floor, New York,
NY 11217, USA

Visit us on the World Wide Web at:
www.americanmedicalpublishers.com

ISBN: 978-1-63927-153-5

Cataloging-in-Publication Data

Gestational diabetes mellitus / edited by Eden Kerr.
p. cm.
Includes bibliographical references and index.
ISBN 978-1-63927-153-5
1. Diabetes in pregnancy. 2. Pregnancy--Complications. I. Kerr, Eden.
RG580.D5 G47 2021
618.3--dc23

Table of Contents

Preface

Gestational diabetes is a clinical condition in which a woman with no diabetes develops high blood sugar levels during pregnancy. This condition increases the risk of a Cesarean section, pre-eclampsia and depression. If unresolved, babies born to mothers with gestational diabetes may be too large, have low sugar levels post-birth and develop jaundice. They may also be at risk of developing type 2 diabetes and being overweight later on in life. Certain risk factors for gestational diabetes include having a family history of type 2 diabetes, polycystic ovarian syndrome, being overweight or having a previous occurrence of gestational diabetes. In order to asses the risk of developing the condition, screening is advisable between 24 and 28 weeks into gestation. The diagnosis is typically done on the basis of blood tests. The condition can be largely prevented with exercise and maintaining a healthy weight prior to pregnancy. This book contains some path-breaking studies in gestational diabetes mellitus. It outlines the diagnostic and therapeutic interventions in the management of gestational diabetes in detail. It will serve as a valuable source of reference for graduate and post graduate students.

This book is a comprehensive compilation of works of different researchers from varied parts of the world. It includes valuable experiences of the researchers with the sole objective of providing the readers (learners) with a proper knowledge of the concerned field. This book will be beneficial in evoking inspiration and enhancing the knowledge of the interested readers.

In the end, I would like to extend my heartiest thanks to the authors who worked with great determination on their chapters. I also appreciate the publisher's support in the course of the book. I would also like to deeply acknowledge my family who stood by me as a source of inspiration during the project.

Editor

1

Lifestyle and health status in a sample of Swedish women four years after pregnancy: a comparison of women with a history of normal pregnancy and women with a history of gestational diabetes mellitus

Margareta Persson[1,2*], Anna Winkvist[3] and Ingrid Mogren[4]

Abstract

Background: Despite the recommendations to continue the regime of healthy food and physical activity (PA) postpartum for women with previous gestational diabetes mellitus (GDM), the scientific evidence reveals that these recommendations may not be complied to. This study compared lifestyle and health status in women whose pregnancy was complicated by GDM with women who had a normal pregnancy and delivery.

Methods: The inclusion criteria were women with GDM (ICD-10: O24.4 A and O24.4B) and women with uncomplicated pregnancy and delivery in 2005 (ICD-10: O80.0). A random sample of women fulfilling the criteria (n = 882) were identified from the Swedish Medical Birth Register. A questionnaire was sent by mail to eligible women approximately four years after the pregnancy. A total of 444 women (50.8%) agreed to participate, 111 diagnosed with GDM in their pregnancy and 333 with normal pregnancy/delivery.

Results: Women with previous GDM were significantly older, reported higher body weight and less PA before the index pregnancy. No major differences between the groups were noticed regarding lifestyle at the follow-up. Overall, few participants fulfilled the national recommendations of PA and diet. At the follow-up, 19 participants had developed diabetes, all with previous GDM. Women with previous GDM reported significantly poorer self-rated health (SRH), higher level of sick-leave and more often using medication on regular basis. However, a history of GDM or having overt diabetes mellitus showed no association with poorer SRH in the multivariate analysis. Irregular eating habits, no regular PA, overweight/obesity, and regular use of medication were associated with poorer SRH in all participants.

Conclusions: Suboptimal levels of PA, and fruit and vegetable consumption were found in a sample of women with a history of GDM as well as for women with normal pregnancy approximately four years after index pregnancy. Women with previous GDM seem to increase their PA after childbirth, but still they perform their PA at lower intensity than women with a history of normal pregnancy. Having GDM at index pregnancy or being diagnosed with overt diabetes mellitus at follow-up did not demonstrate associations with poorer SRH four years after delivery.

* Correspondence: margareta.persson@umu.se
[1]School of Health and Social Studies, Dalarna University, Falun, Sweden
[2]Department of Nursing, Umeå University, SE – 901 87 Umeå, Sweden
Full list of author information is available at the end of the article

Background

Internationally, gestational diabetes mellitus (GDM) affects a rising number of pregnant women in most ethnic groups [1]. Groups of women of different ethical origins present different prevalences of GDM, where Caucasians show the lowest and Asians the highest prevalence of GDM [2]. In a Swedish study, 44.5% of pregnant women with GDM are of non-Nordic origin, even though 25.3% of all women of fertile age are of non-Nordic origin in the population of the study area [3]. Further, the prevalence of GDM is doubled in overweight and is increased six-fold in obese women [4]. The risk of adverse pregnancy and delivery outcomes is increased for women with GDM. Even women with an oral glucose tolerance test below the diagnostic cut-off for GDM have increased risks of adverse pregnancy and delivery outcomes [5].

Within the first five to ten years after a pregnancy complicated by GDM, the cumulative incidence of type 2 diabetes rapidly increases [6]. The risk of developing type 2 diabetes is more than seven-fold for women with previous GDM compared to women with normoglycemic pregnancies [7].

According to a Cochrane review [8], interventions of either diet or exercise alone do not affect the incidence of type 2 diabetes in high-risk populations. Combined diet-and exercise intervention has demonstrated positive effects on blood pressure, body weight, and waist circumference, and also a decrease of the incidence of type 2 diabetes by 37% [8].

Women with previous GDM are recommended lifestyle interventions to prevent overt diabetes mellitus [9]. However, more women gain weight than lose weight postpartum, despite their risk of developing overt diabetes [10]. Perceived barriers to maintain healthy eating and physical activity (PA) postpartum include constraints related to time, finances, child care, work, motivation and fatigue [11].

Lifestyle and health status after pregnancy with GDM, have not previously been studied in a Swedish setting. As shown by Berg et al. [3], a larger proportion of non-Nordic born pregnant women develop GDM, hence comparing the life style and health status after pregnancy for women born in or born outside Sweden would be of interest. This study compared lifestyle and health status approximately four years after childbirth in a random selected sample of women whose pregnancy was complicated by GDM with women who had a normal pregnancy. The specific aims were: 1) to investigate differences in lifestyle; 2) to investigate differences in health outcomes; and 3) to investigate the associations between lifestyle and health outcomes.

Methods

This retrospective study was part of a larger research project investigating health status, quality of life, wellbeing, and lifestyle after normal pregnancy and pregnancy complicated with GDM in Sweden. The study was approved by the Regional Ethical Review Board at Umeå University (Dno: 05-020 M).

Data from the Swedish medical birth register

The Swedish Medical Birth Register (MBR) was established in 1973 and data are collected on almost all pregnancies and deliveries. As it is mandatory for health service providers to report data to the MBR, data for approximately 100 000 deliveries are entered annually [12]. Initially in this project, medical data were retrieved from the MBR by statisticians at the National Board of Health and Welfare, representing a national randomly selected sample of women with delivery during 2005. The sample consisted of 120 women with diet-treated GDM (ICD-10 code: O24.4A), and 120 women with insulin-treated GDM (ICD-10 code O24.4B), and 650 women with normal pregnancy and birth (ICD-10 code: O80.0 and no additional codes), comprising a total sample of 890 women.

The size of the estimated sample (n = 890) was based on the assumption that the prevalence of later poor self-rated health (SRH) would be doubled in women with a history of GDM compared to women with normal pregnancies. Accordingly, we calculated that at least 84 women with a history of GDM (diet or insulin treatment) and 560 women with normal pregnancy would be needed to demonstrate a difference in later poorer SRH at a significance level of 0.05. Presuming a dropout rate of approximately 20% for the follow-up study, a total of 890 women would be necessary to address the issue of SRH.

Procedure, questionnaire and data collection

A flow chart of the complete recruitment procedure is presented in Figure 1. Between May and June 2009, 882 eligible women from the initial sample obtained from the MBR, were mailed an invitation to participate in a questionnaire follow-up study (approximately four years after the index pregnancy). The mail included information about the study, a consent form, a questionnaire and a prepaid envelope. One reminder containing the same material as the first invitation was mailed if needed.

The research team constructed a questionnaire that included quality of life (standard SF-36 form [13-15]), and items regarding medical history, self-reported aspects of dietary intake, and PA. Before data collection, a small pilot study of ten purposively selected women, who recently had given birth, was performed to test the questionnaire. This pilot study resulted in minor changes of the design of the questionnaire and rephrasing of a few questions. In this paper, questionnaire data addressing

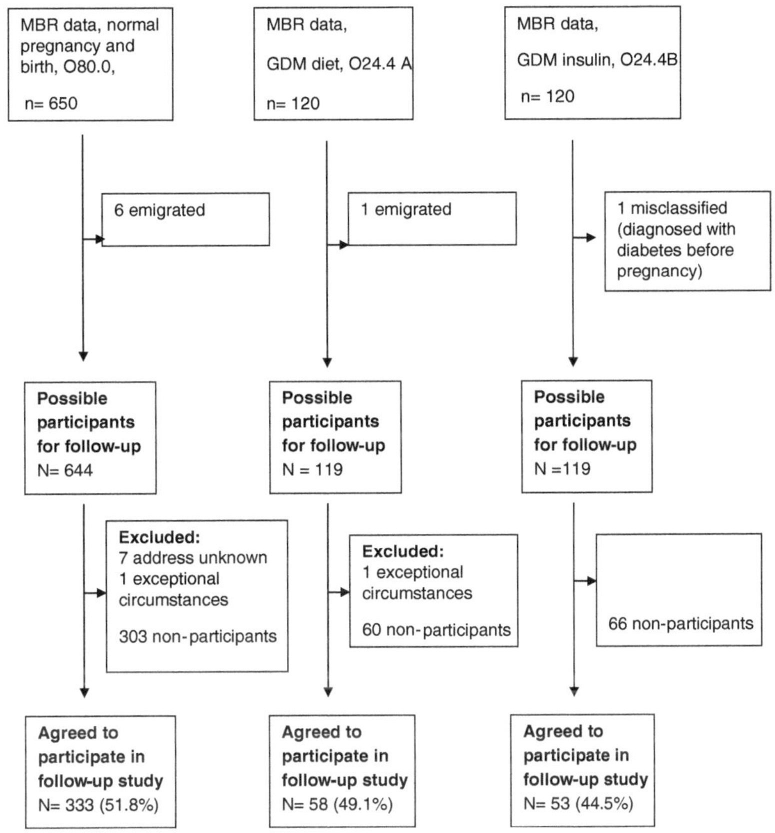

Figure 1 Recruitment procedures of participants in follow-up study.

issues related to lifestyle and health status will be presented.

Variable definitions and processing of data

Self-rated health (SRH)

The respondents were asked to rate their present health as excellent, very good, good, fair or poor. The individual perception of health has shown associations with future mortality. A meta-analysis of 22 studies show that individuals reporting poor SRH on a simple general SRH item have a two-fold increased risk of mortality compared to individuals reporting excellent health [16]. For the analysis, this outcome was categorized as excellent/very good/good (i.e. good health) or fair/poor (i.e. poorer health).

Recommendations of daily intake of vegetables and fruits

The study used the National Food Agency (NFA) recommendation of a daily consumption of 500 g of vegetables and fruits, which is equivalent to three fruits and two large servings of vegetables [17]. In the questionnaire, this information was included as an example of the amounts required to fulfill the recommendation to 100%. The respondents indicated to what extent they fulfilled the recommendation on an "ordinary" day on a 100 mm VAS scale with anchors 0% and 100% of the recommended levels. All responses on the VAS scale were manually measured; for example a value of 60 mm was equivalent to 60%.

Compliance to received dietary advice

The women with a history of GDM responded to statements on how they perceived and adhered to the dietary advice received during and after pregnancy. The statements were for example: "To what extent did you find the dietary advice useful for your situation during pregnancy" and "To what extent did you find the dietary advice important for your situation after child birth". The answers were given on a 100 mm VAS scale with anchors indicating 0% (not at all useful/important) and 100% (very useful/important). All responses were manually measured in the same manner as described above.

Physical activity (PA)

The Swedish national recommendations of PA during pregnancy suggest a minimum of 30 minutes of moderate intensity daily [18]. Respondents were asked to estimate the intensity of their PA (low intensity: able to speak/no heavy breathing during performance; moderate intensity: able to speak with some effort/some heavy breathing; and high intensity: not able to speak/ heavy breathing during performance). The NFA has suggested that this categorization of the intensity of PA is appropriate, when evaluating PA in population studies [19]. In addition, the participants were asked to estimate the frequency of their PA (per week) before pregnancy, during pregnancy and during the six months before the survey. If a respondent answered 3 to 4 times a week, this was calculated as 3.5 times a week for the purpose of the analysis.

The total number of participants with GDM diagnosis (diet-treated and insulin-treated GDM, n = 111) was small: 52.3% (n = 58) were treated with a combination of diet and physical exercise and 47.7% (n = 53) received insulin therapy at the index pregnancy. As no significant differences were found comparing responses of health status or lifestyle, the subgroups were merged when comparing the outcomes to those of the normal pregnancy group.

Further, available data from the MBR were used to compare characteristics of participants and non-participants.

Statistical analysis

An overview of outcomes and potential predictors is presented in Additional file 1. Categorical variables were analyzed using Pearson's Chi^2-test and Fisher's exact test when appropriate. The continuous variables were compared using Student's *t*-test at normal distributions and Mann–Whitney *U*-test when the distribution was skewed, and standard deviation and 25th – 75th percentile are presented respectively. For the analysis of present lifestyle and health status, sixteen women were excluded from the sample. Fourteen women were pregnant and two women had not stated whether they were pregnant or not at the time of the follow-up. This exclusion of these participants was made as pregnancy may contribute to alterations in lifestyle as well as health status. Four of the 14 pregnant women had a history of GDM in their previous pregnancy in 2005; however none of these women had developed overt diabetes mellitus before the current pregnancy.

Univariate logistic regression analyses were used to evaluate the associations between outcomes and possible predictors. Multiple logistic regression analyses were performed by entering predictors found to be significant in the univariate analysis in a stepwise manner. Only the results of the last step of this stepwise analysis are presented in the results section. Significance level was set at $p < 0.05$. Calculations were performed using SPSS for Windows, version 20.0 (IBM, Somers, NY).

To clarify the time period addressed when presenting the findings, the time period will be indicated by using "prior to index pregnancy" to indicate patients' status before index pregnancy, and "during index pregnancy" to indicate patients' status during pregnancy. The patients' status at the follow-up is labelled "present status".

Results

Characteristics of participants

A sample of 444 women (50.8% of all eligible women) agreed to participate in the follow-up study approximately four years after the index pregnancy. Characteristics of the participants and a comparison of characteristics of participants born in and outside of Sweden are presented in Table 1. The women with a history of normal pregnancy (n = 333) were younger, more often born in Sweden, more often reported normal BMI (18.50 – 24.99 kg/m^2), and were more physically active before their index pregnancy than women with a history of GDM (n = 111). Women with normal pregnancies were taller ($p < 0.001$) and had lower body weight ($p = 0.001$); a mean of 1.67 m (SD ± 0.07) and a median body weight of 63.0 kg (25th – 75th percentile: 57.0 – 72.0 kg) respectively compared to women with a history of GDM. These women had a mean maternal height of 1.65 m (SD ± 0.06) and a median body weight of 69.5 kg (25th – 75th percentile: 58.0 – 82.0 kg). However, women with a history of GDM reported less weight gain during their pregnancy compared to women with normal pregnancy. Despite regular PA as part of the treatment of GDM, 36.1% of women with a history of GDM reported performing PA on a regular basis during pregnancy. No significant differences between women with normal pregnancy and women with GDM-affected pregnancy were seen regarding number of pregnancies, number of children born, or marital status. A total of 12.7% of all participants were born outside Sweden; 50.9% from countries in Asia, 30.9% from European countries, 10.9% originated from South America and 7.3% from African countries.

Non-participants

Using available MBR data, the characteristics of the non-participants (n = 429) were compared with those of the participants (n = 444). The non-participants were younger (29.7 yrs., SD ± 5.5) than participants (31.1 yrs., SD ± 4.7) ($p < 0.001$), and had more children (2.1 children, SD ± 1.2) than participants (1.9 children, SD ± 0.9) ($p = 0.027$). No significant differences were observed between non-participants and participants regarding gestational age at birth or marital status. Furthermore, no significant differences were seen in the participation rates between women with normal pregnancies, women with diet-treated GDM and women with insulin-treated GDM. Unfortunately, no register data were available that identified ethnic origin.

Table 1 Characteristics of participants at index pregnancy 2005 presented as women with normal pregnancy and women with pregnancy complicated by gestational diabetes mellitus (GDM) and as born in and outside Sweden

	Normal pregnancy	Pregnancy with GDM	P-value	Participants born in Sweden with normal pregnancy	Participants born in Sweden with pregnancy with GDM	P-value	Participants born outside Sweden with normal pregnancy	Participants born outside Sweden with pregnancy with GDM	P-value
Status prior to index pregnancy 2005	(N = 333)	(N = 111)		(N = 303)	(N = 83)		(N = 29)	(N = 27)	
PCOS diagnosis	5 (1.5%)	8 (7.6%)	0.004 1	4 (1.3%)	6 (7.4%)	0.008[1]	0 (0%)	2 (8.7%)	0.198[1]
Infertility treatment	17 (5.2%)	17 (15.7%)	0.0012	15 (5.0%)	14 (16.9%)	0.001[2]	2 (7.4%)	3 (12.5%)	0.656[1]
Smoking prior to pregnancy	46 (15.4%)	19 (19.0%)	0.3972	42 (15.5%)	16 (21.3%)	0.231[2]	4 (14.8%)	3 (12.5%)	0.811[1]
Heredity of diabetes mellitus	0 (0%)	8 (7.2%)	<0.0011	0 (0%)	4 (4.8%)	0.002[1]	0 (0%)	4 (14.8%)	0.048[1]
Body Mass Index (BMI) prior to pregnancy (kg/m2)									
Mean, (± SD)	23.1 (3.5)	26.2 (5.7)	<0.001[3]	23.2 (3.6)	26.2 (5.5)	<0.001[3]	22.3 (2.2)	26.6 (6.4)	0.002[3]
Median, (25th – 75th percentile)	22.6 (20.7-24.2)	25.1 (21.5-29.8)	<0.001[4]	22.6 (20.8 – 24.3)	25.1 (21.4 - 29.8)	<0.001[4]	21.9 (20.3 – 23.7)	26.3 (21.5 – 30.1)	0.267[4]
Min - max	17.2 – 44.9	17.3 – 44.1		17.2 – 44.9	17.3 – 44.1		18.7 – 27.0	18.1 – 43.8	
Body Mass Index (BMI) classification[5] prior to pregnancy									
Underweight, BMI <18.49	9 (2.8%)	3 (2.8%)	<0.001[2]	9 (3.1%)	2 (2.4%)	<0.001[2]	0	1 (4.0%)	0.004[2]
Normal weight, BMI 18.50-24.99	251 (77.7%)	47 (43.5%)		227 (76.9%)	36 (43.9%)		23 (85.2%)	10 (40.0%)	
Overweight, BMI 25.00-29.99	48 (14.9%)	32 (29.6%)		44 (14.9%)	24 (29.3%)		4 (14.8%)	8 (32.0%)	
Obesity, BMI ≥30.00	15 (4.6%)	26 (24.1%)		15 (5.1%)	20 (24.4%)		0	6 (24.0%)	
Physical activity prior to pregnancy									
No regular physical activity	148 (45.1%)	61 (57.0%)	0.033[2]	134 (44.7%)	40 (49.4%)	0.450[2]	13 (48.1%)	20 (80.0%)	0.0172
Status During Index Pregnancy 2005									
Age									
Yrs (± SD)	31.0 (4.3)	33.5 (5.0)	<0.001[3]	31.0 (±4.3)	33.4 (4.7)	<0.001[3]	30.7 (4.8)	33.7 (6.2)	0.040[3]
Educational level									
Compulsory school	16 (4.8%)	7 (6.4%)	0.655[2]	12 (4.0%)	2 (2.4%)	0.675[2]	4 (13.8%)	5 (19.2%)	0.647[2]
High school/Folk high school	134 (40.4%)	47 (43.1%)		126 (41.6%)	38 (45.8%)		8 (27.6%)	9 (34.6%)	
University	182 (54.8%)	55 (50.5%)		165 (54.5%)	43 (51.8%)		17 (58.6%)	12 (46.2%)	
Parity									
Mean (± SD)	1.3 (0.8)	1.3 (1.3)	0.757[3]	1.3 (0.8)	1.3 (1.1)	0.746[3]	1.4 (1.0)	1.3 (1.7)	0.949[3]
Median, (25th – 75th percentile)	1.0 (1.0 – 2.0)	1.0 (1.0 – 2.0)	0.924[4]	1.0 (1.0 – 2.0)	1.0 (1.0- 2.0)	0.810[4]	1.0 (1.0 – 2.0)	2.0 (1.0 – 3.0)	0.622[4]
Min – Max	0 - 8	0 - 6		0 - 8	0 - 5		0 - 4	0 - 6	

Table 1 Characteristics of participants at index pregnancy 2005 presented as women with normal pregnancy and women with pregnancy complicated by gestational diabetes mellitus (GDM) and as born in and outside Sweden *(Continued)*

Physical activity during pregnancy									
No regular physical activity	178 (55.1%)	69 (63.9%)	0.110^2	158 (53.4%)	48 (60.0%)	0.291^2	19 (73.1%)	20 (74.1%)	0.934^2
Weight gain during pregnancy (kilograms)									
Mean (±SD)	14.8 (6.7)	12.8 (7.8)	0.014^3	14.8 (6.8)	12.2 (7.6)	0.004^3	14.1 (6.0)	14.4 (8.0)	0.863^3

[1]Fishers' test, [2]Chi2-test, [3]Student's *t*-test, [4]Mann–Whitney test, [5]Definitions according to The World Health Organization (http://apps.who.int/bmi/index.jsp?introPage=intro_3.html).

Present lifestyle four years after pregnancy

Reported present lifestyle four years after index pregnancy is shown in Table 2. Regarding Swedish snuff (i.e. oral use of wet tobacco), 7.2% of all participants reported regular use of the substance with no differences between groups. No differences were seen among groups regarding smoking; 18.3% of all participants reported smoking.

Women with a history of GDM reported less compliance to the dietary advice at the time of the follow-up compared to during pregnancy ($p < 0.001$) (Figure 2). On average, participants reached 62.5% of the recommended daily amount of fruit and vegetables, which is equivalent to approximately 310 grams each day. The national recommendation of daily intake of 500 grams of fruit and vegetables was reached by 7.3% of all participants. No differences in reaching recommendations were seen between women with a history of normal pregnancy and women with a history of GDM. A larger proportion of the women with a history of GDM reported drinking alcohol less than once a month or never. However, this difference was only seen among participants born outside Sweden. Women born in Sweden with a history of GDM, had more often irregular eating habits (i.e. skipping meals or frequently eating snacks) compared to women born in Sweden with normal pregnancy ($p = 0.030$). This difference was not found for women born outside Sweden.

Of all participants, 30.9% reported being physically active on a regular basis at all three time periods (prior to pregnancy, during pregnancy, and present status). Significantly fewer women with a history of GDM were physically active at all three time periods compared to women with a history of normal pregnancy (21.8% vs. 33.9%, $p = 0.022$). The risk of being inactive at all three time periods was more than doubled among women born outside Sweden compared to women born in Sweden (OR 2.30, 95% CI: 1.21 – 4.36).

Further, 39.1% of all participants were inactive at the follow-up with no differences between women with a history of normal pregnancy and women with a history of GDM. A significantly larger proportion of women born outside Sweden were inactive at the time of the follow-up compared to women born in Sweden (60.4% vs. 36.3%, $p = 0.001$). Among women being physically active on a regular basis at the time of the follow-up, women with a history of GDM exercised at low intensity to further extent than did women with a history of normal pregnancy. This difference in intensity of PA was not seen among women born outside Sweden.

Health status three to four years after pregnancy

Health status among participants four years after index pregnancy is presented in Table 3. In total, the participants reported an increase of body weight at the follow-up, and no differences were found between groups. However, the individual changes of body weight ranged between losing 47.0 kg and gaining 35.0 kg at the follow-up compared to prior the pregnancy.

In total, 22.7% of all participants reported using medication on a regular basis; 42.3% of the women with a history of GDM compared to 16.2% of women with normal pregnancy ($p < 0.001$). The reported conditions requiring medication were asthma/allergy (6.8%), depression (5.6%), diabetes (3.8%), thyroid conditions (3.6%), pain problems (2.5%), hypertension (0.5%) and other conditions in 1.4% of all participants. Women with a history of GDM reported using analgesics (6.7% vs. 1.5%, $p = 0.007$) and thyroid medication to a higher extent (11.7% vs. 1.8%, $p < 0.001$) than did women with a history of normal pregnancy. Only women with a history of GDM used medication for diabetes mellitus and no differences between groups were found regarding medication for asthma/allergy or depression.

At the time of the follow – up, 19 participants reported a diagnosis of diabetes. All participants with overt diabetes at the follow – up had GDM in their index pregnancy and 16 of them (84.2%) had been treated with insulin during pregnancy.

Fair/ poor SRH, lifestyle, and health status

Forty-three women (9.7%) reported fair or poor SRH at the follow-up. The associations of fair/poor SRH in relation to present lifestyle and health status are presented in Table 4. Reporting fair/poor SRH was related to being born outside Sweden and to lifestyle factors such as irregular eating habits and no regular PA, as well as being overweight or obese, and regular use of medication. In the univariate analysis, an index pregnancy complicated by GDM more than tripled (OR 3.13, 95% CI: 1.64 – 5.97) the risk of reporting fair/poor SRH at the follow-up. However, adjusting for the effects of being born in or outside Sweden, present BMI, sick leave for more than one week since childbirth 2005, medical treatment on regular basis and overt diabetes, we found that this association did not remain significant. Furthermore, being diagnosed with overt diabetes mellitus at the time of the follow-up was not associated with fair/poor SRH neither in the univariate nor multivariate analysis.

Discussion

This study found significant differences between women with normal pregnancy/delivery and women with a pregnancy complicated by GDM with respect to lifestyle and health status approximately four years after childbirth. Furthermore, the study revealed that irregular eating habits, lack of regular PA, being overweight or obese, as well as being on regular medication were all associated with poorer SRH at the follow-up. However, being

Table 2 Life style in participants four years after index pregnancy for women with and without previous GDM and born in or outside Sweden

Present status	Pregnancy without previous GDM (N = 321)	Pregnancy with previousGDM (N = 107)	P-value	Participants born in Sweden without GDM (N = 293)	Participants born in Sweden with GDM (N = 81)	P-value	Participants born outside Sweden without GDM (n = 27)	Participants born outside Sweden with GDM (N = 25)	P-value
Pregnant at follow up (excluded from calculations)	10	4		8	2		2	2	
Smoking									
On daily basis/ Occasionally	60 (18.7%)	21 (18.7%)	1.000[1]	51 (17.4%)	16 (19.8%)	0.626[1]	9 (33.3%)	4 (16.0%)	0.205[2]
Never	261 (81.3%)	90 (81.3%)		242 (82.6%)	65 (80.2%)		18 (66.7%)	21 (84.0%)	
Alcohol habits									
Never	45 (14.0%)	24 (22.4%)	0.007[1]	35 (11.9%)	10 (12.3%)	0.119[1]	10 (37.0%)	14 (56.0%)	0.035[1]
≤ once a month	93 (29.0%)	43 (40.2%)		90 (30.7%)	36 (44.4%)		3 (11.1%)	7 (28.0%)	
2-4 times/ month	142 (44.2%)	27 (25.2%)		131 (44.7%)	25 (30.9%)		10 (37.0%)	2 (8.0%)	
2-3 times/ week	38 (11.8%)	12 (11.2%)		34 (11.6%)	10 (12.0%)		4 (14.8%)	1 (4.0%)	
≥4 times/week	3 (0.9%)	1 (0.9%)		3 (1.0%)	0		0	1 (4.0%)	
Units alcohol at each drinking occasion									
1-2 units	184 (67.2%)	61 (74.4%)	0.215[1]	171 (66.5%)	51 (71.8%)	0.399[1]	12 (75.0%)	9 (90.0%)	0.617[2]
≥3 units	90 (32.8%)	21 (25.6%)		86 (33.5%)	20 (28.2%)		4 (25.0%)	1 (10.0%)	
Eating habits									
3 main courses/day[5]	262 (82.4%)	78 (72.9%)	0.034[1]	245 (84.5%)	60 (74.1%)	0.030[1]	16 (59.3%)	17 (68.0%)	0.512[2]
Irregular habits[6]	56 (17.6%)	29 (27.1%)		45 (15.5%)	21 (25.9%)		11 (40.7%)	8 (32.0%)	
Amount of fruit and vegetables/day									
% of recommended amount, mean (±SD)	63.1% (±25.2)	61.1% (±25.1)	0.494[3]	63.5% (±25.1)	60.4% (±23.0)	0.308[3]	56.4% (±25.1)	62.1% (±31.0)	0.471[3]
Reached recommended amount of fruit and vegetables/day[7]									
Yes	20 (6.3%)	9 (8.4%)	0.451[1]	18 (6.2%)	3 (3.7%)	0.586[2]	1 (3.8%)	5 (20.0%)	0.099[2]
No	298 (93.7%)	98 (91.6%)		273 (93.8%)	78 (96.3%)		25 (96.2%)	20 (80.0%)	
Physical activity on regular basis									
Yes	197 (63.3%)	54 (53.5%)	0.077[1]	186 (64.6%)	47 (60.3%)	0.481[1]	11 (50.0%)	6 (27.3%)	0.215[1]
No	114 (36.7%)	47 (46.5%)		102 (35.4%)	31 (39.7%)		11 (50.0%)	16 (72.7%)	
Frequency of physical activity/week[8]									
No of times/week,									
Mean (±SD)	2.6 (1.6)	2.6 (1.8)	0.759[3]	2.6 (1.5)	2.8 (1.8)	0.490[3]	2.6 (1.3)	2.7 (1.4)	0.910[3]
Median, 25th -75th percentile	2.0 (1.2 - 3.0)	2.0 (1.2 - 3.4)	0.922[4]	2.0 (1.5 – 3.0)	2.0 (1.5 – 3.5)	0.919[4]	2.5 (1.0 – 4.0)	2.5 (1.75 – 3.5)	1.000[4]

Table 2 Life style in participants four years after index pregnancy for women with and without previous GDM and born in or outside Sweden *(Continued)*

Intensity of performed physical activity[8]									
High	57 (29.1%)	5 (9.6%)	0.006[1]	55 (29.7%)	4 (8.5%)	0.007[1]	2 (18.2%)	1 (25.0%)	0.774[2]
Moderate	102 (52.0%)	30 (57.7%)		97 (52.4%)	29 (61.7%)		5 (45.5%)	1 (25.0%)	
Low	37 (18.9%)	17 (32.7%)		33 (17.8%)	14 (29.8%)		4 (36.4%)	2 (50.0%)	
Reached the recommended level of physical activity[8]									
Yes[9]	65 (33.0%)	10 (19.2%)	0.062[2]	61 (32.8%)	10 (21.3%)	0.156[2]	4 (36.4%)	0	0.516[2]
No	132 (67.0%)	42 (80.8%)		125 (67.2%)	37 (78.7%)		7 (63.6%)	4 (100%)	

[1]Chi2-test, [2]Fishers' test, [3]Student's *t*-test, [4]Mann–Whitney test, [5]Breakfast, lunch and dinner with and without 1 – 3 snacks, [6]Skipping courses; ie. reporting irregular eating habits, such as 1 – 2 main courses/ day or frequent snacking and no main courses, [7]500 grams of fruit and vegetables/day, [8]Only participants reporting regular physical activity included in this analysis, [9]≥ 3 times/week at moderate or high intensity.

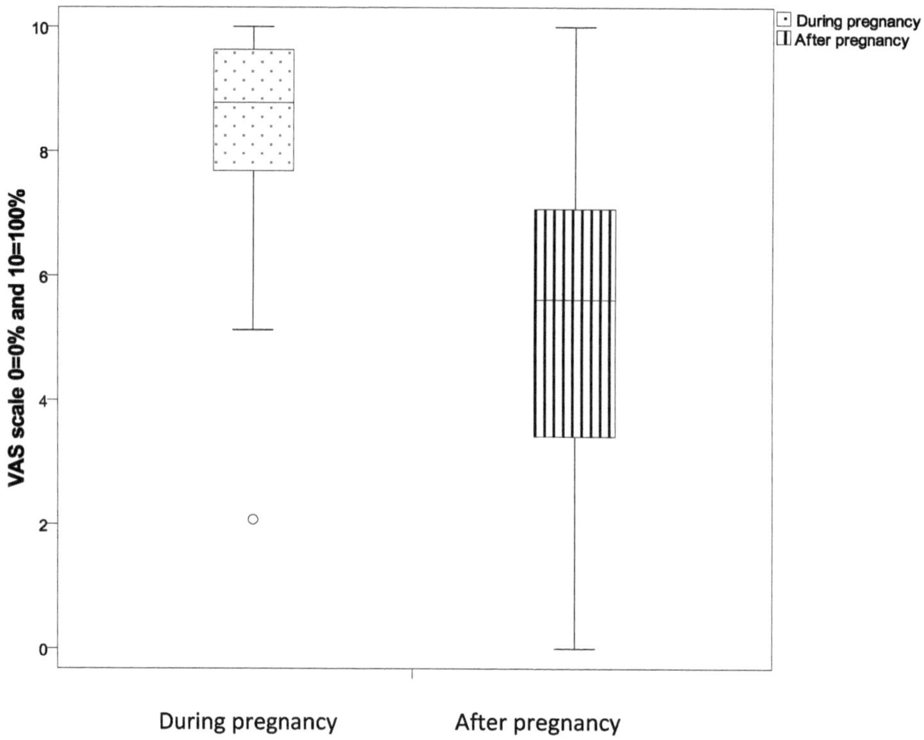

Figure 2 Boxplot presenting reported compliance with dietary advice during and after pregnancy complicated by gestational diabetes mellitus (GDM).

diagnosed with GDM at the index pregnancy or with overt diabetes mellitus at the follow-up showed no association with fair/poor SRH at the time of the follow-up.

Lifestyle four years after pregnancy

Previous research suggests that a diet comprising high quantities of fruits and vegetables, whole grains, poultry, and fish together with less consumption of starchy and processed foods, red meat, and sugar-sweetened drinks may delay the development of type 2 diabetes [20]. In our study, Swedish born women with a history of GDM reported having more irregular meals than women with a history of normal pregnancy, a fact that is of concern. Additionally, irregular eating habits showed a significant association with poorer SRH. Irregular eating habits in relation to development of diabetes are sparsely studied; however, it has been shown that older women with irregular breakfast eating habits are at increased risk for development of diabetes [21]. Further, there is an increased risk of metabolic syndrome when irregular energy intake during breakfast and in between meals is reported [22]. Elsewhere, limited consumptions of fruits and vegetables among women with a history of GDM are also reported. In an Australian survey of postpartum eating habits, 5% of participants with previous GDM consume the recommended amount of vegetables per day and 44% reach the recommended amount of fruit [23].

In a Canadian prospective observational cohort study, women with a history of GDM reported lower pre-pregnancy leisure and sport activity than a control group of women without GDM. One year after childbirth, no difference between groups regarding leisure or sports activity is reported, indicating that women with a history of GDM increase their postpartum PA in the year following birth [24]. A similar pattern was found in our study; the significant pre-pregnancy difference disappeared during pregnancy and after childbirth, which might indicate increased PA among women with a history of GDM. Despite this observed increase in PA, almost half of the participants with previous GDM in our study did not perform regular PA, a finding that differs from some international studies. An Australian study of women with a history of GDM show that 26.5% have a sedentary lifestyle [25]. Our findings are more similar to those reported in a Danish follow-up study of 121 women with previous GDM, where 36-40% of women do not exercise after childbirth [10]. As previously mentioned, a Cochrane review shows that the incidence of type 2 diabetes mellitus in high-risk populations may be decreased by interventions that increase PA and improve diet [8]. Despite some improvements in performance of PA noticed in our study, most women with previous GDM do not seem to change their lifestyle according to recommendations.

Table 3 Health status in participants four years after index pregnancy presented for women with normal pregnancy and women with a history of gestational diabetes mellitus (GDM) and as born in and outside Sweden born in or outside Sweden

Present status	Normal pregnancy 2005 (N = 321)	Pregnancy with GDM 2005 (N = 107)	P-value	Participants born in Sweden with normal pregnancy 2005 (N = 293)	Participants born in Sweden with GDM 2005 (N = 81)	P-value	Participants born outside Sweden with normal pregnancy 2005 (N = 27)	Participants born outside Sweden with GDM 2005 (N = 25)	P-value
Pregnant or missing pregnancy status at follow up (excluded from calculations)	12	4		10	2		2	2	
Overt diabetes mellitus									
Yes	0	19 (17.8%)	<0.001[1]	0	13 (16.0%)	<0.001[1]	0	6 (24.0%)	0.009[1]
No	321 (100%)	88 (82.2%)		293 (100%)	68 (84.0%)		27 (100%)	19 (76.0%)	
Self-rated health at follow-up									
Excellent, very good, good	291 (92.7%)	80 (80.0%)	<0.001[2]	267 (92.4%)	66 (88.0%)	0.225[2]	23 (95.8%)	13 (54.2%)	0.002[1]
Fair, poor	23 (7.3%)	20 (20.0%)		22 (7.6%)	9 (12.0%)		1 (4.2%)	11 (45.8%)	
Body weight at follow-up (kilograms)									
Mean (± SD)	66.5 (11.7)	73.1 (16.7)	<0.001[3]	66.9 (12.0)	73.5 (16.8)	<0.001[3]	62.8 (8.0)	72.1 (16.8)	0.013[3]
Median (25th – 75th percentile)	65.0 (58.0-71.0)	71.0 (60.8–80.5)	0.003[4]	65.0 (58.0–72.0)	73.0 (60.0–81.5)	0.010[4]	65.0 (54.0–68.0)	69.0 (62.0– 81.2)	0.125[4]
(Min –max)	43.0 – 116.0	42.0 – 122.0		43.0 – 116.0	42.0 – 122.0		50.0 – 80.0	48.0 – 109.0	
BMI at follow-up, (kg/m2)									
Underweight, (<18.49)	4 (1.3%)	2 (1.9%)	<0.001[2]	4 (1.4%)	2 (2.5%)	<0.001[2]	0	0	0.013
Normal weight, (18.5-24.99)	229 (72.0%)	48 (45.7%)		208 (71.7%)	37 (45.7%)		20 (74.1%)	10 (41.7%)	
Overweight, (25.0-29.99)	62 (19.5%)	26 (24.8%)		56 (19.3%)	21 (25.9%)		6 (22.2%)	6 (25.0%)	
Obesity, (≥30.0)	23 (7.2%)	29 (27.6%)		22 (7.6%)	21 (25.9%)		1 (3.7%)	8 (33.3%)	
Weight change (pre-pregnancy to follow-up, kilograms)									
Mean (± SD)	+1.6 (5.7)	+1.3 (8.9)	0.736[3]	+1.5 (5.8)	+0.7 (9.4)	0.319[3]	+2.2 (5.4)	+3.6 (6.5)	0.389[3]
Median (25th – 75th percentile)	+1.0 (−1.0 - +3.2)	+1.0 (−2.0 - +6.0)	0.736[4]	+1.0 (−1.0- +3.0)	+1.0 (−2.0- +4.8)	0.931[4]	+1.5 (−1.2- +5.0)	+3.0 (0 - +8.0)	0.328[4]
(Min –max)	−20.0 - + 35.0	−47.0 - + 20.0		−20.0 - + 35.0	−47.0 - + 22.0		−7.0 - + 16.0	−10.0 - + 16.0	
Sick leave for more than one week due to health problems[5]									
Yes	60 (18.8%)	35 (33.3%)	0.002[2]	52 (17.7%)	27 (33.3%)	0.002[2]	8 (29.6%)	8 (33.3%)	0.776[2]
No	260 (81.2%)	70 (66.7%)		241 (82.3%)	54 (66.7%)		19 (70.4%)	16 (66.7%)	
Medication on regular basis[6]									
Yes	52 (16.2%)	45 (42.1%)	<0.001[2]	48 (16.4%)	34 (42.0%)	<0.001[2]	4 (14.8%)	11 (44.0%)	0.032[1]
No	269 (83.8%)	62 (57.9%)		245 (83.6%)	47 (58.0%)		23 (85.2%)	14 (56.0%)	

[1]Fisher's Exact Test, [2]Chi2test, [3]Student's *T*-test, [4]Mann Whitney, [5]Sick leave for longer period than one week requires a medical certificate issued by a physician, [6]Hormonal contraceptives were excluded in the analysis.

Table 4 Odds ratios (ORs) and their 95% confidence intervals (CI) for fair/poor self-rated health (SRH) for women with normal pregnancy and women with a history of gestational diabetes mellitus (GDM) in relation to life style and health status four years after index pregnancy in univariate and stepwise multivariate logistic regression analyses

Present Life Style	Fair/poor SRH (n = 43) No. (%)	Good SRH (n = 386) No. (%)	Univariate OR for poor SRH	95% CI	Multivariate OR* for poor SRH	95% CI			Multivariate OR# for poor SRH	95% CI
Smoking 2009										
No	32 (74.4%)	318 (82.4%)	1.0							
Yes	11 (25.6%)	68 (17.6%)	0.62	0.30 – 1.29						
Alcohol 2009										
Never/≤ once/month	31 (72.1%)	180 (46.6%)	1.0							
≥2-4 times/month	12 (27.9%)	206 (53.4%)	0.34	0.17 – 0.68	0.46	0.22-0.95			0.81	0.34-1.91
Eating habits 2009										
3 main courses	6 (60.5%)	314 (82.0%)	1.0							
Irregular meals	17 (39.5%)	69 (18.0%)	2.98	1.53 – 5.78	2.84	1.36-5.79			2.82	1.22-6.53
Physical activity on regular basis 2009										
Yes	13 (33.3%)	240 (63.8%)	1.0							
No	26 (66.7%)	136 (36.2%)	3.53	1.76 – 7.10	3.01	1.47-6.15			2.86	1.26-6.49
Present health status							Multivariate OR* for poor SRH	95% CI		
Pregnancy 2005										
Normal	23 (53.5%)	302 (78.2%)	1.0							
GDM	20 (46.5%)	84 (21.8%)	3.13	1.64 – 5.97			0.97	0.43-2.19	0.80	0.33-1.98
Born outside Sweden										
No	31 (72.1%)	344 (89.6%)	1.0							
Yes	12 (27.9%)	40 (10.4%)	3.33	1.58 – 7.00			2.61	1.00- 6.77	2.21	0.78-6.24
Body Mass Index 2009										
≤24.99	9 (22.0%)	268 (72.6%)	1.0							
25.0 – 29.99	15 (36.6%)	69 (18.7%)	6.47	2.72 – 15.42			5.25	2.14- 12.86	5.95	2.24-15.83
≥30.0	17 (41.5%)	32 (8.7%)	15.82	6.51 – 38.42			9.94	3.76- 26.29	11.40	3.78-34.34
Sick leave for more than one week since 2005										
No	23 (54.8%)	305 (79.4%)	1.0							
Yes	19 (45.2%)	79 (20.6%)	3.19	1.66 – 6.15			1.80	0.84- 3.85	1.12	0.47-2.65
Medical treatment on regular basis 2009										
No	20 (46.5%)	314 (81.3%)	1.0							
Yes	23 (53.5%)	72 (18.7%)	5.02	2.61 – 9.62			2.97	1.39-6.37	3.18	1.38-7.36

Table 4 Odds ratios (ORs) and their 95% confidence intervals (CI) for fair/poor self-rated health (SRH) for women with normal pregnancy and women with a history of gestational diabetes mellitus (GDM) in relation to life style and health status four years after index pregnancy in univariate and stepwise multivariate logistic regression analyses *(Continued)*

Diabetes diagnosis 2009				
No	40 (93.0%)	371 (96.1%)	1.0	
Yes	3 (7.0%)	15 (3.9%)	1.86	0.52 – 6.68

*Significant variables in the univariate analysis of life style and health status respectively were entered in a stepwise manner. Only last step of stepwise multiple regression analysis is presented. [#]Variables included in the final analysis: alcohol 2009, eating habits 2009, physical activity on regular basis 2009, pregnancy 2005, born outside Sweden, Body Mass Index 2009, and medical treatment on regular basis 2009.

Health status four years after pregnancy

Internationally, differences in self-reported health status for women with a history of normal pregnancy and women with a history of GDM have been reported. In women with previous GDM, a prevalence of 12 – 13.8% fair/poor SRH are reported compared to 7 – 9.3% in women with no GDM [26,27]. In our study, 20% of women with a history of GDM reported fair/poor SRH. However, when adjusting for other risk factors, GDM at index pregnancy was no longer associated with poorer SRH. Being born outside Sweden was found to be associated with poorer SRH; this finding is in agreement with other studies comparing SRH of immigrants and Swedish born individuals [28,29]. However, the SRH status may be affected by other life events mediating the findings. In a qualitative study, women evaluate their whole life situation when answering questions on their SRH, i.e. capturing physical symptoms and emotional problems affecting daily life as well as family functioning, relationship with partner and balancing motherhood and work. Events relating to childbirth were not included in the responses one year after childbirth [30]. Also, poor SRH in pregnancy and six months after childbirth reveal associations with lower levels of social support and friendship network [31].

Previous studies indicate that the cumulative incidence of type 2 diabetes mellitus rapidly increases within the first five years after pregnancy [6]. Other Swedish studies report 11% overt diabetes among women with a history of GDM one to two years postpartum [32] and 30% five years postpartum [33]. Our findings correspond to these results. However, there was no information regarding what type of overt diabetes the women had developed. Hence, there might be biological explanations mediating the development of diabetes not accounted for in this study.

Our findings indicated sub-optimal levels of PA and intake of fruit and vegetables in women with a history of GDM as well as in women with normal pregnancy. Furthermore, irregular eating habits, no regular PA, being overweight or obese and on regular medication showed associations with poorer SRH. Health care providers and societal organizations should initiate counselling and interventions regarding diet and PA for all women postpartum as to remain healthy or improve future health. Further research may address how interventions and counselling aimed to increase PA and improve intake of fruit and vegetables are experienced, especially among women with a history of GDM.

Methodological discussion

The number of non-participants might be considered high in this study; however, the initial sample was based on a random national register selection. A Cochrane review studying strategies to improve the response rate in questionnaires, reveal that the response rate is higher if, for example, hand-written envelopes and shorter questionnaires are used. Also, the response rate decreases when questions addressing sensitive topics are included [34]; i.e. factors that may have contributed to the eligible participants' willingness to participate. One reminder was used for this data collection. Additional reminders may have improved the final response rate. Others describe how the response rate increases continuously with up to four reminders in a questionnaire study [35]. Another explanation to the low participation rate may be that the questionnaire was administrated in Swedish, which may have resulted in fewer immigrants participating. The non-participants were significantly younger and had more children; i.e. a situation that may have skewed some results. These limitations should be considered when evaluating the findings of this study.

The NFA suggests a number of questions to be used as an indicator of quality of diet. The quantity of fruits and vegetables is estimated by reporting numbers of servings per month, week, or day of fruit and vegetables respectively [19]. These NFA questions were not used in this survey; instead the respondents were asked to estimate to what extent they reached the recommendation of fruit and vegetables. Therefore, the reported compliance to recommendations of fruit and vegetables may be less valid compared had the NFA indicators of quality of diet been used. Yet, a review found that the VAS is associated with energy intake well enough to be used as a proxy of energy intake. Further, VAS is predicting with reasonable certainty meal initiation and amount consumed [36].

The respondents recalled some issues regarding pregnancy and postpartum approximately four years before this study. Studies of maternal recall of events related to pregnancy and delivery show high accuracy even several years postpartum [37,38], hence recall bias of such events should not be considered a major limitation of our study. However, during the years following the index pregnancy and delivery, some women may have experienced life events not addressed in the questionnaire that might have affected their lifestyle and health status.

The concept of social desirability (i.e. the tendency of individuals to report themselves in coherence with perceived cultural norms) is associated with overestimation of PA [39] as well as underestimation of energy intake, especially in women [40]. This type of bias may have occurred as there were no objective measures of PA and diet compliance in this population-based study. Additionally, few studies have addressed the reliability of long-term recall of health behaviors. Recall of intense PA is more accurate 10 years later than less intense activities [41]. A more accurate recall regarding more intense activities is also seen 15 years later [42]. Hence, there is little reason to believe that recall bias regarding the more intense PA had a major negative impact on the validity of our findings.

The strength of our study includes the detailed answers provided by the participants, who also represent a variety of women covering all geographical regions of the country, factors that may increase the validity of the results. To address the internal validity of the data, a rigorous control of the accuracy of registered data was performed. Despite the limitations described, our findings agreed with previous studies [43], hence we believe that our study may reflect the lifestyle and health status of women with and without a history of GDM living in similar settings.

Conclusions

These results reveal suboptimal levels of PA, and fruit and vegetable consumption for a sample of women with a history of GDM as well as for women with normal pregnancy approximately four years after index pregnancy. Women with previous GDM seem to increase their PA after childbirth, but still they perform their activity at lower intensity than women with a history of normal pregnancy. Having GDM at index pregnancy or being diagnosed with overt diabetes mellitus at follow-up did not demonstrate associations with poorer SRH four years after delivery.

Competing interests

The authors declare that they have no competing interests.

Authors' contributions

All authors participated in the planning and design of the study. MP, in collaboration with IM, performed the data collection. MP performed the analysis and drafted the manuscript with input from AW and IM. All authors read and approved the final manuscript.

Acknowledgements

Our sincere thanks to all participating women. Additionally, thanks to Britt Granström, who entered all data into SPSS, and to Strategiska Forskningsprogrammet Vård (SFP-Vård) for funding.

Author details

[1]School of Health and Social Studies, Dalarna University, Falun, Sweden. [2]Department of Nursing, Umeå University, SE – 901 87 Umeå, Sweden. [3]Department of Internal Medicine and Clinical Nutrition, Sahlgrenska Academy, University of Gothenburg, Gothenburg, Sweden. [4]Department of Clinical Sciences, Obstetrics and Gynecology, Umeå University, Umeå, Sweden.

References

1. Hunt KJ, Schuller KL. The increasing prevalence of diabetes in pregnancy. Obstet Gynecol Clin North Am. 2007;34(2):173–99. vii.
2. Esakoff TF, Cheng YW, Caughey AB. Screening for gestational diabetes: different cut-offs for different ethnicities? Am J Obstet Gynecol. 2005;193(3 Pt 2):1040–4.
3. Berg M, Adlerberth A, Sultan B, Wennergren M, Wallin G. Early random capillary glucose level screening and multidisciplinary antenatal teamwork to improve outcome in gestational diabetes mellitus. Acta Obstet Gynecol Scand. 2007;86(3):283–90.
4. Cnattingius S, Lambe M. Trends in smoking and overweight during pregnancy: prevalence, risks of pregnancy complications, and adverse pregnancy outcomes. Semin Perinatol. 2002;26(4):286–95.
5. HAPO Study Cooperative Research Group. Hyperglycemia and adverse pregnancy outcomes. N Engl J Med. 2008;358:1991–2002.
6. Kim C, Newton KM, Knopp RH. Gestational diabetes and the incidence of type 2 diabetes: a systematic review. Diabetes Care. 2002;25(10):1862–8.
7. Bellamy L, Casas JP, Hingorani AD, Williams D. Type 2 diabetes mellitus after gestational diabetes: a systematic review and meta-analysis. Lancet. 2009;373(9677):1773–9.
8. Orozco LJ, Buchleitner AM, Gimenez-Perez G, Roque IFM, Richter B, Mauricio D. Exercise or exercise and diet for preventing type 2 diabetes mellitus. Cochrane Database Syst Rev. 2008;3:CD003054.
9. American Diabetes Association (ADA). Standards of medical care in diabetes–2014. Diabetes Care. 2014;37(1):S14–80.
10. Stage E, Ronneby H, Damm P. Lifestyle change after gestational diabetes. Diabetes Res Clin Pract. 2004;63(1):67–72.
11. Nicklas JM, Zera CA, Seely EW, Abdul-Rahim ZS, Rudloff ND, Levkoff SE. Identifying postpartum intervention approaches to prevent type 2 diabetes in women with a history of gestational diabetes. BMC Pregnancy Childbirth. 2011;11:23.
12. Socialstyrelsen (The National Board of Health and Welfare). The Swedish Medical Birth Register. In: Medicinska födelseregistret. http://www.socialstyrelsen.se/register/halsodataregister/medicinskafodelseregistret/inenglish. Assessed 15 Nov 2014
13. Sullivan M, Karlsson J, Ware Jr JE. The Swedish SF-36 health survey–I. Evaluation of data quality, scaling assumptions, reliability and construct validity across general populations in Sweden. Soc Sci Med. 1995;41(10):1349–58.
14. Persson LO, Karlsson J, Bengtsson C, Steen B, Sullivan M. The Swedish SF-36 health survey II. Evaluation of clinical validity: results from population studies of elderly and women in gothenborg. J Clin Epidemiol. 1998;51(11):1095–103.
15. Sullivan M, Karlsson J. The Swedish SF-36 health survey III. Evaluation of criterion-based validity: results from normative population. J Clin Epidemiol. 1998;51(11):1105–13.
16. DeSalvo KB, Bloser N, Reynolds K, He J, Muntner P. Mortality prediction with a single general self-rated health question. A meta-analysis. J Gen Intern Med. 2006;21(3):267–75.
17. Becker W, Hagman U. Mer frukt och grönt, bra för hälsan [More fruit and vegetables, good for the health] [in Swedish]. Vår Föda. 1999;6:24–8.
18. Josefsson A, Bö K. Graviditet [Swedish]. In: Folkhälsoinstitutet. Stockholm: Folkhälsoinstitutet; 2008.
19. Sepp H, Ekelund U, Becker W. Enkätfrågor om kost och fysisk aktivitet bland vuxna - Underlag till urval av frågor i befolkningsinriktade enkäter [In Swedish]. Rapport 21. Stockholm; Sweden: Livsmedelsverket (National Food Administration); 2004. Available at: http://www.livsmedelsverket.se/globalassets/rapporter/2004/rapp-21-hela.pdf?.
20. Esposito K, Kastorini CM, Panagiotakos DB, Giugliano D. Prevention of type 2 diabetes by dietary patterns: a systematic review of prospective studies and meta-analysis. Metab Syndr Relat Disord. 2010;8(6):471–6.
21. Mekary RA, Giovannucci E, Cahill L, Willett WC, van Dam RM, Hu FB. Eating patterns and type 2 diabetes risk in older women: breakfast consumption and eating frequency. Am J Clin Nutr. 2013;98(2):436–43.
22. Pot GK, Hardy R, Stephen AM. Irregular consumption of energy intake in meals is associated with a higher cardiometabolic risk in adults of a British birth cohort. Int J Obesity. 2014;38(12):1518–24.
23. Zehle K, Smith BJ, Chey T, McLean M, Bauman AE, Cheung NW. Psychosocial factors related to diet among women with recent gestational diabetes: opportunities for intervention. Diabetes Educ. 2008;34(5):807–14.
24. Retnakaran R, Qi Y, Sermer M, Connelly PW, Zinman B, Hanley AJ. Gestational diabetes and postpartum physical activity: evidence of lifestyle change 1 year after delivery. Obesity (Silver Spring). 2010;18(7):1323–9.
25. Smith BJ, Cheung NW, Bauman AE, Zehle K, McLean M. Postpartum physical activity and related psychosocial factors among women with recent gestational diabetes mellitus. Diabetes Care. 2005;28(11):2650–4.
26. Kim C, Vahratian A. Self-rated health and health care use among women

with histories of gestational diabetes mellitus. Diabetes Care. 2010;33(1):41–2.
27. Kieffer EC, Sinco B, Kim C. Health behaviors among women of reproductive age with and without a history of gestational diabetes mellitus. Diabetes Care. 2006;29(8):1788–93.
28. Leao TS, Sundquist J, Johansson S, Sundquist K. The influence of age at migration and length of residence on self-rated health among Swedish immigrants: a cross-sectional study. Ethnic Health. 2009;14(1):93–105.
29. Taloyan M, Wajngot A, Johansson S, Tovi J, Sundquist J. Poor self-rated health in adult patients with type 2 diabetes in the town of Södertälje: A cross-sectional study. Scand J Prim Health Care. 2010;28(4):216–20.
30. Schytt E, Waldenstrom U, Olsson P. Self-rated health–what does it capture at 1 year after childbirth? Investigation of a survey question employing thinkaloud interviews. Scand J Caring Sci. 2009;23(4):711–20.
31. Lamarca GA, do Leal MC, Sheiham A, Vettore MV. The association of neighbourhood and individual social capital with consistent self-rated health: a longitudinal study in Brazilian pregnant and postpartum women. BMC Pregnancy Childbirth. 2013;13:1.
32. Anderberg E, Landin-Olsson M, Kalen J, Frid A, Ursing D, Berntorp K. Prevalence of impaired glucose tolerance and diabetes after gestational diabetes mellitus comparing different cut-off criteria for abnormal glucose tolerance during pregnancy. Acta Obstet Gynecol Scand. 2011;90(11):1252–8.
33. Ekelund M, Shaat N, Almgren P, Groop L, Berntorp K. Prediction of postpartum diabetes in women with gestational diabetes mellitus. Diabetologia. 2010;53(3):452–7.
34. Edwards PJ, Roberts I, Clarke MJ, Diguiseppi C, Wentz R, Kwan I, et al. Methods to increase response to postal and electronic questionnaires. Cochrane Database Syst Rev. 2009;3, MR000008.
35. Barclay S, Todd C, Finlay I, Grande G, Wyatt P. Not another questionnaire! Maximizing the response rate, predicting non-response and assessing non-response bias in postal questionnaire studies of GPs. Fam Pract. 2002;19(1):105–11.
36. Stubbs RJ, Hughes DA, Johnstone AM, Rowley E, Reid C, Elia M, et al. The use of visual analogue scales to assess motivation to eat in human subjects: a review of their reliability and validity with an evaluation of new hand-held computerized systems for temporal tracking of appetite ratings. Br J Nutr. 2000;84(4):405–15.
37. Githens PB, Glass CA, Sloan FA, Entman SS. Maternal recall and medical records: an examination of events during pregnancy, childbirth, and early infancy. Birth. 1993;20(3):136–41.
38. Natland ST, Andersen LF, Nilsen TI, Forsmo S, Jacobsen GW. Maternal recall of breastfeeding duration twenty years after delivery. BMC Med Res Methodol. 2012;12:179.
39. Adams SA, Matthews CE, Ebbeling CB, Moore CG, Cunningham JE, Fulton J, et al. The effect of social desirability and social approval on self-reports of physical activity. Am J Epidemiol. 2005;161(4):389–98.
40. Hebert JR, Ma Y, Clemow L, Ockene IS, Saperia G, Stanek 3rd EJ, et al. Gender differences in social desirability and social approval bias in dietary self-report. Am J Epidemiol. 1997;146(12):1046–55.
41. Blair SN, Dowda M, Pate RR, Kronenfeld J, Howe Jr HG, Parker G, et al. Reliability of long-term recall of participation in physical activity by middle-aged men and women. Am J Epidemiol. 1991;133(3):266–75.
42. Smith AW, Cronin KA, Bowles H, Willis G, Jacobs Jr DR, Ballard-Barbash R, et al. Reproducibility of physical activity recall over fifteen years: longitudinal evidence from the CARDIA study. BMC Public Health. 2013;13:180.
43. Jones EJ, Roche CC, Appel SJ. A review of the health beliefs and lifestyle behaviors of women with previous gestational diabetes. J Obstet Gynecol Neonatal Nurs. 2009;38(5):516–26.

2

Maternal vitamin D status, gestational diabetes and infant birth size

Helena H. Hauta-alus[1], Heli T. Viljakainen[1,2*], Elisa M. Holmlund-Suila[1], Maria Enlund-Cerullo[1], Jenni Rosendahl[1], Saara M. Valkama[1], Otto M. Helve[1], Timo K. Hytinantti[1], Outi M. Mäkitie[1,2,3] and Sture Andersson[1]

Abstract

Background: Maternal vitamin D status has been associated with both gestational diabetes mellitus (GDM) and fetal growth restriction, however, the evidence is inconsistent. In Finland, maternal vitamin D status has improved considerably due to national health policies. Our objective was to compare maternal 25-hydroxy vitamin D concentrations [25(OH)D] between mothers with and without GDM, and to investigate if an association existed between maternal vitamin D concentration and infant birth size.

Methods: This cross-sectional study included 723 mother-child pairs. Mothers were of Caucasian origin, and infants were born at term with normal birth weight. GDM diagnosis and birth size were obtained from medical records. Maternal 25(OH)D was determined on average at 11 weeks of gestation in pregnancy and in umbilical cord blood (UCB) at birth.

Results: GDM was observed in 81 of the 723 women (11%). Of the study population, 97% were vitamin D sufficient [25(OH)D ≥ 50 nmol/L]. There was no difference in pregnancy 25(OH)D concentration between GDM and non-GDM mothers (82 vs 82 nmol/L, $P = 0.99$). Regression analysis confirmed no association between oral glucose tolerance test results and maternal 25(OH)D ($P > 0.53$). Regarding the birth size, mothers with optimal pregnancy 25(OH)D (≥ 80 nmol/L) had heavier newborns than those with suboptimal pregnancy 25(OH)D ($P = 0.010$). However, mothers with optimal UCB 25(OH)D had newborns with smaller head circumference than those with suboptimal 25(OH)D ($P = 0.003$), which was further confirmed as a linear association ($P = 0.024$).

Conclusions: Maternal vitamin D concentration was similar in mothers with and without GDM in a mostly vitamin D sufficient population. Associations between maternal vitamin D status and birth size were inconsistent. A sufficient maternal vitamin D status, specified as 25(OH)D above 50 nmol/L, may be a threshold above which the physiological requirements of pregnancy are achieved.

Keywords: Maternal vitamin D status, Newborn vitamin D status, 25-hydroxy vitamin D concentration, Gestational diabetes mellitus, Birth size, Birth weight, Birth length, Head circumference, Ponderal index

Background

Vitamin D deficiency, defined as a circulating 25-hydroxy vitamin D (25(OH)D) concentration below 50 nmol/L, has been common among Finnish pregnant women [1]. However, due to recent changes in national health policies, intake of vitamin D has increased resulting in decreasing rates of vitamin D deficiency [2–5]. Vitamin D deficiency has been associated with gestational diabetes mellitus (GDM) [6], but the evidence is inconsistent [7, 8]. Of all pregnancies, 1–14% are affected by GDM [9], and globally GDM prevalence has been increasing in line with increasing obesity [10]. GDM is the most common pregnancy complication in Europe [11]. In Finland, the prevalence of GDM has increased from 6% in 2008 to 11% in 2014 [12]. GDM increases the risk of adverse pregnancy and neonatal outcomes, and the risk of obesity, metabolic syndrome, diabetes, and cardiovascular disease in later life both of the mother and the child [13].

* Correspondence: heli.viljakainen@helsinki.fi
[1]Children's Hospital, University of Helsinki and Helsinki University Hospital, Biomedicum 2 C, P.O. Box 705, 00020 HUS Helsinki, Finland
[2]Folkhälsan Research Center, Haartmaninkatu 8, P.O.Box 63, 00014 Helsinki, Finland

Fetal growth may have later health implications also within the normal-birth-weight range [14]. Poor maternal vitamin D status has been related to fetal growth restriction [15] but it is unknown whether maternal vitamin D status associates with birth size in infants with normal birth weight.

Many of the findings regarding the relationship between vitamin D deficiency and GDM are based on case-control studies, which may include a potential selection bias. Case-control studies often focus on high-risk groups, for example women who are overweight and sedentary, which are independent risk factors for vitamin D deficiency as well (for example [16]).

The objectives of the present study were to compare 25(OH)D concentration at two consecutive time points between mothers with and without GDM, and to investigate associations between maternal factors and infant's birth size, and the potential role of 25(OH)D concentration therein.

The study is part of the longitudinal Vitamin D Intervention in Infants (VIDI) study.

Methods

Recruitment and study participants

At Kätilöopisto Maternity Hospital, Helsinki, Finland, 987 families were recruited into the VIDI study between January 2013 and June 2014, after delivery during the mother's hospital stay. According to the inclusion criteria, the mothers were of Caucasian origin without regular medication and with singleton pregnancy. Exclusion criteria for the newborns were: nasal continuous positive airway pressure treatment >one day, intravenous glucose infusion, seizures, duration of phototherapy >three days and need for nasogastric tube >one day. The infants were born between 37 + 0 and 42 + 0 weeks of gestation, and newborn's birth weight was appropriate for gestational age (SD-score [SDS] between −2.0 and +2.0). Of the recruited eligible families, 29% (987/3408) agreed to participate in the VIDI study. For the present cross-sectional study, we included mothers who had a record from a community prenatal clinic or baseline questionnaire and both two maternal 25(OH)D measurements. Two infants with a congenital disease (Down syndrome and Rieger syndrome) were excluded. Thus, the total number of subjects was 723. Of the infants, 367 were girls and 356 boys. Number of subjects in each analysis is reported in Tables.

25(OH)D analyses

Maternal pregnancy serum samples for 25(OH)D measurements were collected at community prenatal clinics at gestational weeks 7 to 25 between June 2012 and November 2013 as part of the mothers' normal follow-up [hereafter referred to as pregnancy 25(OH)D]. At birth, umbilical cord blood (UCB) for 25(OH)D measurement was obtained at gestational weeks 37 to 42 between January 2013 and May 2014 [hereafter referred to as UCB 25(OH)D]. Both pregnancy serum and UCB plasma 25(OH)D were analysed simultaneously using the IDS-iSYS fully automated immunoassay system with chemiluminescence detection (Immunodiagnostic Systems Ltd., Bolton, UK). Detailed information on 25(OH)D analysis has been previously reported [5]. The quality and accuracy of the serum 25(OH)D analysis is validated on an ongoing basis by participation in the vitamin D External Quality Assessment Scheme (DEQAS, Charing Cross Hospital, London, UK).

Both 25(OH)D concentrations were corrected by applying a linear regression equation (Oct 2014 value (nmol/L) = [(early 2014 value) − 8.2] / 0.99) provided by the manufacturer because of methodological changes in the IDS-iSYS system between 2014 and 2016 (see Additional file 1). We re-analysed a subsample of 77 samples and verified the correction (adjusted $R^2 = 0.922$, SEE = 9.2 nmol/l).

We employed UCB 25(OH)D to reflect both the maternal vitamin D status at the end of pregnancy and the newborn's vitamin D status at birth [1]. We defined vitamin D deficiency as 25(OH)D < 50 nmol/L, and vitamin D sufficiency as 25(OH)D ≥ 50 nmol/L, since a concentration of ≥50 nmol/L is considered sufficient for bone health [17]. Suboptimal vitamin D status was defined as 25(OH)D < 80 nmol/L, and optimal vitamin D status as 25(OH)D ≥ 80 nmol/L, as has been suggested based on calcium absorption studies [18].

Maternal and newborn data

Maternal data were obtained from a self-administered baseline questionnaire, filled in after delivery, and from medical records. Maternal height (cm) and weight (kg) before pregnancy and parity were collected primarily from the prenatal maternity card or, if missing, from our baseline questionnaire. Gestation was determined by first trimester ultrasound examination. Maternal age was determined at delivery. Parity was categorised into nullipara, secundipara and multipara (>two deliveries). Prepregnancy body mass index (BMI) (kg/m^2) was categorised into underweight (<18.5), normal weight (18.5–24.9), overweight (25.0–29.9) and obese (>30.0).

Prepregnancy weight and weight recorded in prenatal clinics were utilised to calculate gestational weight gain (GWG) (kg). We recorded GWG at first measurement, at approximately the 12th, 20th and 30th gestational weeks, and at last measurement. GWG was adjusted for consecutive gestational week. Concerning the analysis of total GWG, absolute values were used, and women who had their final weight recorded more than three weeks before the delivery were omitted ($n = 7$). Total GWG was categorised into inadequate, adequate and excessive based on national recommendations by prepregnancy

BMI: recommended GWG for underweight mothers was 12.5–18.0 kg, for normal weight 11.5–16.0 kg, for overweight 7.0–11.5 kg, and for obese 5.0–9.0 kg [19].

Education level was graded from one (=comprehensive school/lower secondary education) to six (university degree/first or second stage of tertiary education). Education was re-categorised into 'lower' and 'higher' education (lower = lower or upper secondary or post-secondary non-tertiary education, higher = first or second stage of tertiary education), due to a low number of subjects in other education categories. Prepregnancy smoking status was assessed as number of cigarettes per day. Maternal use of supplements, specific brand names, dosing, and date of commencement were recorded. We calculated the average daily intake of vitamin D from supplementation during the last two months of pregnancy.

Birth size, including birth weight (kg), length (cm), and head circumference (cm), was measured by midwives according to standard procedure. These data and the duration of pregnancy were retrospectively collected from birth records. Birth size measures were transformed into SDS by using Finnish sex-specific normative data for fetal growth [20]. Ponderal index was calculated (birth weight (kg) / birth length $(m)^3$) and standardised into sex-specific z-score.

Assessment of GDM

The diagnosis of GDM was based on a two-hour 75 g oral glucose tolerance test (OGTT). According to the national guidelines, GDM was diagnosed if the OGTT results exceeded cut-offs for one or more values: fasting plasma glucose ≥5.3 mmol/l, 1-h ≥ 10.0 mmol/l and 2-h ≥ 8.6 mmol/l [19]. An OGTT was performed at gestational weeks 10 to 40 between October 2012 and March 2014, and the results were collected from prenatal maternity cards or the hospital laboratory database. In general, screening for GDM depends on a presence of risk factors according to national recommendations [19] and based on these, OGTT was performed on 490 (54.5%) of the participating mothers. None of the pregnant women in our study received insulin therapy nor other regular medication, but mothers with GDM obtained dietary counselling at community prenatal clinics [19].

Statistical analysis

The normality of the variables was visually inspected. Outliers ($n = 18$) of 25(OH)D concentrations were identified with Normal probability plot of residuals, Leverage and Cook's Distance diagnostic tests, and omitted from the analyses. Season with four categories affected maternal 25(OH)D concentrations. Thus, season at pregnancy blood sampling and at birth was coded using dummy variables (with autumn as a reference) in ANCOVA and used as a covariate.

The data included partially missing information. Imputation of missing values for education ($n = 12$) and parity ($n = 2$) were conducted using the median value in subgroups by GDM status. Missing data on prepregnancy smoking as number of cigarettes daily were imputed as a median value (= zero) by GDM status according to smoking status ($n = 22$). Imputation of missing values for GWG at 12 gestational weeks was conducted using a mean value of two consecutive measurements ($n = 12$). Missing values of other variables were not imputed. Maternal characteristics in Table 1 are described only as un-imputed values.

Independent sample t-tests, Mann-Whitney U-tests, repeated measures ANOVA or the Pearson Chi-Square test, when appropriate, were applied to compare maternal characteristics between GDM and non-GDM mothers. The difference in 25(OH)D between GDM and non-GDM mothers was investigated with ANCOVA adjusted for season, maternal age, education and prepregnancy BMI. Association between pregnancy 25(OH)D and OGTT results/birth weight, and between UCB 25(OH)D and head circumference at birth were tested with univariate linear regression. Prevalence of vitamin D deficiency in non-GDM and GDM mothers were tested with Fisher's Exact test.

Newborn birth size was investigated in categories of maternal prepregnancy BMI (underweight, normal weight, overweight, obese), GWG (inadequate, adequate, excessive), prepregnancy smoking status (yes, no), maternal education (higher, lower), parity (nullipara, secundipara, multipara), GDM status (yes, no), vitamin D status (suboptimal, optimal) in pregnancy and in UCB, with ANCOVA with Bonferroni correction when applicable, and adjusted for maternal height. Changing covariates appearing in the ANCOVA models were: prepregnancy BMI, GWG at last measurement, smoking, education, parity, GDM and 25(OH)D concentrations. Using both 25(OH)D concentrations as covariates in the GWG analysis induced a multicollinearity problem based on Cook's Distance and Levene's test, but excluding these covariates from the model did not change the results.

Results are shown as means or adjusted means with SD or SEM. The means and medians were similar in both vitamin D concentrations. Associations were considered significant at $P < 0.05$. All statistical analyses were conducted using the IBM SPSS program for Windows, version 22 (IBM, Chicago, IL, USA).

Results

In the study population 97% were vitamin D sufficient [25(OH)D > 50 nmol/L] in both mothers and newborns, while optimal vitamin D status [25(OH)D above 80 nmol/L] was seen in 52% of the mothers and 45% of the newborns.

Table 1 Maternal characteristics in GDM and non-GDM mothers. *P*-values refer to differences between the groups

Maternal characteristics	*n*	Non-GDM	*n*	GDM	*p* value
Age at delivery (y)	642	31.4 ± 4.3	81	32.7 ± 4.5	0.018
Level of education[a]	632	5.0 ± 1.3	79	4.7 ± 1.4	0.051
Parity	640	1.5 ± 0.7	81	1.5 ± 0.7	0.275
Prepregnancy smoking, number of cigarettes daily	625	1.2 ± 3.7	76	2.0 ± 4.6	0.064
Alcohol consumption before pregnancy, portion/wk.	625	1.9 ± 2.0	78	2.3 ± 3.5	0.755
Prepregnancy height (cm)	642	166.3 ± 6.0	81	165.9 ± 5.4	0.398
Prepregnancy weight (kg)	631	63.5 ± 10.2	81	72.1 ± 13.5	<0.001
Prepregnancy BMI (kg/m^2)	639	23.0 ± 3.5	81	26.2 ± 4.8	<0.001
Duration of gestation at OGTT (wk)	323	26.3 ± 4.3	80	25.9 ± 5.9	0.774
Duration of gestation at pregnancy blood sampling (wk)	642	11.3 ± 1.9	81	11.2 ± 2.2	0.089
Duration of gestation at delivery (wk)	642	40.2 ± 1.1	81	40.1 ± 1.1	0.410
Pregnancy 25(OH)D (nmol/L)	642	81.9 ± 19.5	81	80.0 ± 21.2	0.417
UCB 25(OH)D (nmol/L)	642	80.1 ± 20.0	81	78.4 ± 18.8	0.448
Supplemental vitamin D intake during pregnancy (µg/d)	621	15.5 ± 16.6	76	13.5 ± 10.8	0.162
Cumulative gestational weight gain at[b] (kg)					0.093
first measurement	580	1.7 ± 0.5	74	1.6 ± 0.5	
12th gestational week	580	3.8 ± 1.0	74	3.6 ± 1.1	
20th gestational week	580	6.3 ± 0.8	74	6.2 ± 0.8	
30th gestational week	580	9.7 ± 0.5	74	9.7 ± 0.4	
last measurement	580	13.8 ± 0.4	74	13.7 ± 0.3	

GDM gestational diabetes mellitus, *25(OH)D* 25-hydroxy vitamin D, *UCB* umbilical cord blood
Values are means ± SD
[a]Scale from 1 = lower secondary education to 6 = first or second stage of tertiary education
[b]Values are adjusted for duration of gestation

Majority (95%) of the mothers took vitamin D supplements during pregnancy, most of them were highly educated (75% had at least a bachelor level education), and 73% had normal weight before pregnancy.

Vitamin D status and GDM

In our cohort GDM was present in 81 of the 723 women (11%). The comparison of maternal characteristics of GDM and non-GDM mothers is summarised in Table 1. Pregnancy 25(OH)D concentration was measured on average at 11 weeks of gestation, and GDM was diagnosed on average at 26 weeks of gestation in both GDM and non-GDM mothers. Mothers with GDM were older ($P = 0.018$), heavier and had higher prepregnancy BMI (P for both <0.001), and their educational level was at borderline of significance ($P = 0.051$) lower compared with mothers without GDM. No differences between the groups were observed in several other characteristics, including GWG, duration of gestation, and supplemental vitamin D intake.

We investigated whether pregnancy 25(OH)D concentration differed between mothers with ($n = 81$) and without GDM ($n = 639$) (Fig. 1) in a crude model and in a model adjusted for season, maternal age, education and prepregnancy BMI. Adjusted analysis confirmed no difference in mean ± SEM pregnancy 25(OH)D concentration between GDM and non-GDM mothers (81.7 ± 2.3 vs 81.7 ± 0.8 nmol/L, $P = 0.99$). Similarly in UCB, the adjusted analysis showed no difference in 25(OH)D concentrations in infants born to women with and without GDM (79.1 ± 2.3 vs 80.1 ± 0.8 nmol/L, $P = 0.69$) (Fig. 1). These results remained when only those who had undergone OGTT were included: pregnancy and UCB 25(OH)D concentrations were similar in GDM ($n = 80$) and non-GDM mothers ($n = 323$) ($P = 0.94$ and $P = 0.43$, respectively).

We further tested for possible associations between pregnancy 25(OH)D concentration and OGTT results with a univariate regression model. We observed no association between pregnancy 25(OH)D and fasting plasma glucose (B -0.00; 95% CI -0.00, 0.00; $P = 0.54$), 1-h glucose (B 0.00; 95% CI -0.01, 0.01; $P = 0.53$) or 2-h glucose (B -0.00; 95% CI -0.01, 0.01; $P = 0.54$).

The prevalence of vitamin D deficiency [25(OH)D < 50 nmol/L] during pregnancy was similar between mothers with or without GDM [4.9% (4/81) vs 3.3% (21/642), $P = 0.51$]. However, more GDM mothers were vitamin D deficient at the delivery compared with non-GDM mothers [7.4% (6/81) vs 2.8% (18/642) ($P = 0.042$)]. However, of

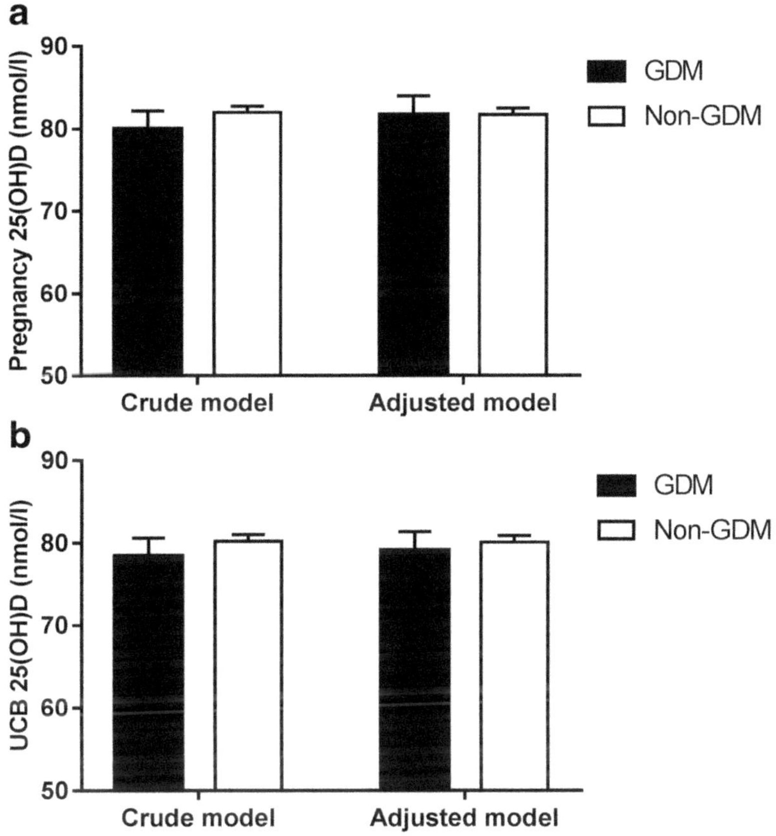

Fig. 1 Maternal vitamin D status and gestational diabetes mellitus. Adjusted mean ± SEM values of pregnancy 25(OH)D (**a**) and UCB 25(OH)D concentration (nmol/L) (**b**) in GDM and non-GDM mothers. Adjustments are for season, maternal age, education and prepregnancy BMI. Maternal 25(OH)D concentrations were similar between non-GDM and GDM mothers. Abbreviations: 25(OH)D, 25-hydroxy vitamin D; UCB, umbilical cord blood; GDM, gestational diabetes mellitus

these six deficient GDM-mothers five (83%) were smokers, and correspondingly in non-GDM mothers four out of eighteen were smokers (24%) ($P = 0.018$).

Maternal 25(OH)D and newborn birth size

The effect of maternal factors on birth size in fully adjusted models is presented in Table 2 and Fig. 2. Neither pregnancy 25(OH)D nor UCB 25(OH)D concentrations were related to birth length or ponderal index. As compared to mothers with suboptimal pregnancy 25(OH)D, mothers with optimal pregnancy 25(OH)D had heavier newborns ($P = 0.010$), but this positive association was not verified in linear regression (B 0.00; 95% CI -0.00, 0.01; $P =$ 0.16). Newborn head circumference was larger in those with suboptimal UBC 25(OH)D compared with mothers with optimal UCB 25(OH)D ($P = 0.003$). Further, linear regression confirmed the inverse association between UCB 25(OH)D and head circumference (B -1.74; 95% CI -3.25, −0.23; $P =$ 0.024). These results did not change after adjusting for mode of delivery (vaginal, vacuum assisted or caesarean section). Prepregnancy BMI, GWG, and parity had independent effects on birth size (Table 2 and Fig. 2).

Discussion

The primary focus of this work was to determine whether 25(OH)D concentration differs between mothers with and without GDM, and whether vitamin D status affects birth size in normal-birth-weight infants. GDM was diagnosed in 11% of mothers in our cohort. Almost all mother-child pairs (97%) were vitamin D sufficient [25(OH)D ≥ 50 nmol/L], and about half of the mother-child pairs had optimal vitamin D status [25(OH)D ≥ 80 nmol/L]. Maternal 25(OH)D concentrations were similar in GDM and non-GDM mothers. Interestingly, pregnancy vitamin D status associated positively with birth weight, but an inverse association was observed between newborn vitamin D status and head circumference at birth.

Lu et al. (2016) concluded in their meta-analysis that maternal vitamin D insufficiency (< 50 nmol/L or <75 nmol/L) was associated with greater risk of GDM [6]. However, they suggested that this applied only in developed countries and when no adjustments for confounders were made [6]. In our study, maternal vitamin D concentrations were similar in non-GDM and GDM

Table 2 Independent effect of maternal factors on birth size[a]

	Birth weight (SDS)		Birth length (SDS)	Head circumference (SDS)[b]	Ponderal index (z-score)[c]
Maternal factors	*n*	*p* value	*p* value	*p* value	*p* value
Prepregnancy BMI		**0.020**	0.201	0.364	0.719
Underweight	19	−0.49 ± 0.17	−0.36 ± 0.19	−0.34 ± 0.22	−0.12 ± 0.23
Normal weight	494	−0.30 ± 0.03	−0.23 ± 0.04	−0.14 ± 0.04	−0.01 ± 0.05
Overweight	117	−0.13 ± 0.07	−0.12 ± 0.08	−0.04 ± 0.09	0.08 ± 0.09
Obese	44	−0.05 ± 0.12	−0.01 ± 0.13	0.03 ± 0.14	0.08 ± 0.16
Gestational weight gain		**<0.001**	**0.006**	0.186	0.505
Inadequate	164	−0.43 ± 0.06	−0.37 ± 0.07	−0.23 ± 0.07	−0.05 ± 0.08
Adequate	261	−0.28 ± 0.05	−0.20 ± 0.05	−0.11 ± 0.06	−0.02 ± 0.06
Excessive	242	−0.12 ± 0.05	−0.09 ± 0.06	−0.05 ± 0.06	0.07 ± 0.07
Prepregnancy smoking		**0.021**	0.227	0.093	0.173
Yes	101	−0.43 ± 0.08	−0.30 ± 0.09	−0.27 ± 0.10	−0.13 ± 0.11
No	573	−0.23 ± 0.03	−0.18 ± 0.04	−0.09 ± 0.04	0.03 ± 0.04
Maternal education		0.972	0.670	0.721	0.634
Higher	513	−0.26 ± 0.03	−0.19 ± 0.04	−0.11 ± 0.04	−0.00 ± 0.05
Lower	161	−0.26 ± 0.06	−0.23 ± 0.07	−0.14 ± 0.08	0.04 ± 0.08
Parity		**<0.001**	**<0.001**	**0.007**	**0.027**
Nullipara	431	−0.40 ± 0.04	−0.32 ± 0.04	−0.20 ± 0.05	−0.05 ± 0.05
Secundipara	185	−0.03 ± 0.05	−0.05 ± 0.06	−0.03 ± 0.07	0.18 ± 0.07
Multipara	58	0.04 ± 0.10	0.22 ± 0.11	0.17 ± 0.12	−0.07 ± 0.13
Gestational diabetes mellitus	0.063		0.559	0.351	0.075
Yes	76	−0.10 ± 0.09	−0.15 ± 0.10	−0.02 ± 0.11	0.21 ± 0.12
No	598	−0.28 ± 0.03	−0.21 ± 0.03	−0.13 ± 0.04	−0.02 ± 0.04
Pregnancy 25(OH)D concentration		**0.010**	0.095	0.398	0.236
Suboptimal (<80 nmol/L)	333	−0.34 ± 0.04	−0.26 ± 0.05	−0.15 ± 0.05	−0.04 ± 0.06
Optimal (≥80 nmol/L)	341	−0.19 ± 0.04	−0.15 ± 0.05	−0.09 ± 0.05	0.05 ± 0.06
UCB 25(OH)D concentration	0.149		0.486	**0.003**	0.234
Suboptimal (<80 nmol/L)	369	−0.22 ± 0.04	−0.18 ± 0.04	−0.02 ± 0.05	0.05 ± 0.05
Optimal (≥80 nmol/L)	305	−0.31 ± 0.04	−0.23 ± 0.05	−0.24 ± 0.05	−0.05 ± 0.06

25(OH)D 25-hydroxy vitamin D, *UCB* umbilical cord blood
Values are adjusted mean ± SEM. *p* value is in bold when statistically significant
[a] Adjusted for maternal height and other listed maternal factors as changing covariates
[b] Two values are missing from analyses
[c] Adjusted for gestational age

mothers, and there was no linear association between vitamin D concentrations and OGTT results. However, we observed that vitamin D deficiency at delivery was more prevalent in mothers with GDM compared with non-GDM mothers, but this was not marked during pregnancy. This finding was possibly confounded by smoking, which was more prevalent in the deficient GDM mothers compared with deficient non-GDM mothers. Nevertheless due to small number of deficient mothers we could not investigate this reliably. In accordance with other studies, our results imply that in a vitamin D sufficient population, the association between 25(OH)D and GDM may not exist [8, 21, 22]. Similarly, Josefson et al. (2016) stated that maternal fasting glucose or GDM status was not associated with pregnancy 25(OH)D, which in their study was on average 93 nmol/L [23].

GDM is a multifactorial disease involving various risk factors, for example lifestyle factors, obesity, rapid weight gain and predisposing genetic factors. Furthermore, some of these factors are related to or co-exist with poor vitamin D status [24, 25], which further increases the challenge when dissecting independent effect. It is possible that in previous studies where no adjustment for confounding factors was performed, the association between 25(OH)D and GDM reflects shared factors such as an unhealthy lifestyle or adiposity [26].

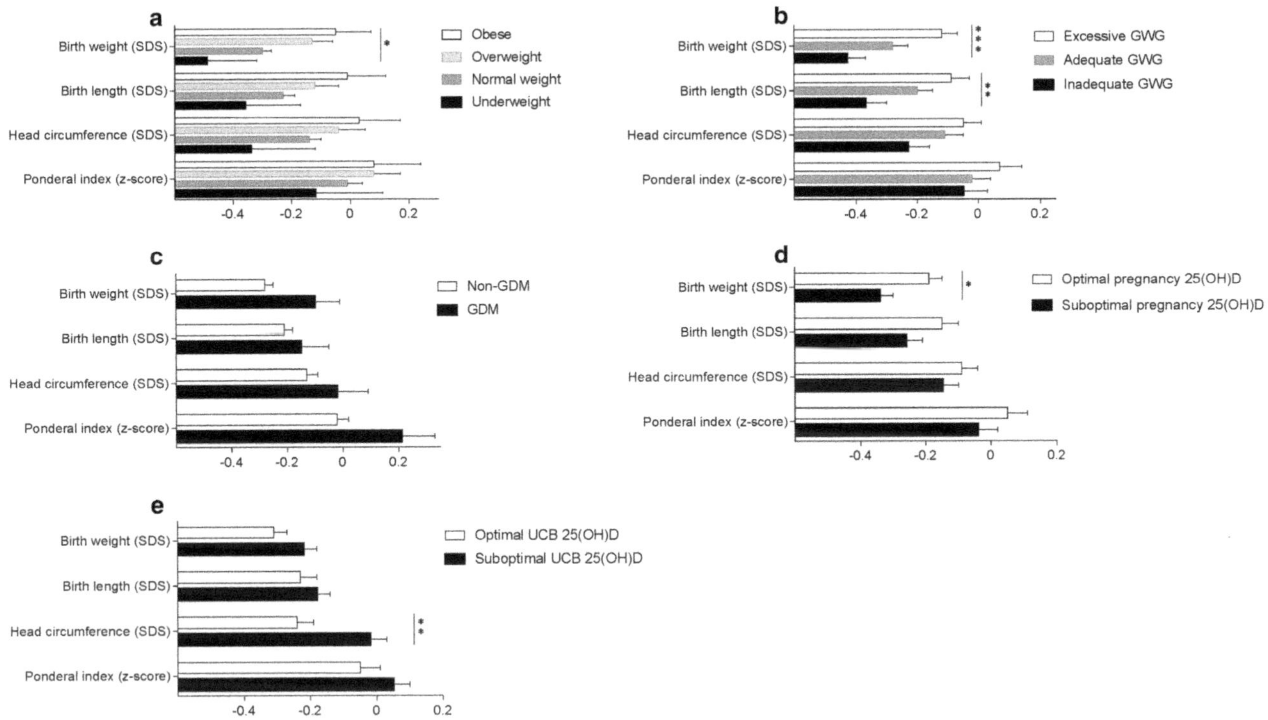

Fig. 2 Maternal factors and birth size. Adjusted mean ± SEM values of birth weight, length, head circumference SD-scores and ponderal index z-score between (**a**) maternal prepregnancy BMI groups of underweight, normal weight, overweight and obese; (**b**) mothers' inadequate GWG, adequate GWG and excessive GWG; (**c**) GDM and non-GDM mothers; (**d**) suboptimal and optimal pregnancy 25(OH)D; and (**e**) suboptimal and optimal UCB 25(OH)D. Statistical significance is denoted by $^{*}P < 0.05$, $^{**}P < 0.01$ and $^{***}P < 0.001$. Abbreviations: GWG, gestational weight gain; GDM, gestational diabetes mellitus; 25(OH)D, 25-hydroxy vitamin D; suboptimal, UCB, umbilical cord blood; 25(OH)D < 80 nmol/L; optimal 25(OH)D ≥ 80 nmol/L

Yet, contrary to many studies, associations between high 25(OH)D and GDM have been reported [27, 28]. Although a biological mechanism between low vitamin D status and diabetes is plausible [29], only a few interventions have been conducted, and these have not proved an effect of vitamin D supplementation on risk of GDM [30].

Maternal vitamin D status associated with birth size: pregnancy 25(OH)D showed a positive association towards birth weight, but UCB 25(OH)D an inverse association with head circumference, while only the inverse association with head circumference was verified with linear model. Harvey et al. (2014) concluded that modest evidence exist for a positive relation between maternal vitamin D status and birth weight [31]. Some earlier studies have shown that severe maternal vitamin D deficiency associates with smaller head circumference at birth [32, 33], yet some have not [34, 35]. In agreement with our findings, others have discovered that mothers with higher vitamin D concentration have infants with smaller head circumference at birth [36, 37]. However, the clinical relevance, if any, of the inverse relationship between maternal vitamin D status and head circumference at birth remains unexplained. It is unknown whether this reflects differences in brain size or in skull bones' structure, and needs to be explored in future studies. The mean difference in head circumference was 0.22 SD units between the groups with optimal and suboptimal UCB 25OHD. A possible explanation for this might be a U-shaped association between maternal vitamin D concentration and fetal outcomes in a population with sufficient vitamin D status. We have previously suggested the U-shaped association between 25(OH)D concentration and inflammatory biomarkers in cord blood [5].

We have collected a homogenous cohort of Caucasian mothers from the capital region of Finland representing mothers without regular medication and their newborns who were born at term with normal birth weight. In many previous studies, participants had various ethnic backgrounds which could affect both vitamin D status and their risk of GDM [7, 38]. A strength of the present study lies in the recruitment of subjects, which took place in a single hospital, enabled standardised data collection and covered all seasons. However, a multi-centre study might have resulted in a wider variety of socioeconomic backgrounds.

A challenge in previous studies on vitamin D status and GDM has been the lack of relevant adjustments, for example adjustments for BMI and smoking status [6]. In the present study, we have systematically investigated confounders between groups, and adjusted for those when applicable. The threshold for defining vitamin D deficiency and the diagnostic criteria for GDM vary between studies, which might affect the results and complicate the comparison of studies. A further limitation is that the OGTT was not performed on all mothers, and a slight possibility exists that the actual prevalence of GDM might be underestimated. Yet, our main results were repeated in a subgroup analysis of only those women to whom an OGTT was performed. In addition, the prevalence of GDM was in accordance with the national statistics [12]. However, in a cross-sectional setting causal relationships cannot be determined.

Conclusion

In summary, maternal vitamin D concentration was similar in mothers with and without GDM in a vitamin D sufficient population. Furthermore, we found an inverse association between UCB 25(OH)D and infant head circumference. The clinical relevance of this finding remains unsolved and needs to be considered in future studies. Sufficient maternal vitamin D status, specified as 25(OH)D above 50 nmol/L, seems a threshold value, above which the physiological requirements of pregnancy are achieved. Our findings suggest that an adequate maternal vitamin status have been achieved in Finland. However, randomised controlled trials are required in specific risk groups of vitamin D deficiency to clarify if vitamin D supplementation affects the risk of GDM.

Abbreviations

25(OH)D: 25-hydroxy vitamin D concentration; GDM: Gestational diabetes mellitus; GWG: Gestational weight gain; UCB: Umbilical cord blood

Acknowledgements

We are grateful to our research nurses Sirpa Nolvi, Rhea Paajanen, Nea Boman and Päivi Turunen for their assistance in data collection. Laboratory technician Sari Lindén is acknowledged for her valuable work. We acknowledge the midwives and laboratory technicians at Kätilöopisto Maternity Hospital for obtaining umbilical cord blood samples. We are grateful to Professor Kari Teramo, MD, PhD, (Department of Obstetrics and Gynaecology, University of Helsinki and Helsinki University Hospital) for his valuable comments on the manuscript. Most importantly, we thank all the families that participated in this study.

Funding

Research project funding sources are Academy of Finland, Governmental Subsidy for Clinical Research, Foundation for Pediatric Research, Finska Läkaresällskapet, Folkhälsan Research Foundation, Sigrid Jusélius Foundation, Stiftelsen Dorothea Olivia, Karl Walter och Jarl Walter Perkléns Minne, and Päivikki and Sakari Sohlberg Foundation.

Authors' contributions

The authors' contributions are as follows: HHH, HTV, OMM and SA designed the study; HHH, HTV, EMH, ME, JR, SMV, TKH and OMH participated in acquisition of the data; HHH analysed the data; HHH and HTV wrote the first draft of the manuscript. All of the authors critically revised the manuscript and approved the final version.

Competing interests

The authors declare that they have no competing interests.

Author details

[1]Children's Hospital, University of Helsinki and Helsinki University Hospital, Biomedicum 2 C, P.O. Box 705, 00020 HUS Helsinki, Finland. [2]Folkhälsan Research Center, Haartmaninkatu 8, P.O.Box 63, 00014 Helsinki, Finland. [3]Center for Molecular Medicine, Karolinska Institute and Clinical Genetics, Karolinska University Hospital, 171 76 Solna, Stockholm, Sweden.

References

1. Viljakainen HT, Saarnio E, Hytinantti T, Miettinen M, Surcel H, Makitie O, Andersson S, Laitinen K, Lamberg-Allardt C. Maternal vitamin D status determines bone variables in the newborn. J Clin Endocrinol Metab. 2010;95(4):1749–57.
2. Itkonen ST, Lamberg-Allardt C. Food fortification as a means to increase vitamin D intake. Br J Nutr. 2016;115(11):2075–6.
3. Cashman KD, Dowling KG, Skrabakova Z, Kiely M, Lamberg-Allardt C, Durazo-Arvizu RA, Sempos CT, Koskinen S, Lundqvist A, Sundvall J, Linneberg A, Thuesen B, Husemoen LL, Meyer HE, Holvik K, Gronborg IM, Tetens I, Andersen R. Standardizing serum 25-hydroxyvitamin D data from four Nordic population samples using the vitamin D standardization program protocols: shedding new light on vitamin D status in Nordic individuals. Scand J Clin Lab Invest. 2015;75(7):549–61.
4. Raulio S, Erlund I, Männistö S, Sarlio-Lähteenkorva S, Sundvall J, Tapanainen H, Vartiainen E, Virtanen S. Successful nutrition policy: improvement of vitamin D intake and status in Finnish adults over the last decade. Eur J Pub Health. 2016; doi:10.1093/eurpub/ckw154.
5. Rosendahl J, Holmlund-Suila E, Helve O, Viljakainen H, Hauta-Alus H, Valkama S, Enlund-Cerullo M, Hytinantti T, Tervahartiala T, Sorsa T, Makitie O, Andersson S. 25-hydroxyvitamin D correlates with inflammatory markers in cord blood of healthy newborns. Pediatr Res. 2017; doi:10.1038/pr.2017.9.
6. Lu M, Xu Y, Lv L, Zhang M. Association between vitamin D status and the risk of gestational diabetes mellitus: a meta-analysis. Arch Gynecol Obstet. 2016;293(5):959–66.
7. Burris HH, Camargo CA Jr. Vitamin D and gestational diabetes mellitus. Curr Diab Rep. 2014;14(1):451. -013-0451-3
8. Loy SL, Lek N, Yap F, Soh SE, Padmapriya N, Tan KH, Biswas A, Yeo GS, Kwek K, Gluckman PD, Godfrey KM, Saw SM, Muller-Riemenschneider F, Chong YS, Chong MF, Chan JK. Growing up in Singapore towards healthy outcomes (GUSTO) study group: Association of Maternal Vitamin D Status with glucose tolerance and caesarean section in a multi-ethnic Asian cohort: the growing up in Singapore towards healthy outcomes study. PLoS One. 2015;10(11):e0142239.
9. American Diabetes Association. Diagnosis and Classification of Diabetes. Diabetes Care. 2013;36(Supplement 1):S67–74.
10. Ferrara A. Increasing prevalence of gestational diabetes mellitus: a public health perspective. Diabetes Care. 2007;30(Suppl 2):S141–6.
11. Buckley BS, Harreiter J, Damm P, Corcoy R, Chico A, Simmons D, Vellinga A, Dunne F, Core Investigator DALI. Group: gestational diabetes mellitus in Europe: prevalence, current screening practice and barriers to screening. A review. Diabet Med. 2012;29(7):844–54.
12. Vuori E, Gissler M. Official Statistics of Finland. Health 2015. National Institute for Health and Welfare: Perinatal statistics: parturients, deliveries and newborns 2014. 2015;19:5.
13. Damm P, Houshmand-Oeregaard A, Kelstrup L, Lauenborg J, Mathiesen ER, Clausen TD. Gestational diabetes mellitus and long-term consequences for mother and offspring: a view from Denmark. Diabetologia. 2016;59(7):1396–9.
14. Harder T, Rodekamp E, Schellong K, Dudenhausen JW, Plagemann A. Birth weight and subsequent risk of type 2 diabetes: a meta-analysis. Am J Epidemiol. 2007;165(8):849–57.
15. Weinert LS, Silveiro SP. Maternal-fetal impact of vitamin d deficiency: a critical review. Matern Child Health J. 2015;19(1):94–101.
16. Thuesen B, Husemoen L, Fenger M, Jakobsen J, Schwarz P, Toft U, Ovesen L, Jorgensen T, Linneberg A. Determinants of vitamin D status in a general population of Danish adults. Bone. 2012;50(3):605–10.
17. Henry HL, Bouillon R, Norman AW, Gallagher JC, Lips P, Heaney RP, Vieth R, Pettifor JM, Dawson-Hughes B, Lamberg-Allardt CJ, Ebeling PR. 14th vitamin D workshop consensus on vitamin D nutritional guidelines. J Steroid Biochem Mol Biol. 2010;121(1–2):4–6.

18. Heaney RP, Dowell MS, Hale CA, Bendich A. Calcium absorption varies within the reference range for serum 25-hydroxyvitamin D. J Am Coll Nutr. 2003;22(2):142–6.
19. Kaaja R, Alenius H, Kinnunen T, Komulainen J, Peränen N, Rönnemaa T, Saramies J, Soukka H, Teramo K, Vuorela P, Vääräsmäki M. 2013 [current care guidelines - gestational diabetes] Käypä hoito -suositus - Raskausdiabetes. Available from: http://www.kaypahoito.fi/web/english/guidelineabstracts/guideline?id=ccs00047. Accessed 15 May 2016.
20. Pihkala J, Hakala T, Voutilainen P, Raivio K. Characteristic of recent fetal growth curves in Finland. Duodecim. 1989;105(18):1540–6.
21. Burris HH, Rifas-Shiman SL, Kleinman K, Litonjua AA, Huh SY, Rich-Edwards JW, Camargo CA Jr, Gillman MW. Vitamin D deficiency in pregnancy and gestational diabetes mellitus. Am J Obstet Gynecol. 2012;207(3):182.e1–8.
22. Schneuer FJ, Roberts CL, Guilbert C, Simpson JM, Algert CS, Khambalia AZ, Tasevski V, Ashton AW, Morris JM, Nassar N. Effects of maternal serum 25-hydroxyvitamin D concentrations in the first trimester on subsequent pregnancy outcomes in an Australian population. Am J Clin Nutr. 2014;99(2):287–95.
23. Josefson JL, Reisetter A, Scholtens DM, Price HE, Metzger BE, Langman CB, HAPO Study Cooperative. Research group: maternal BMI associations with maternal and cord blood vitamin D levels in a north American subset of hyperglycemia and adverse pregnancy outcome (HAPO) study participants. PLoS One. 2016;11(3):e0150221.
24. Pereira-Santos M, Costa PR, Assis AM, Santos CA, Santos DB. Obesity and vitamin D deficiency: a systematic review and meta-analysis. Obes Rev. 2015;16(4):341–9.
25. Vimaleswaran KS, Berry DJ, Lu C, Tikkanen E, Pilz S, Hiraki LT, Cooper JD, Dastani Z, Li R, Houston DK, Wood AR, Michaelsson K, Vandenput L, Zgaga L, Yerges-Armstrong LM, McCarthy MI, Dupuis J, Kaakinen M, Kleber ME, Jameson K, Arden N, Raitakari O, Viikari J, Lohman KK, Ferrucci L, Melhus H, Ingelsson E, Byberg L, Lind L, Lorentzon M, Salomaa V, Campbell H, Dunlop M, Mitchell BD, Herzig KH, Pouta A, Hartikainen AL, Genetic investigation of anthropometric traits-GIANT consortium, Streeten EA, Theodoratou E, Jula A, Wareham NJ, Ohlsson C, Frayling TM, Kritchevsky SB, Spector TD, Richards JB, Lehtimaki T, Ouwehand WH, Kraft P, Cooper C, Marz W, Power C, Loos RJ, Wang TJ, Jarvelin MR, Whittaker JC, Hingorani AD, Hypponen E. causal relationship between obesity and vitamin D status: bi-directional Mendelian randomization analysis of multiple cohorts. PLoS Med. 2013;10(2):e1001383.
26. Autier P, Boniol M, Pizot C, Mullie P, Vitamin D. Status and ill health: a systematic review. Lancet Diabetes Endocrinol. 2014;2(1):76–89.
27. Nobles CJ, Markenson G, Chasan-Taber L. Early pregnancy vitamin D status and risk for adverse maternal and infant outcomes in a bi-ethnic cohort: the behaviors affecting baby and you (B.A.B.Y.) study. Br J Nutr. 2015;114(12):2116–28.
28. Farrant HJ, Krishnaveni GV, Hill JC, Boucher BJ, Fisher DJ, Noonan K, Osmond C, Veena SR, Fall CH, Vitamin D. Insufficiency is common in Indian mothers but is not associated with gestational diabetes or variation in newborn size. Eur J Clin Nutr. 2009;63(5):646–52.
29. Mathieu C, Vitamin D. Diabetes: where do we stand? Diabetes Res Clin Pract. 2015;108(2):201–9.
30. De-Regil LM, Palacios C, Lombardo LK, Pena-Rosas JP, Vitamin D. Supplementation for women during pregnancy. Cochrane Database Syst Rev. 2016;1:CD008873.
31. Harvey NC, Holroyd C, Ntani G, Javaid K, Cooper P, Moon R, Cole Z, Tinati T, Godfrey K, Dennison E, Bishop NJ, Baird J, Cooper C, Vitamin D. Supplementation in pregnancy: a systematic review. Health Technol Assess. 2014;18(45):1–190.
32. Miliku K, Vinkhuyzen A, Blanken LM, McGrath JJ, Eyles DW, Burne TH, Hofman A, Tiemeier H, Steegers EA, Gaillard R, Jaddoe VW. Maternal vitamin D concentrations during pregnancy, fetal growth patterns, and risks of adverse birth outcomes. Am J Clin Nutr. 2016;103(6):1514–22.
33. Song SJ, Si S, Liu J, Chen X, Zhou L, Jia G, Liu G, Niu Y, Wu J, Zhang W, Zhang J, Vitamin D. Status in Chinese pregnant women and their newborns in Beijing and their relationships to birth size. Public Health Nutr. 2013;16(4):687–92.
34. Kiely M, O'Donovan SM, Kenny LC, Hourihane JO, Irvine AD, Murray DM, Vitamin D. Metabolite concentrations in umbilical cord blood serum and associations with clinical characteristics in a large prospective mother-infant cohort in Ireland. J Steroid Biochem Mol Biol. 2017;167:162–8.
35. Shor DB, Barzel J, Tauber E, Amital H. The effects of maternal vitamin D on neonatal growth parameters. Eur J Pediatr. 2015;174(9):1169–74.
36. Rodriguez A, Garcia-Esteban R, Basterretxea M, Lertxundi A, Rodriguez-Bernal C, Iniguez C, Rodriguez-Dehli C, Tardon A, Espada M, Sunyer J, Morales E. Associations of maternal circulating 25-hydroxyvitamin D3 concentration with pregnancy and birth outcomes. BJOG. 2015;122(12):1695–704.
37. Hanieh S, Ha TT, Simpson JA, Thuy TT, Khuong NC, Thoang DD, Tran TD, Tuan T, Fisher J, Biggs BA. Maternal vitamin D status and infant outcomes in rural Vietnam: a prospective cohort study. PLoS One. 2014;9(6):e99005.
38. Hunt KJ, Schuller KL. The increasing prevalence of diabetes in pregnancy. Obstet Gynecol Clin N Am. 2007;34(2):173–99. vii

3

The short-term economic burden of gestational diabetes mellitus in Italy

Michela Meregaglia[1*†], Livia Dainelli[2†], Helen Banks[1], Chiara Benedetto[3], Patrick Detzel[2] and Giovanni Fattore[1,4]

Abstract

Background: The incidence of Gestational Diabetes Mellitus (GDM) is rising in all developed countries. This study aimed at assessing the short-term economic burden of GDM from the Italian healthcare system perspective.

Methods: A model was built over the last pregnancy trimester (i.e., from the 28th gestational week until childbirth included). The National Hospital Discharge Database (2014) was accessed to estimate delivery outcome probabilities and inpatient costs in GDM and normal pregnancies (i.e., euglycemia). International Classification of Disease-9th Revision-Clinical Modification (ICD9-CM) diagnostic codes and Diagnosis-Related Group (DRG) codes were used to identify GDM cases and different types of delivery (i.e., vaginal or cesarean) within the database. Neonatal outcomes probabilities were estimated from the literature and included macrosomia, hypoglycemia, hyperbilirubinemia, shoulder dystocia, respiratory distress, and brachial plexus injury. Additional data sources such as regional documents, official price and tariff lists, national statistics and expert opinion were used to populate the model. The average cost per case was calculated at national level to estimate the annual economic burden of GDM. One-way sensitivity analyses and Monte Carlo simulations were performed to quantify the uncertainty around base case results.

Results: The amount of pregnancies complicated by GDM in Italy was assessed at 54,783 in 2014 using a prevalence rate of 10.9%. The antenatal outpatient cost per case was estimated at €43.7 in normal pregnancies compared to €370.6 in GDM patients, which is equivalent to a weighted sum of insulin- (14%; €1034.6) and diet- (86%; €262.5) treated women's costs. Inpatient delivery costs were assessed at €1601.6 and €1150.3 for euglycemic women and their infants, and at €1835.0 and €1407.7 for GDM women and their infants, respectively. Thus, the overall cost per case difference between GDM and normal pregnancies was equal to €817.8 (+ 29.2%), resulting in an economic burden of about €44.8 million in 2014 at national level. Probabilistic sensitivity analysis yielded a cost per case difference ranging between €464.9 and €1164.8 in 80% of simulations.

Conclusions: The economic burden of GDM in Italy is substantial even accounting for short-term medical costs only. Future research also addressing long-term consequences from a broader societal perspective is recommended.

Keywords: Gestational diabetes mellitus (GDM), Hospital discharge database (HDD), Delivery outcomes, Costs, Italy

Background

Gestational Diabetes Mellitus (GDM) is defined as "any degree of glucose intolerance with onset or first recognition during pregnancy" and represents one of the most common complications [1]. GDM is associated with higher risk for adverse pregnancy outcomes as well as an increased probability of developing future type 2 diabetes mellitus in both mother and infant [2–5].

In Italy, a 75-gr oral glucose tolerance test (OGTT) for GDM is recommended at weeks 16–18 and/or at week 24–28 of pregnancy according to pre-defined risk factors including age, body mass index (BMI), family history of type 2 diabetes, previous history of GDM, and ethnicity [6]. According to the criteria promoted by the International Association of Diabetes and Pregnancy Study Groups (IADPSG) in 2010 [7], GDM prevalence was recently assessed at around 11% in Italy [8, 9]. This rate is 25% higher than the value estimated ten years before with the old criteria and may affect both the pre- and post-natal healthcare burden in the near future [8–12].

* Correspondence: michela.meregaglia@unibocconi.it
[†]Equal contributors
[1]CERGAS (Centre for Research on Health and Social Care Management), Bocconi University, Via Roentgen 1, 20136 Milan, Italy

The prevalence rate is aligned with data from other countries, where GDM is estimated to affect between 1% and 15% of pregnancies depending on ethnicity and diagnostic criteria adopted [12]. The aim of this study was to estimate the economic burden of GDM over the last pregnancy tem in Italy compared to normal pregnancies (i.e., euglycemia) from a national healthcare system perspective.

Methods

A model covering a period of three months (around 90 days) ranging from the 28th gestational week until childbirth (included) was built in Microsoft Excel (2013) and Tree Age Pro (2015).

Data sources

Data from the Italian National Hospital Discharge Database (HDD) provided by the Ministry of Health were accessed in order to obtain information about the women's characteristics and types of childbirth in GDM and normal pregnancies [13]. The database covers all hospitalizations in any public or private healthcare facility in any part of Italy. Women who gave birth were identified through specific Diagnosis-Related Group (DRG) codes (370–375) for birth or using International Classification of Disease-9th Revision-Clinical Modification (ICD9-CM) diagnostic codes that indicated childbirth (details are available on request) where resulting DRG codes were outside the expected range (e.g., for severe complications requiring surgery). GDM cases were discerned in the HDD using the ICD9-CM code 648.8, either in the birth admission or through linking the identification (ID) number of the mother to admissions during a three-month period prior to delivery. DRG codes (370–375) were used to discriminate among the different delivery methods and calculate the corresponding probabilities and costs in GDM and euglycemia (excluding those admissions for childbirth with other DRG codes). A separate database of the infants' hospitalizations for birth was extracted, which was used to estimate the average hospitalization costs of infants affected by neonatal complications frequently associated with GDM as compared to a normal newborn's cost.

Probabilities of GDM-related neonatal outcomes were obtained from the literature since it was not possible to identify children born to GDM mothers. In HDD, about one third of the newborns lack a unique ID code (i.e., unique IDs, assigned after birth, are not always included in the birth discharge record); the date of birth, age in days and residence are not provided; and no code exists to link infants with their mothers in the dataset. After a review of the literature, we agreed to rely on a large retrospective study of 36,241 women with and without GDM that allowed all risk varying according to the presence or not of macrosomia (i.e., birthweight ≥4 kg) [14]. Indeed, GDM is an established risk factor for macrosomia, which is in turn associated with several adverse neonatal outcomes [2]. The probability of giving birth to a normal infant was obtained by difference in the model. The number of births in 2014 (502,596) as reported by official statistics [15] was used as a 'proxy' of the number of pregnant women in the same period, although their number might be slightly different due to multiple pregnancies and stillbirths.

Cost analysis

The cost analysis was conducted from the perspective of the Italian National Health Service. Italy has a tax-based system funded mainly through reimbursement tariffs using DRGs for hospital care and national/regional tariffs for outpatient services and materials (with some use of additional subsidies from individual regions to their hospitals and patient co-payments for medications and outpatient services). In this study, antenatal outpatient and inpatient delivery costs broken down between mother and infant were calculated in GDM and euglycemia, respectively; DRG tariffs were used as a 'proxy' for inpatient costs. No discounting was applied as the time horizon was shorter than one year.

Mothers' delivery costs were calculated as DRG tariffs adjusted for the length of stay (LOS). In detail, a cost per admission day was obtained for each delivery method by dividing the official tariff by the average LOS in days across all women in labor identified in the HDD. Then, the daily cost was multiplied by the average LOS in GDM and euglycemic women, respectively, in order to obtain the average cost of a delivery stay in the two women's groups. In this cost calculation, we excluded 'outliers' defined as admissions with a LOS above the 99° percentile in the HDD.

From the infant's perspective, no cost values were assigned to macrosomia as such, but only to the events that followed; we calculated the average cost of admissions reporting each complication considered in the model adjusted for the LOS. For example, the cost associated with respiratory distress represented the average reimbursement tariff of all admissions reporting ICD9-CM diagnostic code 769 (neonatal respiratory distress) in the HDD 2014. In the model, the cost of a normal childbirth was assessed at €560 (DRG 391).

An average cost per case was obtained in GDM and euglycemia, respectively, as the sum of the products of probabilities and costs attached to each maternal and neonatal event considered in the model. Therefore, the annual economic burden of GDM in Italy for the year 2014 was estimated by multiplying the number of GDM cases (using a prevalence rate of 10.9% [8]) by the difference in cost per case between GDM and euglycemia [2].

Sensitivity analyses

We conducted both deterministic and probabilistic sensitivity analyses in order to test the robustness of base case results. One-way sensitivity analyses were applied by varying (± 20%) the probabilities retrieved from the literature (i.e., infant complications) and all inpatient costs in the model. In probabilistic sensitivity analysis (i.e., Monte Carlo simulations), probabilities were modeled using a beta distribution and costs using a gamma distribution.

Results

Mother's characteristics

After exclusions for lack of a unique (blinded) ID (44,402, 9.1%) and accounting for multiple pregnancies in one year (122), the characteristics of the 445,812 pregnant women uniquely identified in the database and delivering in 2014 were preliminarily investigated and presented in Table 1. Women with a GDM diagnosis were more likely to be in advanced maternal age, overweight - BMI ≥25 Kg/m^2 and/or obese - BMI ≥30 Kg/m^2 (ICD9-CM: 649.1; 278.0), have a nationality other than Italian and a lower educational level compared to euglycemic ones.

Antenatal outpatient costs

The screening and treatment path for GDM, as recommended by Italian guidelines, is reported in Fig. 1 [6]. In this study, we assumed all GDM diagnoses occurred at the 28th week of gestation. Accordingly, Table 2 summarizes resources consumption and costs associated with the different blood glucose states during the last pregnancy trimester. Insulin-treated GDM patients (14%) [16] perform a blood glucose test four times a day (i.e., fasting, and 1 h after breakfast, lunch, and dinner) with a portable glucometer, while those under a special diet and exercise regimen only can limit testing to two surveys per day [10, 17]. In case of variable consumption frequencies (e.g., once or twice a day), the lowest bound (e.g., once a day) was conservatively adopted to estimate the costs. The cost of insulin therapy was assessed by referring to the most prescribed drug (i.e., insulin aspart) for GDM in Italy. Additional visits and exams, including a visual field test for eye complications, were reported in GDM women during pregnancy [17]. The cost of one oral 75-g OGTT was included to account for an extra test prescribed to GDM women shortly after delivery [6].

Inpatient costs

Maternal events resulting in hospitalization in the model represented the different delivery options as described by the DRG system (codes: 370–375); the corresponding probabilities were retrieved from the HDD for normal pregnancies and those complicated by GDM, respectively (Table 3). The analysis was performed on 442,285 deliveries after excluding 3650 records with other DRG codes.

The health events considered for infants were hypoglycemia (blood glucose < 35 mg/dL), hyperbilirubinemia (total serum bilirubin > 5 mg/dL), respiratory distress, shoulder dystocia and brachial plexus injury as reported by the study from Esakoff et al. [14]; the risk of macrosomia was retrieved instead by an Italian study [18] (Table 4).

Inpatient costs estimated for each event considered in the model are reported in Table 5. For neonatal complications, a unique cost value was reported since the database does not allow to distinguish between children born from GDM and euglycemic mothers.

Overall costs

As reported in Table 6, the base case analysis yielded a cost per GDM case equal to €3613.4 divided into antenatal outpatient (€370.6) and inpatient costs for mother (€1835.0) and infant (€1407.7).

GDM outpatient costs corresponded to a weighted sum of insulin- and diet-treated women's costs and were on average €326.9 higher than in euglycemic women. Similarly, total inpatient costs (mother and infant) in GDM (€3242.8) outweighed those in normal pregnancies (€2751.9). Overall, each pregnancy affected by GDM cost 29.2% more than a pregnancy without GDM, with a cost per case difference of €817.8. The number of

Table 1 Mother's characteristics by euglycemic status

	GDM (*N* = 11,540)		Euglycemia (*N* = 434,272)		Source
Age (mean ± SD)	33.7 ± 5.4		31.6 ± 5.6		[13]
Advanced age (≥35)	5369	46.5%	140,238	32.3%	[13]
Overweight/Obesity	276	2.4%	1190	0.3%	[13]
Foreign citizenship	3920	34.0%	82,433	19.0%	[13]
University degree[a]	1370	13.3%	61,349	15.1%	[13]

[a]Education level was reported in 416,079 of records (93.3%)

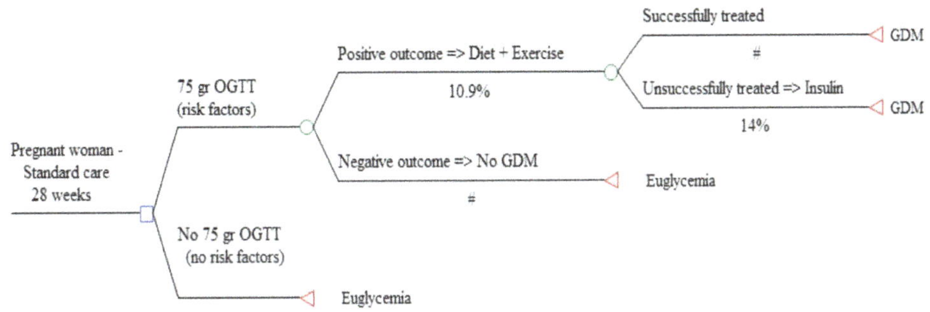

Fig. 1 Screening and treatment path for GDM. The figure shows the generic framework of GDM screening path as recommended by Italian guidelines. The square node on the far left symbolizes the choice between the two screening options; circles represent chance events. The symbol # indicates that probabilities of that branch are complementary to those of the parallel branch. Triangles represent the terminal nodes

pregnancies affected by GDM was estimated at 54,783 (out of 502,596 births) in 2014, resulting in an extra cost of around €44.8 million for the Italian National Health Service.

Sensitivity analyses

In Table 7 we showed the effects of varying selected parameters on the inpatient cost per case difference between GDM and euglycemia. The largest impact on Δ cost/case was obtained by varying ±20% the cost of cesarean section without complications in GDM, which yielded an interval of the cost difference equal to €324.1 - €657.7.

Figure 2 displays Monte Carlo probability distributions (1000 iterations) of the expected inpatient cost per case in euglycemic and GDM women, respectively. The possible values ranged between €2326.6 and €3206.6 in euglycemia and €2792.0 and €3890.4 in GDM. However, 80% of the expected cost values were included in the range €2577.7 - €2915.7 in euglycemia and €3053.7 - €3415.6 in GDM. Under these simulations, inpatient cost per case difference between GDM and euglycemia might vary between €138.0 and €837.9 which, summed with the outpatient cost/case difference (€326.9), would give an overall cost/case difference range of €464.9 - €1164.8.

Discussion

Main findings

There is a lack of research on the burden associated with GDM in many countries, masking its potential importance for policy-makers. To our knowledge, this is the first study to estimate the economic consequences of GDM in Italy.

This analysis showed that pregnant women affected by GDM are more likely to present established risk factors

Table 2 Antenatal outpatient costs by mother's euglycemic status

Category	Resource	Consumption			Code	Unit cost (€)	Total costs per case (€)			Source
		GDM (Diet)	*GDM (Insulin)*	*Euglycemia*			*GDM (Diet)*	*GDM (Insulin)*	*Euglycemia*	
Screening	OGTT 75 g	2	2	1	90.26.4	2.38	4.76	4.76	2.38	[6]
Self-monitoring blood glucose kit	Glucometer	Yes	Yes	No	–	Free of charge	0.0	0.0	0.0	Expert opinion
	Test strip	2/day	4/day	No	–	0.55	99.0	198.0	0.0	[10, 17, 23]
	Finger stick	2/day	4/day	No	–	0.10	18.0	36.0	0.0	[24]
Insulin therapy	Insulin (shot)	No	1–2 shots/day	No	–	6.34	0.0	570.6	0.0	[17, 25]
	Needle	No		No	–	0.14	0.0	12.6	0.0	[24]
	Syringe	No		No	–	0.11	0.0	9.9	0.0	[24]
Visits and exams	Obstetric visit	Every 3–4 weeks	Every 1–2 weeks	Every 5–6 weeks	89.26	20.66	62.0	124.0	41.3	Expert opinion; [26]
	Obstetric ultrasound	2 (at 32th week and 36th week)		No	88.78.2	30.99	62.0	62.0	0.0	Expert opinion; [17]
	Visual field test	1		No	95.05	16.78	16.8	16.8	0.0	[17]
Total costs							262.5	1034.6	43.7	

Table 3 Delivery options probabilities by mother's euglycemic status

DRG	Description	Euglycemia (N = 430,851)		GDM (N = 11,434)		Source
370	Caesarean section with CC	11,437	2.6%	538	4.7%	[13]
371	Caesarean section without CC	145,212	33.7%	4019	35.2%	[13]
372	Vaginal delivery with CC	9447	2.2%	447	3.9%	[13]
373	Vaginal delivery without CC	260,036	60.3%	6287	55.0%	[13]
374	Vaginal delivery with sterilization and/or dilatation and curettage	4274	1.0%	125	1.1%	[13]
375	Vaginal delivery with other interventions but sterilization and/or dilatation and curettage	445	0.1%	18	0.2%	[13]

such as obesity, advanced maternal age, non-Italian citizenship, and low educational level and to experience adverse pregnancy outcomes. Even accounting for short-term medical costs only, the yearly economic burden of GDM was substantial (€44.8 million) in 2014. At the outpatient level, a relevant difference in cost (+ 748%) was observed between GDM and euglycemic women, while in terms of hospitalization, mother and infant costs were respectively 14.6% and 22.3% higher than in euglycemia. These results remained robust after performing both deterministic and probabilistic sensitivity analysis.

Strengths and limitations

The main strength of this study was the availability of administrative data on hospital discharges for all women who delivered in 2014 in Italy. As a check on the reliability of the data, we measured an infant mortality rate of 3.3 per 1000 live births, which is in line with the rate of 3.1 in published data for Italy [15]. However, our database contained fewer women (445,812) uniquely identified as giving births than those reported by official statistics (502,596), likely due to exclusions for incomplete (blinded) ID codes and inconclusive diagnostic and DRG coding. We also found wide, unexplained variation in the percentage of women with a GDM diagnosis among regions (from 0.5% in Aosta Valley to 6.1% in Tuscany) and a low overall GDM rate (< 3%) in hospital delivery records, even though clinical studies [8, 9] and expert opinion estimated the prevalence to be 10% or more in Italy. This inconsistency (and presumed under-reporting) is likely due to variation among regions in coding practices and number of diagnostic code fields reported at discharge, plus a lack of financial incentive to consistently record secondary diagnoses. This is a main limiting factor in using administrative data rather than medical records for research purposes.

This analysis also presented a few additional limitations. First, the costs associated to GDM were likely to be underestimated for several reasons. For example, we only considered the public expenditure for GDM, while out-of-pocket expenses for extra visits and exams, nutritional supplements, food substitution and physical activity may be substantial. Moreover, we did not consider that GDM can be diagnosed at an earlier pregnancy stage (16th–18th week) in high-risk women, nor that it may be under diagnosed in women without any of the risk factors required to perform the OGTT test. We also disregarded that women can be admitted at the hospital during the pre-delivery period for complications related to GDM, and that patient compliance in performing daily glucose tests or assuming the prescribed therapies may not be perfect.

Second, the data sources for mother's and infant's events were very different, since for the latter it was not possible to derive GDM-related probabilities from the HDD due to the unknown mother's glycemic status; in particular, we referred to a single study [14] reporting perinatal outcomes in infants born in San Francisco before 2006. Until now, no study has reported all the neonatal outcomes of interest for Italy through a comparison between GDM and non-GDM women, thus it was not possible to refer to a more recent and country-specific study. However, some of the outcomes reported by the reviewed study [14]

Table 4 Neonatal events probabilities by mother's euglycemic status

	Macrosomia	Hypoglycemia	Hyperbilirubinemia	Shoulder dystocia	Respiratory distress	Brachial plexus injury	Normal newborn
Euglycemia	Yes (7.4%)	2.4%	7.6%	6.0%	1.7%	0.7%	81.6%
	No	1.2%	9.1%	0.9%	1.2%	0.1%	87.5%
GDM	Yes (8.7%)	5.3%	13.2%	10.5%	4.0%	2.6%	64.4%
	No	2.6%	10.4%	1.6%	1.5%	0.2%	83.7%
Source	[18]	[14]	[14]	[14]	[14]	[14]	Own calculation

Table 5 Inpatient costs (€) of mother's and neonatal events

	Code(s)	Event	Cost (€)		Source
			Euglycemia	GDM	
Mother	370[a]	Caesarean section with CC	2774.5	2938.5	[13]
	371[a]	Caesarean section without CC	2084.3	2373.0	[13]
	372[a]	Vaginal delivery with CC	1610.3	1802.8	[13]
	373[a]	Vaginal delivery without CC	1269.3	1385.2	[13]
	374[a]	Vaginal delivery with sterilization and/or dilatation and curettage	2116.0	2330.9	[13]
	375[a]	Vaginal delivery with other interventions but sterilization and/or dilatation and curettage	2842.0	3265.9	[13]
Infant	769[b]	Respiratory distress	24,337.8		[13]
	775.0/775.6[b]	Hypoglycemia	6571.8		[13]
	774.2/774.6[b]	Hyperbilirubinemia	2854.2		[13]
	767.6[b]	Brachial plexus injury	1671.9		[13]
	660.4[b]	Shoulder dystocia	1407.6		[13]
	391[a]	Normal newborn	560.0		[13]

[a]DRG; [b]ICD9-CM

were aligned with the values indicated in the Italian literature; for example, in GDM, fetal distress was estimated at 3.4% and hypoglycemia at 2.5% in the study by Lapolla et al. [18]; unfortunately, the authors did not provide these figures for normal pregnancies.

Third, we adopted a national reference for reimbursement tariffs to model costs, although tariffs may vary at the regional level in Italy. The inter-regional unitary tariff for DRGs is the best available estimate of hospitalization costs across regions, although it represents an approximation of real costs; the production cost, indeed, is only one of the variables used for setting tariffs [19]. Thus, we performed sensitivity analysis on inpatient costs to consider any potential variations.

Interpretation

According to the literature, the GDM rate is growing rapidly worldwide with a consequent large healthcare cost increase [20]. A cluster-randomized trial from Finland [21] reported that mean healthcare costs, including both inpatient and outpatient care before and after delivery, were 25% higher in women diagnosed with GDM (€6432) than among euglycemic women (€5143) in the 2007–2009 period. Moreover, women affected by GDM were more likely to be in advanced maternal age, overweight or obese and with a low educational level.

A recent modeling study [2] conducted in the US estimated a short-term cost of GDM of $1.8 billion in 2014 (corresponding to around €1.5 billion) using a prevalence rate of 5.5%, which might underestimate the real GDM burden since the US did not adopt the IADSPG criteria [22]. The average additional cost per case was $15,593 (around €13,700).

Due to differences in methodological approaches and healthcare financing systems, findings from previous studies were hardly comparable with ours; however, they confirmed a substantial economic burden of GDM at least in developed countries. This study, unlike the Finnish one, did not adopt an experimental design, and relied instead on heterogeneous data sources to estimate the costs of GDM in Italy; however, by using administrative data, we could review a much larger sample of observations that those generally available in empirical studies.

Table 6 Mother's and infant's cost per case (€) by mother's euglycemic status

	Outpatient	Inpatient		Inpatient cost/case	Total cost/case
	Mother	Mother	Infant		
Euglycemia	43.7	1601.6	1150.3	2751.9	2795.6
GDM	370.6	1835.0	1407.7	3242.8	3613.4
Diet (86%)	262.5	–	–	–	–
Insulin (14%)	1034.6	–	–	–	–
Delta	326.9	233.4	257.4	490.9	817.8

Table 7 One-way sensitivity analysis on the inpatient costs per case (€)

	Cost/case (euglycemia)	Cost/case (GDM)	Δ cost/case
Base case	2751.8	3242.7	490.9
Costs (€)			
Hypoglycemia			
−20%	2734.9	3205.4	470.5
+ 20%	2768.8	3280.0	511.2
Respiratory distress			
− 20%	2691.6	3159.1	467.5
+ 20%	2812.1	3326.3	514.2
Cesarean section with CC (GDM)			
− 20%	2751.8	3215.0	463.2
+ 20%	2751.8	3270.4	518.6
Cesarean section without CC (GDM)			
− 20%	2751.8	3075.9	324.1
+ 20%	2751.8	3409.5	657.7
Vaginal delivery without CC (GDM)			
− 20%	2751.8	3090.3	338.5
+ 20%	2751.8	3395.0	643.2
Cesarean section without CC (euglycemia)			
− 20%	2611.4	3242.7	631.3
+ 20%	2892.3	3242.7	350.4
Vaginal delivery without CC (euglycemia)			
− 20%	2598.6	3242.7	644.1
+ 20%	2905.1	3242.7	337.6
Probabilities			
Hyperbilirubinemia (GDM/no macrosomia)			
− 20%	2751.8	3199.1	447.3
+ 20%	2751.8	3286.3	534.5
Hypoglycemia (GDM/no macrosomia)			
− 20%	2751.8	3214.2	462.4
+ 20%	2751.8	3271.2	519.4
Respiratory distress (GDM/no macrosomia)			
− 20%	2751.8	3177.6	425.8
+ 20%	2751.8	3307.8	556.0
Hyperbilirubinemia (euglycemia/no macrosomia)			
− 20%	2713.2	3242.7	529.5
+ 20%	2790.5	3242.7	452.2
Respiratory distress (euglycemia/no macrosomia)			
− 20%	2699.0	3242.7	543.7
+ 20%	2804.7	3242.7	438.0

Conclusions

This study should be interpreted as a first step towards further research in diabetes in pregnancy and highlights the need of collecting additional data regarding GDM in Italy and elsewhere. Parameters included in this model are likely to be used in future cost-effectiveness analyses of novel GDM treatments or preventive interventions targeted to women of childbearing age. Our analysis

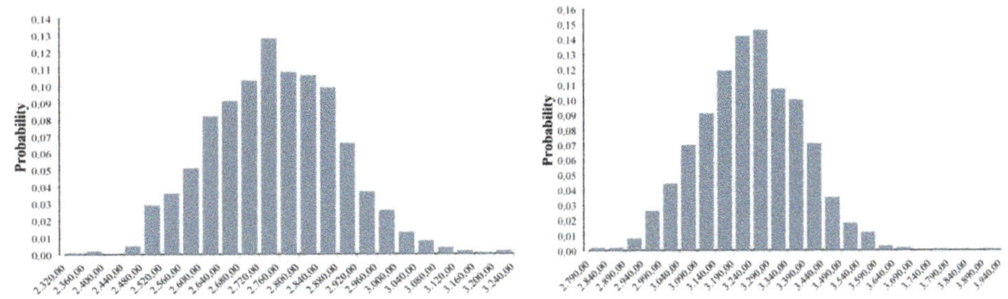

Fig. 2 Monte Carlo probability distributions in euglycemia (left) and GDM (right). The figure shows Monte Carlo probability distribution (1000 iterations) of the expected inpatient cost per case in euglycemia (left) and GDM (right). The most likely value (the highest bar in the histogram) corresponds to the base case result

focused on the gestational period only, but long-term consequences of GDM in mother (i.e., type 2 diabetes) and infant (i.e., type 2 diabetes, congenital malformations, obesity, and cardiovascular diseases) are likely to increase the estimated economic burden. Thus, additional studies investigating GDM-related effects over mothers' and infants' lifetimes are also needed.

Abbreviations

BMI: Body mass index; DRG: Diagnosis-Related Group; GDM: Gestational Diabetes Mellitus; HDD: Hospital Discharge Database; IADPSG: International Association of Diabetes and Pregnancy Study Groups; ICD9-CM: International Classification of Disease-9th Revision-Clinical Modification; ID: (unique) identifier; OGTT: oral glucose tolerance test

Acknowledgments

The authors gratefully thank the Italian Ministry of Health who provided the data for this study. They also thank Dr. Irma Silva Zolezzi and Dr. Sara Colombo Mottaz (Nestlé Research Center, Switzerland) for project guidance and support, and Prof. Phil Baker (University of Leicester, UK) for his precious suggestions. Lastly, they are grateful to Mr. Marco Stegani (CERGAS, Bocconi University) for indispensable assistance in extracting and classifying patients in the National Hospital Discharge Database.

Funding

The study was funded by the Nestlé Research Centre (Switzerland), which was involved in the study design, in the interpretation of data and in the writing of the manuscript.

Authors' contributions

LD and PD conceived the study. LD, MM, PD and GF designed it. GF, MM, and LD contributed to the data collection. GF, HB and MM had full access to all data from the Ministry of Health and were responsible for the integrity of these data. MM, LD and HB performed the statistical analyses and drafted the article. PD and GF contributed to the interpretation of the data and the critical revision of the manuscript. CB provided independent clinical advice. All authors reviewed and approved the final version of the article.

Competing interests

The authors declare that they have no competing interests.

Author details

[1]CERGAS (Centre for Research on Health and Social Care Management), Bocconi University, Via Roentgen 1, 20136 Milan, Italy. [2]Nestlé Research Center, Nestec SA, Route du Jorat 57, 1000 Lausanne, Switzerland. [3]Department of Gynecology & Obstetrics, S. Anna Hospital, University of Turin, Via Ventimiglia 3, 10126 Turin, Italy. [4]Department of Policy Analysis and Public Management, Bocconi University, Via Roentgen 1, 20136 Milan, Italy.

References

1. American Diabetes Association. Diagnosis and classification of diabetes mellitus. Diabetes Care. 2009;32(1):S62–7.
2. Lenoir-Wijnkoop I, Van Der Beek EM, Garssen J, Nuijten MJ, Uauy RD. Health economic modeling to assess short-term costs of maternal overweight, gestational diabetes, and related macrosomia–a pilot evaluation. Front Pharmacol. 2015;6:103. https://doi.org/10.3389/fphar.2015.00103.
3. Jiménez-Moleón JJ, Bueno-Cavanillas A, De D Luna-del-Castillo J, Garcia-Martiin M, Lardelli-Claret P, Gálvez-Vargas R. Impact of different levels of carbohydrate intolerance on neonatal outcomes classically associated with gestational diabetes mellitus. Eur J Obstet Gynecol Reprod Biol. 2002;102(1):36–41.
4. Holder T, Giannini C, Santoro N, Pierpont B, Shaw M, Duran E, Caprio S, Weiss R. A low disposition index in adolescent offspring of mothers with gestational diabetes: a risk marker for the development of impaired glucose tolerance in youth. Diabetologia. 2014;57(11):2413–20.
5. Verier-Mine O. Outcomes in women with a history of gestational diabetes. Screening and prevention of type 2 diabetes. Literature review. Diabetes Metab. 2010;36(6 Pt 2):595–616.
6. Ministry of Health (2011), Istituto Superiore di Sanità, CeVEAS (Centro per la valutazione dell'efficacia dell'assistenza sanitaria). Linee Guida Gravidanza Fisiologica (Aggiornamento 2011). Available at: http://www.salute.gov.it/imgs/c_17_pubblicazioni_1436_allegato.pdf. Accessed 2 Feb 2016.
7. International Association of Diabetes and Pregnancy Study Groups Consensus Panel (Metzger BE, Gabbe SG, Persson B, Buchanan TA, Catalano PA, Damm P, Dyer AR, Leiva Ad, Hod M, Kitzmiler JL, Lowe LP, McIntyre HD, Oats JJ, Omori Y, Schmidt MI). International association of diabetes and pregnancy study groups recommendations on the diagnosis and classification of hyperglycemia in pregnancy. Diabetes Care 2010; 33(3): 676–682.
8. Lacaria E, Lencioni C, Russo L, Romano M, Lemmi P, Battini L, Del Prato S, Bertolotto A, Di Cianni G. Selective screening for GDM in Italy: application and effectiveness of National Guidelines. J Matern Fetal Neonatal Med. 2015;28(15):1842–4.
9. Di Cianni G, Gualdani E, Berni C, Meucci A, Roti L, Lencioni C, Lacaria E, Seghieri G, Francesconi P. Screening for gestational diabetes in Tuscany, Italy. A population study. Diabetes Res Clin Pract. 2017;132:149–56.
10. Capula C, Chiefari E, Vero A, Arcidiacono B, Iiritano S, Puccio L, Pullano V, Foti DP, Brunetti A, Vero R. Gestational diabetes mellitus: screening and outcomes in southern Italian pregnant women. ISRN Endocrinol. 2013;2013:387495. https://doi.org/10.1155/2013/387495.
11. Di Cianni G, Lacaria E, Lencioni C, Russo L, Bertolotto A. Applicazione delle Linee Guida Nazionali per lo Screening del Diabete Gestazionale: efficacia e criticità. G It Diabetol Metabol. 2015;35:157–60.
12. Lapolla A, Dalfrà MG, Ragazzi E, De Cata AP, Fedele D. New International Association of the Diabetes and Pregnancy Study Groups (IADPSG) recommendations for diagnosing gestational diabetes compared with

former criteria: a retrospective study on pregnancy outcome. Diabet Med. 2011;28(9):1074–7.

13. Archivio Nazionale dati SDO, Ministero della salute, Direzione Generale della Programmazione Sanitaria, Ufficio VI. Data for analysis was provided upon written request and approval from the Italian Ministry of Health. A description of the database is available at: http://www.salute.gov.it/portale/p5_1_1.jsp?lingua=italiano&id=126.
14. Esakoff TF, Cheng YW, Sparks TN, Caughey AB. The association between birthweight 4000g or greater and perinatal outcomes in patients with and without gestational diabetes mellitus. Am J Obstet Gynecol 2009; 200: 672. e1–672672.e4.
15. ISTAT (Anno 2014). Natalità e fecondità della popolazione residente. Available at: http://www.istat.it/it/archivio/140132. Accessed 20 Jan 2016.
16. Corrado F, Pintaudi B, D'Anna R, Santamaria A, Giunta L, Di Benedetto A. Perinatal outcome in a Caucasian population with gestational diabetes and preexisting diabetes first diagnosed in pregnancy. Diabetes Metab. 2016; 42(2):122–5.
17. Friuli Venezia-Giulia, Regione Autonoma. Il diabete gestazionale. Documento di indirizzo per la gestione del diabete gestazionale (2014). Available at: http://www.ass1.sanita.fvg.it/opencms/export/sites/ass1/it/_materiale_informativo/docs/documento_gestione_diabete_gestazionale.pdf. Accessed 3 Feb 2016.
18. Lapolla A, Dalfrà MG, Bonomo M, Parretti E, Mannino D, Mello G, Di Cianni G. Scientific committee of GISOGD group. Gestational diabetes mellitus in Italy: a multicenter study. Eur J Obstet Gynecol Reprod Biol. 2009;145:149–53.
19. Fattore G, Torbica A. Inpatient reimbursement system in Italy: how do tariffs relate to costs? Health Care Manag Sci. 2006;9(3):251–8.
20. Ferrara A. Increasing prevalence of gestational diabetes mellitus a public health perspective. Diabetes Care. 2007;30(Supplement 2):S141–6.
21. Kolu P, Raitanen J, Rissanen P, Luoto R. Healthcare costs associated with gestational diabetes mellitus among high-risk women – results from a randomized trial. BMC Pregnancy Childbirth. 2012;12:71.
22. Brown FM, Wyckoff J. Application of one-step IADPSG versus two-step diagnostic criteria for gestational diabetes in the real world: impact on health services, clinical care, and outcomes. Current Diabetes Reports. 2017; 17(10):85.
23. Veneto, Regione. Deliberazione della giunta regionale n. 43 del 28 gennaio 2014. Available at: http://bur.regione.veneto.it/BurvServices/pubblica/DettaglioDgr.aspx?id=268004. Accessed 3 Feb 2016.
24. Veneto, Regione. Bollettino Ufficiale della Regione del Veneto n. 58 del 12 luglio 2013. Accessed 3 Feb 2016.
25. Emilia-Romagna, Regione. Farmaci AVR 2015. Available at: http://intercenter.regione.emilia-romagna.it. Accessed 3 Feb 2016.
26. Ministry of Health (2012). Decreto 18 ottobre 2012. Remunerazione delle prestazioni di assistenza ospedaliera per acuti, assistenza ospedaliera di riabilitazione e di lungodegenza post acuzie e di assistenza specialistica ambulatoriale. Available at: http://www.trovanorme.salute.gov.it/norme/renderPdf.spring?seriegu=SG&datagu=28/01/2013&redaz=13A00528&artp=1&art=1&subart=1&subart1=10&vers=1&prog=001. Accessed 13 Gen 2016.

4

Impact of adopting the 2013 World Health Organization criteria for diagnosis of gestational diabetes in a multi-ethnic Asian cohort

Claudia Chi[1*†], See Ling Loy[2,3†], Shiao-Yng Chan[1,4,5], Cherie Choong[1], Shirong Cai[5], Shu E. Soh[4,6], Kok Hian Tan[7], Fabian Yap[3,8,9], Peter D. Gluckman[4,10], Keith M. Godfrey[11,12], Lynette Pei-Chi Shek[6,13], Jerry Kok Yen Chan[2,3], Michael S. Kramer[5,14,15] and Yap-Seng Chong[1,4,5]

Abstract

Background: We assessed the impact of adopting the 2013 World Health Organization (WHO) diagnostic criteria on the rates of gestational diabetes (GDM), pregnancy outcomes and identification of women at future risk of type 2 diabetes.

Methods: During a period when the 1999 WHO GDM criteria were in effect, pregnant women were universally screened using a one-step 75 g 2-h oral glucose tolerance test at 26–28 weeks' gestation. Women were retrospectively reclassified according to the 2013 criteria, but without the 1-h glycaemia measurement. Pregnancy outcomes and glucose tolerance at 4–5 years post-delivery were compared for women with GDM classified by the 1999 criteria alone, GDM by the 2013 criteria alone, GDM by both criteria and without GDM by both sets of criteria.

Results: Of 1092 women, 204 (18.7%) and 142 (13.0%) were diagnosed with GDM by the 1999 and 2013 WHO criteria, respectively, with 27 (2.5%) reclassified to GDM and 89 (8.2%) reclassified to non-GDM when shifting from the 1999 to 2013 criteria. Compared to women without GDM by both criteria, cases reclassified to GDM by the 2013 criteria had an increased risk of neonatal jaundice requiring phototherapy (relative risk (RR) = 2.78, 95% confidence interval (CI) 1.32, 5.86); despite receiving treatment for GDM, cases reclassified to non-GDM by the 2013 criteria had higher risks of prematurity (RR = 2.17, 95% CI 1.12, 4.24), neonatal hypoglycaemia (RR = 3.42, 95% CI 1.04, 11.29), jaundice requiring phototherapy (RR = 1.71, 95% CI 1.04, 2.82), and a higher rate of abnormal glucose tolerance at 4–5 years post-delivery (RR = 3.39, 95% CI 2.30, 5.00).

Conclusions: Adoption of the 2013 WHO criteria, without the 1-h glycaemia measurement, reduced the GDM rate. Lowering the fasting glucose threshold identified women who might benefit from treatment, but raising the 2-h threshold may fail to identify women at increased risk of adverse pregnancy and future metabolic outcomes.

Keywords: Gestational diabetes mellitus, Glucose tolerance, Pregnancy outcomes, Type 2 diabetes, World Health Organization

* Correspondence: claudia_chi@nuhs.edu.sg
†Equal contributors
[1]Department of Obstetrics & Gynaecology, National University Hospital, Singapore 119074, Singapore
Full list of author information is available at the end of the article

Background

Gestational diabetes mellitus (GDM), defined as any degree of glucose intolerance with onset or first recognition during pregnancy [1], is associated with adverse outcomes in mothers and offspring [2, 3]. However, international uniformity for the ascertainment and diagnosis of GDM has not been reached and has remained a contentious issue [4]. In 2010, the International Association of Diabetes and Pregnancy Study Group (IADPSG) proposed a new set of diagnostic criteria for GDM [5] based on the graded dose-response associating maternal glycaemia with pregnancy outcomes reported in the Hyperglycaemia and Adverse Pregnancy Outcomes (HAPO) Study [2]. It was recommended that GDM be diagnosed if one or more of the following criteria are met: fasting plasma glucose (FPG) 5.1–6.9 mmol/L, 1-h plasma glucose (PG) ≥ 10. 0 mmol/L or 2-h PG 8.5–11.0 mmol/L [5, 6]; whilst those with FPG ≥ 7.0 mmol/L or 2-h PG ≥ 11.1 mmol/L are diagnosed with diabetes in pregnancy [6]. The thresholds for GDM diagnosis were the glucose values at which the odds for birth weight, cord C peptide concentration and percentage of newborns with neonatal body fat greater than the 90th centile reached 1.75 times the odds of these outcomes at the mean glucose values of the entire study cohort of pregnant women who were deemed not to have pre-existing diabetes [5]. In contrast, the earlier 1999 WHO GDM diagnostic criteria were based on the thresholds used to define diabetes mellitus or impaired glucose tolerance outside pregnancy (FPG > 7.0 mmol/L, 2-h PG ≥7.8 mmol/L) [7], whilst the original O'Sullivan and Mahan criteria (FPG ≥5.8 mmol/L, 1-h PG ≥10.6 mmol/L, 2-h PG ≥9.2 mmol/L, 3-h PG ≥8.1 mmol/L) was aimed primarily to identify women at increased risk of developing future type 2 diabetes mellitus [8].

In 2013, the World Health Organization (WHO) endorsed and adopted the IADPSG diagnostic criteria for GDM in an attempt to achieve a universal standard for the diagnosis of GDM [6]. Nevertheless, the use of these new criteria in GDM screening remains controversial as no evidence from prospective randomized studies have shown improved maternal and fetal outcomes with their adoption [9]. In addition, differences in GDM prevalence and in the relative diagnostic importance of FPG, 1-h PG and 2-h PG were observed across the geographically-diverse centres of the HAPO study [10]. Therefore, the WHO has recommended further evaluation of the impact of adopting the 2013 criteria in diverse settings and ethnic groups [6].

In comparison to the 1999 WHO criteria [7], the 2013 criteria used a lower threshold for FPG but a higher threshold for the 2 h PG and the addition of a 1-h PG [6]. A shift from the 1999 WHO criteria to the new 2013 WHO criteria may lead to diagnosis of more cases with increased FPG and/or increased 1-h PG but "miss" cases with slightly increased 2-h PG (i.e. those between 7.8 mmol/L and 8. 4 mmol/L). It is therefore important to document the fraction of newly-diagnosed GDM cases and "missed" GDM cases, and to assess their pregnancy outcomes and subsequent metabolic risk. Such information may impact screening strategies and affect the proportion of pregnant women who receive GDM treatment and are followed-up after delivery for future development of type 2 diabetes mellitus.

People of Chinese (74.3%), Malay (13.3%) and Indian (9.1%) ethnicity make up the majority of the population in Singapore [11]. Based on the latest report from the International Diabetes Federation, people of Chinese and Indian ethnicity comprise the world's largest populations at risk of developing type 2 diabetes mellitus [12]. Because of its ageing and increasingly sedentary population, Singapore presages health problems that other Asian countries are likely to face in the decades ahead [13]. The prevalence of type 2 diabetes mellitus in Singapore has been forecasted to double from 7.3% in 1990 to 15.0% in 2050 [13]. Furthermore, Singapore has one of the highest GDM rates in the world [10].

Women with GDM are at high risk of developing type 2 diabetes mellitus [14]. It is therefore important to study the prevalence of GDM in ethnicities most heavily affected by diabetes. In this study, we used prospectively collected data from a multi-ethnic group of Asian women participating in the Growing Up in Singapore Towards healthy Outcomes (GUSTO) cohort study [15] to compare the prevalence of GDM based on the 1999 and 2013 WHO criteria across three Asian ethnicities, and assess the impact of GDM reclassification switching from the older to the newer criteria on pregnancy outcomes and on glucose tolerance of women 4–5 years after delivery.

Methods

Study design and participants

GUSTO is an on-going Asian mother-offspring cohort study [15]. It is conducted according to the guidelines laid down in the Declaration of Helsinki. Ethical approval was obtained from the Centralised Institutional Review Board of SingHealth (reference 2009/280/D) and the Domain Specific Review Board of Singapore National Healthcare Group (reference D/09/021). Informed written consent was obtained from all participants.

Between June 2009 and September 2010, 1247 pregnant women aged 18 and above were recruited during the first trimester of pregnancy (< 14 weeks' gestation based on a first trimester dating ultrasound scan) from KK Women's and Children's Hospital (KKH) and National University Hospital (NUH), the two major public maternity units in Singapore. The recruited women were Singapore citizens or permanent residents from three different ethnic groups (Chinese, Malay, and Asian Indian) with homogenous parental ethnic background. Women receiving chemotherapy or psychotropic drugs or with type 1 diabetes mellitus were excluded. For this study we also excluded women with multiple pregnancies, resulting in 1237 women.

Data collection

Recruited women returned to the hospitals at 26–28 weeks' gestation for a follow-up study visit. Detailed interviews and measurements were conducted in the clinics at recruitment and at 26–28 weeks' gestation. Data on socioeconomic status, family history, obstetric history and smoking status were collected. Family history of diabetes mellitus was based only on first-degree relatives. Smoking status was defined as smoking during the current pregnancy.

Self-reported pre-pregnancy weight and measured booking weight at the first antenatal clinic visits (≤14 weeks' gestation) were ascertained. Height was measured with a portable stadiometer (Seca 213, Hamburg, Germany) at 26–28 weeks' gestation. Body mass index (BMI) was determined using the formula of weight (kg)/ height (m^2). Since early pregnancy BMI at the first clinic visit was free from recall bias, was strongly correlated with pre-pregnancy BMI ($r = 0.96$, $p < 0.001$) and had fewer missing values (0.7%), it was used in all analyses. Gestational weight gain (GWG) was computed as the difference between booking weight and the measured weight at 26–28 weeks' gestation and expressed as gestational age-specific z-score based on the reference of [16].

Data on pregnancy outcomes were retrieved from the hospital case notes, discharge summaries and electronic medical records by trained health personnel.

Oral glucose tolerance test

Women underwent a 75-g oral glucose tolerance test (OGTT) after an overnight fast (8 to 10 h) at 26–28 weeks' gestation and at 4–5 years after delivery. Plasma glucose concentrations at 0 and 120 min following the oral glucose load were measured by colorimetry [Advia 2400 Chemistry system (Siemens Medical Solutions Diagnostics) and Beckman LX20 Pro analyser (Beckman Coulter)]. GDM was diagnosed using the 1999 WHO criteria: ≥7.0 mmol/L for FPG and/ or ≥ 7.8 mmol/L for 2-h PG [7]. Women with GDM were subsequently managed with dietary advice with or without insulin treatment according to standard protocols in both hospitals. Following an OGTT 4–5 years after delivery, type 2 diabetes mellitus (DM), impaired fasting glucose (IFG) and impaired glucose tolerance (IGT) were diagnosed using the 2006 WHO criteria: FPG ≥7.0 mmol/L or 2-h PG ≥11.1 mmol/L for DM; FPG 6.1 to 6.9 mmol/L and 2-h PG < 7.8 mmol/L for IFG; and FPG < 7.0 mmol/L and 2-h PG ≥7.8 and < 11.1 mmol/L for IGT [17].

GDM diagnostic criteria

GDM was diagnosed using the 1999 WHO criteria (≥7.0 mmol/L for FPG and/ or ≥ 7.8 mmol/L for 2-h PG) [7] during the GUSTO pregnancy period and retrospectively the 2013 WHO criteria (≥5.1 mmol/L for FPG and/ or ≥ 8.5 mmol/L for 2-h PG) [6] was applied for the purposes of this specific study. The 1-h PG included in the 2013 WHO criteria was not measured in our study, as it was not part of the routine OGTT performed at that time. Women were reclassified into four mutually exclusive groups using the 1999 and 2013 WHO GDM diagnostic criteria. Group 1 included women who were classified as non-GDM by both criteria (FPG < 5.1 mmol/L and 2-h PG < 7.8 mmol/L); Group 2 included women who were diagnosed as GDM by the 1999 WHO criteria but reclassified as normal by the 2013 WHO criteria (FPG < 5.1 mmol/L but 2-h PG between ≥7.8 and < 8.5 mmol/L); Group 3 included women who were normal by the 1999 WHO criteria but reclassified as GDM by the 2013 WHO criteria (FPG between ≥5.1 and < 7.0 mmol/L but 2-h PG < 7.8 mmol/L); Group 4 included women who were GDM by both criteria (FPG ≥7.0 mmol/L and/ or 2-h PG ≥8.5 mmol/L).

Outcome measures

Maternal outcomes included requirement for insulin, induction of labour, caesarean delivery, instrumental vaginal delivery, hypertensive disorders (including chronic hypertension, pregnancy-induced hypertension and pre-eclampsia in the index pregnancy), as well as abnormal glucose tolerance (type 2 DM, IFG and IGT) at 4–5 years after delivery.

Foetal outcomes included gestational age at birth, preterm birth (< 37 completed weeks), Apgar scores at 1 min and 5 min, birth weight-for-gestational-age (birth-weight-for-GA) z-score, small-for-gestational-age (SGA) birth, large-for-gestational-age (LGA) birth, macrosomia (> 4 kg), shoulder dystocia, hypoglycaemia, neonatal jaundice requiring phototherapy and neonatal intensive care unit (NICU) admission. Gestational age was determined based on ultrasound scan measurements at 7–12 weeks. A customized birth weight-for-GA centile chart based on GUSTO data was derived according to Mikolajczyk et al. [18] using solely gestational age for customization. SGA and LGA birth were defined, respectively, as <10th and > 90th centile using the customized birth weight-for-GA centile chart. Hypoglycaemia was defined as a capillary blood glucose ≤2.5 mmol/L.

Statistical analysis

Statistical analyses were performed using SPSS software, Version 20 (USA) and StataCorp Stata Statistical Software, Release 13 (USA). Categorical data are presented as frequencies and percentages, while continuous data are presented as means and SDs. Comparisons of maternal characteristics and outcomes between groups were performed using Pearson's Chi-square or Fisher's exact tests, as appropriate, for categorical variables and independent t-tests for continuous variables. Differences in GDM rates between paired proportions were assessed using McNemar's test. Modified poisson regression [19] was used to obtain adjusted relative risks (RRs) and 95% confidence intervals (CIs) associated with each GDM classification group for categorical outcomes, while linear regression was used for continuous outcomes with non-GDM women defined as the reference group. Potential confounding variables were identified from the literature [20, 21] and included maternal age, ethnicity, education, body mass index, gestational weight gain, parity, family history of diabetes and type of conception. Additional adjustment for infant sex was performed for LGA and birth weight-for-GA z-score outcomes and adjustment for SGA birth was performed for neonatal hypoglycaemia and jaundice requiring phototherapy.

According to the 2013 WHO criteria, diabetes in pregnancy, as opposed to GDM, is diagnosed when FPG ≥7.0 mmol/L or 2-h PG ≥11.1 mmol/L [6]. In our study, nine women fell into this category. Therefore we also conducted a sensitivity analysis restricting the samples to those with FPG < 7.0 mmol/L and 2-h PG < 11.1 mmol/L ($n = 1083$ for assessing pregnancy outcomes; $n = 648$ for assessing glucose tolerance at 4–5 years post-delivery).

Results

Of the 1237 women with singleton pregnancies, 1092 (88.3%) underwent OGTT at 26–28 weeks' gestation. The remaining 145 (11.7%) women either missed their 26–28 weeks study visit, declined testing or had type 2 diabetes mellitus. No significant differences were observed between the 1092 women who had OGTT and the 145 women who did not have OGTT in terms of ethnicity, age, BMI, GWG, education, parity, family history of diabetes, smoking during pregnancy and type of conception.

Table 1 shows the numbers and proportions of women diagnosed with GDM based on the 1999 and 2013 WHO criteria, and reclassification of GDM using the different criteria. Use of the 2013 WHO criteria, (without the 1-h PG) reduced the overall GDM rate from 18.7% ($n = 204$) to 13.0% ($n = 142$) based on universal screening. The greatest reduction in the rate of GDM was observed among Chinese women (from 20.3% to 11.8%; $p < 0.001$), with the same trend among Indians (from 23.8% to 18.5%; $p = 0.064$) but little change among Malay women (from 11.5% to 11.9%; $p > 0.950$). Overall, 89 women with GDM (8.2% of total, and 43.6% of GDM cases based on the 1999 WHO criteria) were reclassified to non-GDM, while 27 (2.5% of total) women without GDM by the 1999 WHO criteria were reclassified to GDM with the 2013 WHO criteria. The diagnosis of GDM remained unchanged in 115 (10.5% of total) women who were diagnosed with GDM by both the 1999 and 2013 WHO criteria.

Table 2 compares the characteristics and pregnancy outcomes among the four groups. Baseline characteristics and pregnancy outcomes of women reclassified from GDM to non-GDM (Group 2), from non-GDM to GDM (Group 3) and GDM by both the 1999 and 2013 WHO criteria (Group 4) were compared against women who were non-GDM by both criteria (Group 1). In comparison to Group 1, those in Group 2 were older (32.2 vs 30.2 years, $p = 0.001$) and were more likely to have received higher education (46.1% vs 32.5%, $p = 0.010$). Women in Group 3 had a higher BMI (28.0 vs 23.3 kg/m^2, $p < 0.001$) and were more likely to be multiparous (74.1% vs 52.9%, $p = 0.030$) and have a positive family history of diabetes (59.3% vs 28.1%, $p < 0.001$). Women in Group 4 were older (32.7 vs 30.2 years, $p < 0.001$), had a higher BMI (25.5 vs 23.3 kg/m^2, $p < 0.001$), lower GWG z-score (− 1.1 vs − 0.8, $p = 0.024$) and more likely to conceive through in vitro fertilization (14.8% vs 5.9%, $p < 0.001$).

Compared to Group 1, a higher proportion of cases in Group 2 had labour induction (50.0% vs 34.9%, $p = 0.011$), instrumental vaginal delivery (15.8% vs 7.9%, $p = 0.049$), prematurity (12.4% vs. 6.1%, $p = 0.025$), shoulder dystocia (2.4% vs 0.1%, $p = 0.025$), neonatal hypoglycaemia (7.3% vs 1.9%, $p = 0.011$) and neonatal jaundice requiring phototherapy (20.2% vs

Table 1 Rates of GDM and the reclassification of the diagnosis of GDM using the 1999 and 2013 WHO criteria

	GDM based on 1999 WHO criteria	GDM based on 2013 WHO Criteria[a]	Non-GDM based on both 1999 and 2013 WHO criteria[a] (Group 1)	Reclassified from GDM to non-GDM using 2013 WHO criteria[a] (Group 2)	Reclassified from non-GDM to GDM using 2013 WHO criteria (Group 3)	GDM based on both 1999 and 2013 WHO criteria (Group 4)
	n (%)	*n* (%)	*n* (%)	*n* (%)	*n* (%)	*n* (%)
Chinese ($n = 625$)	127 (20.3)	74 (11.8)[b]	490 (78.4)	61 (9.8)	8 (1.3)	66 (10.6)
Malay ($n = 278$)	32 (11.5)	33 (11.9)	234 (84.2)	11 (4.0)	12 (4.3)	21 (7.6)
Indian ($n = 189$)	45 (23.8)	35 (18.5)	137 (72.5)	17 (9.0)	7 (3.7)	28 (14.8)
Total ($n = 1092$)	204 (18.7)	142 (13.0)[b]	861 (78.8)	89 (8.2)	27 (2.5)	115 (10.5)

GDM gestational diabetes mellitus, *WHO* World Health Organization

[a]without the 1-h plasma glucose measure

[b]differences in GDM rates based on 1999 vs 2013 WHO criteria; $P < 0.001$ based on McNemar's test

Table 2 Characteristics and pregnancy outcomes of women

	Group 1: Non-GDM based on both 1999 and 2013 WHO criteria ($n = 861$)	Group 2: Reclassified from GDM to non-GDM using 2013 WHO criteria ($n = 89$)	Group 3: Reclassified from non-GDM to GDM using 2013 WHO criteria ($n = 27$)	Group 4: GDM based on both 1999 and 2013 WHO criteria ($n = 115$)	*P* value (Group 2 vs. 1)	*P* value (Group 3 vs. 1)	*P* value (Group 4 vs. 1)
Characteristics							
Age, years [mean (SD)]	30.2 (5.1)	32.2 (4.9)	31.2 (5.4)	32.7 (4.6)	0.001	0.348	< 0.001
Body mass index, kgm^{-2} [mean (SD)]	23.3 (4.6)	24.0 (4.5)	28.0 (5.7)	25.5 (4.9)	0.195	< 0.001	< 0.001
Gestational weight gain, z-score [mean (SD)]	−0.8 (1.1)	−0.8 (0.9)	−0.9 (1.2)	−1.1 (1.1)	0.581	0.792	0.024
Education, *n* (%)							
None/ primary/ secondary	573 (67.5)	48 (53.9)	20 (80.0)	70 (60.9)	0.010	0.187	0.157
Tertiary	276 (32.5)	41 (46.1)	5 (20.0)	45 (39.1)			
Multiparous, *n* (%)	450 (52.9)	46 (51.7)	20 (74.1)	70 (60.9)	0.821	0.030	0.109
Positive family history of diabetes, *n* (%)	242 (28.1)	28 (31.5)	16 (59.3)	39 (33.9)	0.504	< 0.001	0.197
Smoking during pregnancy, *n* (%)	23 (2.7)	2 (2.3)	1 (3.8)	1 (0.9)	> 0.950	0.517	0.346
Type of conception, *n* (%)							
Natural	810 (94.1)	83 (93.3)	25 (92.6)	98 (85.2)	0.757	0.673	< 0.001
in vitro fertilization	51 (5.9)	6 (6.7)	2 (7.4)	17 (14.8)			
Maternal Outcomes							
Insulin requirement, *n* (%)	0	5 (5.6)	0	12 (10.4)	< 0.001	–	< 0.001
Induction of labour, *n* (%)	260 (34.9)	36 (50.0)	9 (42.9)	51 (51.5)	0.011	0.448	0.001
Caesarean section, *n* (%)	242 (30.1)	32 (40.0)	11 (40.7)	34 (30.6)	0.069	0.239	0.915
Instrumental delivery, *n* (%)	48 (7.9)	9 (15.8)	0	4 (4.9)	0.049	0.626	0.346
Hypertension and/ or preeclampsia, *n* (%)	57 (6.6)	5 (5.6)	3 (11.1)	16 (13.9)	0.716	0.420	0.005
Neonatal Outcomes							
Gestation at birth, weeks [mean (SD)]	38.4 (1.4)	38.2 (1.4)	38.1 (1.3)	37.9 (2.2)	0.078	0.200	0.008
Prematurity, *n* (%)	52 (6.1)	11 (12.4)	2 (7.4)	13 (11.3)	0.025	0.680	0.038
Apgar score at 1 min [mean (SD)]	8.9 (0.6)	8.8 (0.6)	8.6 (1.6)	8.8 (0.8)	0.297	0.379	0.179
Apgar score at 5 min [mean (SD)]	9.0 (0.1)	9.0 (0.1)	8.9 (0.6)	9.0 (0.3)	0.456	0.369	0.569
	0.1 (1.1)	0.1 (1.1)	0.7 (1.2)	0.5 (1.6)	0.861	0.006	0.012

Table 2 Characteristics and pregnancy outcomes of women *(Continued)*

	Group 1: Non-GDM based on both 1999 and 2013 WHO criteria ($n = 861$)	Group 2: Reclassified from GDM to non-GDM using 2013 WHO criteria ($n = 89$)	Group 3: Reclassified from non-GDM to GDM using 2013 WHO criteria ($n = 27$)	Group 4: GDM based on both 1999 and 2013 WHO criteria ($n = 115$)	*P* value (Group 2 vs. 1)	*P* value (Group 3 vs. 1)	*P* value (Group 4 vs. 1)
Birth weight-for-gestational age, z-score [mean (SD)]							
Small for gestational age, *n* (%)	91 (10.7)	10 (11.2)	1 (3.7)	11 (9.6)	0.881	0.348	0.706
Large for gestational age, *n* (%)	124 (14.6)	14 (15.7)	6 (22.2)	25 (21.7)	0.776	0.271	0.047
Macrosomia, *n* (%)	15 (1.8)	1 (1.1)	1 (3.7)	2 (1.7)	> 0.950	0.397	> 0.950
Shoulder dystocia, *n* (%)	1 (0.1)	2 (2.4)	0	0	0.025	> 0.950	> 0.950
Hypoglycaemia, *n* (%)	15 (1.9)	6 (7.3)	1 (3.8)	18 (16.2)	0.011	0.413	< 0.001
Neonatal jaundice requiring phototherapy, *n* (%)	86 (11.2)	17 (20.2)	7 (26.9)	22 (20.2)	0.015	0.024	0.007
Neonatal intensive care unit admission, *n* (%)	30 (3.6)	5 (5.7)	2 (7.7)	6 (5.2)	0.368	0.247	0.427

GDM gestational diabetes mellitus, *WHO* World Health Organization, *P* value based on independent t-test, Pearson's Chi-square or Fisher's exact test, as appropriate

11.2%, $p = 0.015$). Newborns of women in Group 3 had a higher mean birth weight-for-GA z-score (0.7 vs 0.1, $p = 0.006$) and were more likely to have jaundice requiring phototherapy (26.9% vs 11.2%, $p = 0.024$) compared to those born to women in Group 1. Treatment with insulin was given to 5.6 and 10.4% of women in Groups 2 and 4, respectively. A higher proportion of cases in Group 4 had labour induction (51.5% vs 34.9%, $p = 0.001$), hypertensive disorders (13.9% vs 6.6%, $p = 0.005$), prematurity (11.3% vs 6.1%, $p = 0.038$), neonatal hypoglycaemia (16.2% vs 1.9%, $p < 0.001$) and neonatal jaundice requiring phototherapy (20.2% vs 11.2%, $p = 0.007$) compared to women in Group 1. Women in Group 4 delivered at an earlier mean gestation (37.9 vs 38.4 weeks, $p = 0.008$) and their newborns had a higher mean birth weight-for-GA z-score (0.5 vs 0.1, $p = 0.012$) compared to women in Group 1. There were no difference in the proportions of SGA births in Groups 2, 3 and 4 compared to Group 1 (Table 2).

Table 3 shows the RRs for associations between GDM reclassification groups and pregnancy outcomes after adjustment for confounding variables. The risks of prematurity, neonatal hypoglycaemia and jaundice requiring phototherapy were 2.17 times (95% CI 1.12, 4.24), 3.42 times (95% CI 1.04, 11.29) and 1.71 times (95% CI 1.04, 2.82) higher, respectively, among women in Group 2 than among those in Group 1, respectively. An increased risk of neonatal jaundice requiring phototherapy [RR = 2.78 (95% CI 1.32, 5.86)] was also observed among newborns of women in Group 3 compared to those in Group 1. Cases in Group 4 had increased risks of prematurity [RR = 2.06 (95% CI 1.10, 3.84)], LGA birth [RR = 1.60 (95% CI 1.07, 2.39)] and neonatal hypoglycaemia [RR = 11.23 (95% CI 4.98, 25.32)]. An increased birth weight-for-GA z-score was observed in women in Group 4 [0.35 (95% CI 0.12, 0.59)] compared with those in Group 1, but not in Groups 2 or 3.

Table 4 shows the prevalence of abnormal glucose tolerance in the subset of women who consented to an OGTT at 4–5 years after delivery. Women who underwent OGTT at 4–5 years after delivery were older ($p < 0.001$) and more likely to be multiparous ($p = 0.025$) than those who did not; these were adjusted for in subsequent analyses. Of the 653 women who underwent OGTT, 124 (19.0%) had abnormal glucose tolerance, with higher proportions observed among women in Groups 2 (42.6%) and 4 (45.2%) ($p < 0.001$) (Table 4). Women in Groups 2 and 4 had three-fold increased adjusted risks of developing abnormal glucose tolerance by 4–5 years after delivery compared to women in Group 1 [Group 2: RR = 3.39 (95% CI 2.30, 5.00); Group 4: RR = 2.87 (95% CI 1.93, 4.27)]. However, the trend of an increased risk for women in Group 3 was not statistically significant, perhaps due to the small number [Group 3: RR 1.90 (95% CI 0.88, 4.11)].

In the sensitivity analyses, with the exclusion of women classified with diabetes in pregnancy by the 2013 WHO criteria ($n = 9$), the results remained similar with minimal changes in the effect estimates for the relationship between GDM reclassification groups and risks of pregnancy outcomes (See, Additional file 1: Table S1; See, Additional file 2: Table S2) and abnormal glucose development postnatally (See, Additional file 3: Table S3).

Discussion

In the multi-ethnic Asian GUSTO cohort, we found that the adoption of the 2013 WHO criteria, without the 1-h PG, reduced the GDM rate from 18.7 to 13.0%, but with marked ethnic variation. The reduction was specifically observed in Chinese and Indian women but remained unchanged among Malay women. This reduction would lead to "missing" almost half (44%) of the cases which may benefit from GDM intervention during pregnancy to reduce maternal and neonatal morbidity, and from postpartum surveillance for primary prevention and early diagnosis of type 2 diabetes mellitus.

The adoption of the 2013 WHO GDM diagnostic criteria substantially increased the prevalence of GDM in the Caucasian population [22, 23] compared to the 1999 WHO GDM diagnostic criteria. However, reported changes in GDM rates have varied across studies of Asian populations. The 2013 WHO criteria diagnosed more GDM cases in the studies by Pan et al. [21] from China (7.7% vs. 6.8%, $n = 17{,}808$) and Gilder et al. [24] from Thailand (10.1% vs. 6.6%, $n = 228$), a similar proportion of

Table 3 Associations between reclassification of gestational diabetes mellitus diagnosis and pregnancy outcomes

Pregnancy outcomes	Group 1	Group 2		Group 3		Group 4	
		RR (95% CI)	P	RR (95% CI)	P	RR (95% CI)	P
Hypertension/ preeclampsia[a]	reference	0.80 (0.35, 1.84)	0.596	1.19 (0.46, 3.09)	0.724	1.54 (0.88, 2.70)	0.126
Prematurity[a]	reference	2.17 (1.12, 4.24)	0.023	0.70 (0.10, 4.87)	0.716	2.06 (1.10, 3.84)	0.023
Large for gestational age[b]	reference	1.23 (0.75, 2.03)	0.411	1.14 (0.62, 2.12)	0.667	1.60 (1.07, 2.39)	0.021
Hypoglycaemia[c]	reference	3.42 (1.04, 11.29)	0.044	2.40 (0.31, 18.63)	0.402	11.23 (4.98, 25.32)	< 0.001
Neonatal jaundice requiring phototherapy[c]	reference	1.71 (1.04, 2.82)	0.034	2.78 (1.32, 5.86)	0.007	1.61 (0.98, 2.66)	0.060

RR = relative risk; CI = confidence interval

[a] Model 1: adjusted for maternal age, ethnicity, education, body mass index, gestational weight gain, parity and family history of diabetes, type of conception

[b] Model 2: adjusted for same variables as in model 1 + neonatal sex

[c] Model 3: adjusted for same variables as in model 1 + small-for-gestational-age birth

Table 4 Abnormal glucose tolerance development of women by 4 to 5 years after delivery ($n = 653$)

Diabetes status	Group 1: Non-GDM based on both 1999 and 2013 WHO criteria ($n = 498$)	Group 2: Reclassified from GDM to non-GDM using 2013 WHO criteria ($n = 61$)	Group 3: Reclassified from non-GDM to GDM using 2013 WHO criteria ($n = 21$)	Group 4: GDM based on both 1999 and 2013 WHO criteria ($n = 73$)	*P* value
Normal, *n* (%)	439 (67.2)	35 (5.4)	15 (2.3)	40 (6.1)	< 0.001
Abnormal[a] *n* (%)	59 (9.0)	26 (4.0)	6 (0.9)	33 (5.1)	

GDM gestational diabetes mellitus, *WHO* World Health Organization
[a]Abnormal status included diabetes mellitus (FG ≥7.0 mmol/l or PG ≥11.1 mmol/l), impaired fasting glucose (FG 6.1 to 6.9 mmol/l and PG < 7.8 mmol/l) and impaired glucose tolerance (FG < 7.0 mmol/l and PG ≥7.8 and < 11.1 mmol/l). Abnormal, $n = 124$ (19.0%)

GDM cases in the study by Sagili et al. [25] from India (12.6% vs. 12.4%, $n = 1231$), and fewer GDM cases in studies by Tran et al. [26] from Vietnam (20.4% vs. 24.3%, $n = 2772$) and Yew et al. [20] from Singapore (21.1% vs. 28.8%, $n = 855$). These disparities and data from our study and others' [27] support the notion of variation in glycaemic responses to a glucose load in pregnancy among different Asian ethnicities. Pregnant women from East Asia and South Asia have been found to be more insulin-resistant, with poorer homeostatic model assessment (HOMA) β-cell function, than Western Europeans [28], leading to different rates of GDM. Other contributory factors to the variations in the reported change in GDM rates include differences in the study setting (community vs. tertiary-care hospital) and type of screening approach (universal vs. risk-based and one-step vs. two-step screening).

The lower overall GDM rate we observed with a shift from the 1999 to the 2013 WHO criteria mainly resulted from the marked reduction (20.3 to 11.8%) in GDM rate among Chinese women. Only a small proportion (1.3%) of Chinese women had a FPG between 5.1 and 6.9 mmol/L which moved them into the GDM category, while a significantly larger proportion (9.8%) had a 2-h PG between 7.8 and 8.4 mmol/L, moving them out of the GDM category. Similarly, amongst the 15 HAPO centres internationally, Hong Kong Chinese participants had one of the lowest proportion (26%; range 24–74%) of GDM diagnosed by FPG but the highest proportion (29%; range 6–29%) of GDM diagnosed by the 2-h PG [10]. We also observed a similar pattern among women of Indian ethnicity. This is consistent with the findings of several studies on Indian women showing the majority of GDM were detected not by the FPG but by the 2-h PG threshold of ≥7.8 mmol/L based on the 1999 WHO Criteria [25, 29, 30]. Hence the 2-h PG is important in Chinese and Indian women and raising the 2-h PG fails to detect many cases that may benefit from identification and treatment to reduce adverse outcomes.

The benefits of screening for and treating GDM have been demonstrated by two randomized controlled trials. The Australian Carbohydrate Intolerance Study in Pregnant Women (ACHOIS) trial found treatment of GDM women as defined by the 1999 WHO criteria reduced the risk (RR of 0.33, 95% CI 0.14–0.75) of serious perinatal complications (defined as shoulder dystocia, bone fracture, nerve palsy and death) [31]. The second trial from the Maternal Fetal Medicine Units (MFMU) network in the US reported that treatment of mild GDM (FPG < 5.3 mmol/L) reduced mean birth weight and the number of LGA infants [32]. In our study, women who fulfilled the 1999 WHO criteria for GDM received treatment. We are therefore unable to assess the true impact on pregnancy outcomes solely due to change in the 2-h PG threshold. However, treatment of GDM in Group 2 would almost certainly have underestimated the difference in the observed outcomes compared to Group 1. The diagnosis of GDM in Groups 2 and 4 was associated with higher rates of labour induction, as this was part of the standard clinical management of GDM, but it did not result in a significantly higher rate of caesarean delivery compared with the non-GDM cases (Group 1). Women with a 2-h PG in the range of 7.8–8.4 mmol/L (Group 2) would be regarded as normal using the 2013 WHO criteria 2-h PG threshold. We found that five (5.6%) women in Group 2 received insulin treatment, probably reflecting a degree of hyperglycaemia during pregnancy that did not respond to dietary intervention alone; eleven (12.4%) and two (2.4%) offspring of mothers in this group experienced preterm birth and shoulder dystocia at delivery, respectively. Furthermore, the offspring of mothers in this group were at 3.4-fold increased risk of neonatal hypoglycaemia and 1.7-fold increased risk of neonatal jaundice requiring phototherapy compared to those whose mothers did not have GDM by both sets of criteria, even after adjusting for demographic and clinical covariates. Knowledge of the diagnosis of GDM might have created a bias towards the diagnosis of neonatal hypoglycaemia and neonatal jaundice through increased surveillance. However, these complications are likely to be in part related to relative foetal hyperglycaemia in utero, as there was no difference in the proportion of SGA births, a known cofounder in the development of these complications, in Group 2 compared to Group 1.

The FPG threshold of 7.0 mmol/L in the 1999 WHO GDM criteria is regarded as being too high as it is the same as the diagnostic cut-off for type 2 diabetes mellitus in non-pregnant adults [6]. In our study women with FPG between 5.1 and 6.9 mmol/L (Group 3) would be reclassified from non-GDM to GDM under the 2013 criteria. In the absence of treatment, their offspring were at

2.8-fold increased risk of developing jaundice requiring phototherapy compared to non-GDM women by both criteria (Group 1). Although higher percentages of women in Group 3 had hypertensive disorders in pregnancy and LGA infants, the differences were not statistically significant compared with Group 1, perhaps reflecting the small number of women in this group. Nonetheless our results suggest that lowering the FPG threshold might be important in reducing hyperglycaemia-related adverse maternal and neonatal outcomes.

The main strength of our study is our ability to assess the impact of GDM reclassification on identifying women at future risk of type 2 diabetes mellitus. To the best of our knowledge, our study is the first to compare later maternal metabolic outcome based on different GDM diagnostic criteria. In a previous meta-analysis, women who have had GDM using a variety of older diagnostic criteria have been shown to have at least a seven-fold increased risk of developing later type 2 diabetes compared with those who had a normoglycaemic pregnancy [14]. In our study we observed that women with GDM by both criteria (Group 4) were at three-fold increased risk of developing abnormal glucose tolerance within a relatively short interval of 4–5 years after delivery compared to women with no GDM by both criteria. More importantly, women who would not have been identified as GDM by the 2013 criteria but only by the 1999 criteria were also at significantly increased risk (similarly high at three-fold) of abnormal glucose tolerance. The adoption of the 2013 WHO criteria would have failed to identify these women who could benefit from timely intervention to reduce their risk of developing later type 2 diabetes mellitus. Other strengths of our study include its multi-ethnic Asian sample and prospective cohort study design.

Our study also has several limitations. The lack of a 1-h PG value could potentially underestimate the prevalence of GDM using the 2013 criteria by not identifying women with an isolated abnormal 1-h PG. In the HAPO survey, 39% of Singaporean women were diagnosed with GDM based on 1-h PG of ≥10.0 mmol/L [10], whilst a study on South Indians found 14% had elevated 1-h PG value [29]. It is currently not known whether women identified as GDM through an isolated raised 1-h PG value in the 2013 WHO criteria would have had different pregnancy outcomes from those identified using the FPG or 2-h PG thresholds. Moreover, women with an isolated raised 1-h PG would come from Group 1; hence the removal of these cases from the control group could conceivably result in further exaggeration of the difference in pregnancy and metabolic outcomes compared with Groups 2, 3 and 4. However, in the absence of a randomised prospective trial of universal screening comparing the utility of the 1999 with the 2013 WHO criteria, the comparison made in our study provides the best estimates of the consequences of using these two different sets of criteria.

The 2013 WHO criteria represent an important initiative to achieve internationally accepted criteria for the diagnosis of GDM [6]. However, the challenge is that any dichotomous classification of normal vs abnormal glucose tolerance in pregnancy fails to account for the fact that maternal glycaemia shows a continuous, monotonic association with adverse pregnancy outcomes [2]. Furthermore, clear differences in the patterns of insulin resistance, glucose tolerance, and rates of GDM among different ethnic groups have been demonstrated in our and other studies [10, 27].

In 2015, the UK National Institute of Health and Care Excellence (NICE) adopted a different set of GDM diagnostic criteria after considering its own health economic evidence and recommended an intermediate FPG threshold of 5.6 mmol/L (between both WHO criteria) but kept the 2-h PG threshold at ≥7.8 mmol/L as in the 1999 criteria [33]. However, power limitations prevent us from assessing the impact of adopting the NICE recommendation in our cohort as it would have reclassified only seven women from non-GDM to GDM.

Conclusion

In summary, a shift from the 1999 WHO criteria to the 2013 WHO criteria without a 1-h PG measurement, reduced the rate of GDM in this multi-ethnic Asian cohort. Lowering the fasting threshold as per the new WHO criteria identified women who might benefit from GDM treatment, but raising the 2-h threshold, without the 1-h value, would "miss" women at increased risk of adverse pregnancy and metabolic outcomes. In the absence of the 1-h PG measurements, our data support lowering the FPG but not changing the 2-h PG threshold for our population. Further studies are needed to guide the development of effective strategies for screening and identification of women at risk of adverse pregnancy outcomes and long-term metabolic complications particularly in countries experiencing an epidemic of diabetes, like Singapore.

Additional files

Additional file 1: Table S1. Modified poisson regression models of the associations between reclassification of gestational diabetes mellitus diagnosis and pregnancy outcomes, with the inclusion of women without diabetes in pregnancy.

Additional file 2: Table S2. Linear regression models of the associations between reclassification of gestational diabetes mellitus diagnosis and birth weight-for-GA, with the inclusion of women without diabetes in pregnancy.

Additional file 3: Table S3. Abnormal glucose tolerance development of women by 4 to 5 years after delivery, with the inclusion of women without diabetes in pregnancy.

Abbreviations

ACHOIS: Australian carbohydrate intolerance study in pregnant women; BMI: Body mass index; CI: Confidence interval; DM: Diabete mellitus; FG: Fasting glucose; FPG: Fasting plasma glucose; GA: Gestational age; GDM: Gestational diabetes mellitus; GUSTO: Growing up in singapore towards healthy outcomes; GWG: Gestational weight gain; HAPO: Hyperglycaemia and adverse pregnancy outcome; HOMA: Homeostatic model assessment; IADPSG: International association of diabetes and pregnancy study group; IFG: Impaired fasting glucose; IGT: Impaired glucose tolerance; LGA: Large-for-gestational-age; MFMU: Maternal fetal medicine unit; NICE: National institute of health care excellence; NICU: Neonatal intensive care unit; OGTT: Oral glucose tolerance test; PG: Plasma glucose; RR: Relative risk; SD: Standard deviation; SGA: Small-for-gestational-age; WHO: World Health Organisation

Acknowledgements

We would like to thank the study subjects and their families for their participation. We also thank the GUSTO study group, which includes Allan Sheppard, Amutha Chinnadurai, Anne Eng Neo Goh, Anne Rifkin-Graboi, Anqi Qiu, Arijit Biswas, Bee Wah Lee, Birit F.P. Broekman, Boon Long Quah, Borys Shuter, Chai Kiat Chng, Cheryl Ngo, Choon Looi Bong, Christiani Jeyakumar Henry, Cornelia Yin Ing Chee, Yam Thiam Daniel Goh, Doris Fok, E Shyong Tai, Elaine Tham, Elaine Quah Phaik Ling, Evelyn Chung Ning Law, Evelyn Xiu Ling Loo, Falk Mueller-Riemenschneider, George Seow Heong Yeo, Helen Chen, Heng Hao Tan, Hugo P S van Bever, Iliana Magiati, Inez Bik Yun Wong, Ivy Yee-Man Lau, Izzuddin Bin Mohd Aris, Jeevesh Kapur, Jenny L. Richmond, Joanna D. Holbrook, Joanne Yoong, Joao N. Ferreira., Jonathan Tze Liang Choo, Jonathan Y. Bernard, Joshua J. Gooley, Kenneth Kwek, Krishnamoorthy Niduvaje, Kuan Jin Lee, Leher Singh, Lieng Hsi Ling, Lin Lin Su, Ling-Wei Chen, Lourdes Mary Daniel, Marielle V. Fortier, Mark Hanson, Mary Foong-Fong Chong, Mary Rauff, Mei Chien Chua, Melvin Khee-Shing Leow, Michael Meaney, Mya Thway Tint, Neerja Karnani, Ngee Lek, Oon Hoe Teoh, P. C. Wong, Paulin Tay Straughan, Pratibha Agarwal, Queenie Ling Jun Li, Rob M. van Dam, Salome A. Rebello, Seang-Mei Saw, S. Sendhil Velan, Seng Bin Ang, Shang Chee Chong, Sharon Ng, Sok Bee Lim, Stella Tsotsi, Chin-Ying Stephen Hsu, Sue Anne Toh, Swee Chye Quek, Victor Samuel Rajadurai, Walter Stunkel, Wayne Cutfield, Wee Meng Han, Wei Wei Pang, Yin Bun Cheung, Yiong Huak Chan and Yung Seng Lee.

Funding

This research is supported by the Singapore National Research Foundation under its Translational and Clinical Research (TCR) Flagship Programme and administered by the Singapore Ministry of Health's National Medical Research Council (NMRC), Singapore- NMRC/TCR/004-NUS/2008; NMRC/TCR/012-NUHS/2014. Additional funding is provided by the Singapore Institute for Clinical Sciences, Agency for Science Technology and Research (A*STAR), Singapore. KMG is supported by the National Institute for Health Research through the NIHR Southampton Biomedical Research Centre and by the European Union's Seventh Framework Programme (FP7/2007–2013), project EarlyNutrition under grant agreement n°289346. JKYC received salary support from the Ministry of Health's National Medical Research Council, Singapore (NMRC/CSA(SI)/008/2016). The funding bodies had no influence on the study design, data collection, analysis, interpretation and content of the manuscript.

Authors' contributions

KHT, FY, PDG, KMG, LPCS and YSC designed the GUSTO cohort study. CC1 and SLL participated in the conception and design of this substudy. SLL, SC, CC2 and SES participated in the data management and statistical analyses. CC1, SLL, SYC, KMG, JKYC, MSK and YSC interpreted the findings and revised drafts of the paper. All authors contributed to interpretation of the data, critically revised the article for important intellectual content and approved the final manuscript.

Competing interests

FY, PDG, KMG and YSC have received reimbursement for speaking at conferences sponsored by companies selling nutritional products. SYC, PDG, KMG and YSC are part of an academic consortium that has received research funding from Abbott Nutrition, Nestlé and Danone. Other authors declared that they have no competing interests.

Author details

[1]Department of Obstetrics & Gynaecology, National University Hospital, Singapore 119074, Singapore. [2]Department of Reproductive Medicine, KK Women's and Children's Hospital, Singapore 229899, Singapore. [3]Duke-NUS Medical School, Singapore 169857, Singapore. [4]Singapore Institute for Clinical Sciences, Agency for Science, Technology and Research (A*STAR), Singapore 117609, Singapore. [5]Department of Obstetrics & Gynaecology, Yong Loo Lin School of Medicine, National University of Singapore, National University Health System, Singapore 119228, Singapore. [6]Department of Paediatrics, Yong Loo Lin School of Medicine, National University of Singapore, Singapore 119228, Singapore. [7]Department of Maternal Fetal Medicine, KK Women's and Children's Hospital, Singapore 229899, Singapore. [8]Department of Paediatrics, KK Women's and Children's Hospital, Singapore 229899, Singapore. [9]Lee Kong Chian School of Medicine, Nanyang Technological University, Singapore 636921, Singapore. [10]Liggins Institute, University of Auckland, Auckland 1142, New Zealand. [11]Medical Research Council Lifecourse Epidemiology Unit, University of Southampton, Southampton SO16 6YD, UK. [12]National Institute for Health Research Southampton Biomedical Research Centre, University of Southampton and University Hospital Southampton National Health Service Foundation Trust, Southampton SO16 6YD, UK. [13]Khoo Teck Puat-National University Children's Medical Institute, National University Hospital, National University Health System, Singapore 119074, Singapore. [14]Department of Pediatrics, McGill University Faculty of Medicine, 845 Rue Sherbrooke Ouest, Montreal, QC H3A 0G4, Canada. [15]Department of Epidemiology, Biostatistics and Occupational Health, McGill University Faculty of Medicine, 845 Rue Sherbrooke Ouest, Montreal, QC H3A 0G4, Canada.

References

1. American Diabetes Association. Diagnosis and classification of diabetes. Diabetes Care. 2014;37(Suppl 1):S81–90.
2. Metzger BE, Lowe LP, Dyer AR, Trimble ER, Chaovarindr U, Coustan DR, et al. Hyperglycemia and adverse pregnancy outcomes. N Engl J Med. 2008;358: 1991–2002.
3. Retnakaran R, Qi Y, Sermer M, Connelly PW, Hanley AJ, Zinman B. Glucose intolerance in pregnancy and future risk of pre-diabetes or diabetes. Diabetes Care. 2008;31:2026–31.
4. Weinert LS. International Association of Diabetes and Pregnancy Study Groups recommendations on the diagnosis and classification of hyperglycemia in pregnancy: comment to the International Association of Diabetes and Pregnancy Study Groups Consensus Panel. Diabetes Care. 2010;33:e97.
5. International Association of Diabetes Pregnancy Study Groups Consensus Panel, Metzger BE, Gabbe SG, Persson B, Buchanan TA, Catalano PA, et al. International Association of Diabetes and Pregnancy Study Groups recommendations on the diagnosis and classification of hyperglycemia in pregnancy. Diabetes Care. 2010;33:676–82.
6. World Health Organization. Diagnostic criteria and classification of hyperglycaemia first detected in pregnancy: a World Health Organization guideline. Diabetes Res Clin Pract. 2014;103:341–63.
7. Alberti KG, Zimmet PZ. Definition, diagnosis and classification of diabetes mellitus and its complications. Part 1: diagnosis and classification of diabetes mellitus provisional report of a WHO consultation. Diabet Med. 1998;15:539–53.

8. O'sullivan JB, Mahan CM. Criteria for oral glucose tolerance test in pregnancy. Diabetes. 1964;13:278–85.
9. Cundy T, Ackermann E, Ryan EA. Gestational diabetes: new criteria may triple the prevalence but effect on outcomes is unclear. BMJ. 2014;348:g1567.
10. Sacks DA, Hadden DR, Maresh M, Deerochanawong C, Dyer AR, Metzger BE, et al. Frequency of gestational diabetes mellitus at collaborating centers based on IADPSG consensus panel-recommended criteria: the hyperglycemia and adverse pregnancy outcome (HAPO) study. Diabetes Care. 2012;35:526–8.
11. Department of Statistics Singapore. Population Trends 2015. Department of Statistics, Ministry of Trade & Industry, Republic of Singapore. http://www.singstat.gov.sg/publications/publications-and-papers/population-and-population-structure/population-trends. Accessed 23 Feb 2016.
12. International Diabetes Federation. Diabetes Atlas. 7th. Brussels: International Diabetes Federation. 2015. http://www.diabetesatlas.org/. Accessed 17 Feb 2016.
13. Phan TP, Alkema L, Tai ES, Tan KH, Yang Q, Lim WY, et al. Forecasting the burden of type 2 diabetes in Singapore using a demographic epidemiological model of Singapore. BMJ Open Diabetes Res Care. 2014;2:e000012.
14. Bellamy L, Casas JP, Hingorani AD, Williams D. Type 2 diabetes mellitus after gestational diabetes: a systematic review and meta-analysis. Lancet. 2009; 373:1773–9.
15. Soh SE, Tint MT, Gluckman PD, Godfrey KM, Rifkin-Graboi A, Chan YH, et al. Cohort profile: growing up in Singapore towards healthy outcomes (GUSTO) birth cohort study. Int J Epidemiol. 2014;43:1401–9.
16. Hutcheon JA, Platt RW, Abrams B, Himes KP, Simhan HN, Bodnar LM. A weight-gain-for-gestational-age z score chart for the assessment of maternal weight gain in pregnancy. Am J Clin Nutr. 2013;97:1062–7.
17. World Health Organization. Definition and diagnosis of diabetes mellitus and intermediate hyperglycemia. Switzerland: report of a WHO/IDF consultation; 2006.
18. Mikolajczyk RT, Zhang J, Betran AP, Souza JP, Mori R, Gulmezoglu AM. A global reference for fetal-weight and birthweight percentiles. Lancet. 2011; 377:1855–61.
19. Zou G. A modified poisson regression approach to prospective studies with binary data. Am J Epidemiol. 2004;159:702–6.
20. Yew TW, Khoo CM, Thai AC, Kale AS, Yong EL, Tai ES. The prevalence of gestational diabetes mellitus among Asian females is lower using the new 2013 World Health Organization diagnostic criteria. Endocr Pract. 2014;20:1064–9.
21. Pan L, Leng J, Liu G, Zhang C, Liu H, Li M, et al. Pregnancy outcomes of Chinese women with gestational diabetes mellitus defined by the IADPSG's but not by the 1999 WHO's criteria. Clin Endocrinol. 2015;83:684–93.
22. Moses RG, Morris GJ, Petocz P, San Gil F, Garg D. The impact of potential new diagnostic criteria on the prevalence of gestational diabetes mellitus in Australia. Med J Aust. 2011;194:338–40.
23. O'Sullivan EP, Avalos G, O'Reilly M, et al. Atlantic diabetes in pregnancy (DIP): the prevalence and outcomes of gestational diabetes mellitus using the new diagnostic criteria. Diabetologia. 2011;54:1670–5.
24. Gilder ME, Zin TW, Wai NS, Ner M, Say PS, Htoo M, et al. Gestational diabetes mellitus prevalence in Maela refugee camp on the Thai-Myanmar border: a clinical report. Glob Health Action. 2014;7:23887.
25. Sagili H, Kamalanathan S, Sahoo J, Lakshminarayanan S, Rani R, Jayalakshmi D, et al. Comparison of different criteria for diagnosis of gestational diabetes mellitus. Indian J Endocrinol Metab. 2015;19:824–8.
26. Tran TS, Hirst JE, Do MA, Morris JM, Jeffery HE. Early prediction of gestational diabetes mellitus in Vietnam: clinical impact of currently recommended diagnostic criteria. Diabetes Care. 2013;36:618–24.
27. Chu SY, Abe K, Hall LR, Kim SY, Njoroge T, Qin C. Gestational diabetes mellitus: all Asians are not alike. Prev Med. 2009;49:265–8.
28. Morkrid K, Jenum AK, Sletner L, Vardal MH, Waage CW, Nakstad B, et al. Failure to increase insulin secretory capacity during pregnancy-induced insulin resistance is associated with ethnicity and gestational diabetes. Eur J Endocrinol. 2012;167:579–88.
29. Nallaperumal S, Bhavadharini B, Mahalakshmi MM, Maheswari K, Jalaja R, Moses A, et al. Comparison of the World Health Organization and the International Association of Diabetes and Pregnancy Study Groups criteria in diagnosing gestational diabetes mellitus in south Indians. Indian J Endocrinol Metab. 2013;17:906–9.
30. Seshiah V, Balaji V, Shah SN, Joshi S, Das AK, Sahay BK, et al. Diagnosis of gestational diabetes mellitus in the community. J Assoc Physicians India. 2012;60:15–7.
31. Crowther CA, Hiller JE, Moss JR, McPhee AJ, Jeffries WS, Robinson JS, et al. Effect of treatment of gestational diabetes mellitus on pregnancy outcomes. N Engl J Med. 2005;352:2477–86.
32. Landon MB, Spong CY, Thom E, Carpenter MW, Ramin SM, Casey B, et al. A multicenter, randomized trial of treatment for mild gestational diabetes. N Engl J Med. 2009;361:1339–48.
33. National institute for Health and Care Excellence. Diabetes in pregnancy: management from preconception to the postnatal period. 2015. https://www.nice.org.uk/guidance/ng3. Accessed 17 Feb 2016.

Enablers and barriers for women with gestational diabetes mellitus to achieve optimal glycaemic control – a qualitative study using the theoretical domains framework

Ruth Martis[1], Julie Brown[1], Judith McAra-Couper[2] and Caroline A. Crowther[1*]

Abstract

Background: Glycaemic target recommendations vary widely between international professional organisations for women with gestational diabetes mellitus (GDM). Some studies have reported women's experiences of having GDM, but little is known how this relates to their glycaemic targets. The aim of this study was to identify enablers and barriers for women with GDM to achieve optimal glycaemic control.

Methods: Women with GDM were recruited from two large, geographically different, hospitals in New Zealand to participate in a semi-structured interview to explore their views and experiences focusing on enablers and barriers to achieving optimal glycaemic control. Final thematic analysis was performed using the Theoretical Domains Framework.

Results: Sixty women participated in the study. Women reported a shift from their initial negative response to accepting their diagnosis but disliked the constant focus on numbers. Enablers and barriers were categorised into ten domains across the three study questions. Enablers included: the ability to attend group teaching sessions with family and hear from women who have had GDM; easy access to a diabetes dietitian with diet recommendations tailored to a woman's context including ethnic food and financial considerations; free capillary blood glucose (CBG) monitoring equipment, health shuttles to take women to appointments; child care when attending clinic appointments; and being taught CBG testing by a community pharmacist. Barriers included: lack of health information, teaching sessions, consultations, and food diaries in a woman's first language; long waiting times at clinic appointments; seeing a different health professional every clinic visit; inconsistent advice; no tailored physical activities assessments; not knowing where to access appropriate information on the internet; unsupportive partners, families, and workplaces; and unavailability of social media or support groups for women with GDM. Perceived judgement by others led some women only to share their GDM diagnosis with their partners. This created social isolation.

Conclusion: Women with GDM report multiple enablers and barriers to achieving optimal glycaemic control. The findings of this study may assist health professionals and diabetes in pregnancy services to improve their care for women with GDM and support them to achieve optimal glycaemic control.

Keywords: Gestational diabetes mellitus, Pregnant women, Self-management, Dietary advice, Exercise, Health literacy, Theoretical domains framework

* Correspondence: c.crowther@auckland.ac.nz
[1]Liggins Institute, The University of Auckland, Private Bag 92019, Auckland 1142, New Zealand
Full list of author information is available at the end of the article

Background

In New Zealand one in eleven pregnant women is diagnosed with gestational diabetes mellitus (GDM) [1]. Maternal hyperglycaemia associated with GDM is a potentially serious complication that can result in short- and long-term health risks for the woman and her baby [2–5]. Optimal blood glucose regulation within recommended glycaemic targets using lifestyle changes and/or pharmacological treatments aims to reduce or prevent the adverse outcomes associated with GDM [6–8]. A woman's perceptions of GDM may influence whether she embraces any lifestyle changes, complies with the recommended treatment, and achieves optimal blood glucose control [9].

The New Zealand Health and Disability Commissioner has identified that consumer (a health system user) involvement is a priority in health decision making [10]. Legislation such as the Health and Disability Commissioner Act 1994 [11], and the Health and Disability Services Consumers' Rights 1996 Code [12] support this. International organisations including Cochrane and the World Health Organisation (WHO) concur [13, 14]. They recommend that for any research involving consumers, their experiences should be investigated to support the research results [11–14].

In 2015 the National Institute for Health and Care Excellence (NICE) published an up-dated guideline for 'Diabetes in pregnancy: management from preconception to the postnatal period' and recommended that further robust qualitative studies were needed to explore enablers and barriers for women with GDM to maintain optimal glycaemic blood control [15]. Increased understanding of the enablers and barriers for women with GDM may help facilitate behaviour change and assist health care professionals to support women with GDM more effectively to overcome the barriers identified and support the enablers.

The use of the Theoretical Domains Framework (TDF), which informed data analysis, is an effective tool to identify enablers and barriers and to understand, inform and facilitate effective behavioural change and health service provision [16–18]. TDF was developed using an expert consensus process and validation to identify psychological and organisational theory relevant to behaviour change [16–19]. The most recent validated version of the TDF includes 14 domains and their component constructs [20] (Table 1). The TDF has been used in health care to identify factors influencing health practitioner's clinical behaviour and behaviour change [20–22] but is increasingly being used to identify enablers and barriers for the consumer (user of health care) to understand their experiences and views to adherence of treatment and lifestyle changes [23–26].

The aims of this study were to explore the views and experiences of women with GDM with a focus on enablers and barriers to achieving optimal CBG control. Initially women were asked about how they felt and reacted when they were first diagnosed with GDM and if these impressions changed over time. To achieve the aims of the study, three broad questions were explored with participating women:

1. What is it like for a woman to monitor their CBG concentrations?
2. What affects a woman's capillary CBG concentrations and how does she maintain optimal CBG control with this knowledge?
3. What support have women found helpful/not helpful in learning about and maintaining optimal CBG control?

Methods

Study design and procedure

This was a qualitative descriptive study and thematic content analysis as informed by Braun and Clarke and the Theoretical Domains Framework was used to analyse the data [16, 20, 27, 28]. Semi-structured interviews enabled women with GDM to express their views and experiences in their own words [29, 30]. Women could choose to be interviewed face-to-face, or to be telephoned. Women were made aware that the interview was not an assessment of their knowledge about GDM and that they could stop the interview at any time. They were advised that all their information would be kept confidential. All women chose a pseudonym at the end of the interview for de-identifying their data and for use when disseminating the results.

This qualitative study was nested within the TARGET Trial (Optimal Glycaemic Targets for Gestational Diabetes), a stepped wedge randomised controlled trial (Australian New Zealand Trial Registry: ACTRN12615000282583), which is assessing less tight and tighter glycaemic targets for women with GDM and the effect on maternal and perinatal morbidities. The study was approved by the New Zealand Health and Disability Ethics committee (HDEC) Ref. 14/NTA/163, research registration number 1965. Locality agreements were obtained from Canterbury and Counties Manukau District Health Boards (DHB).

Study setting

Two New Zealand tertiary hospitals participated, one from the South Island (Canterbury DHB)) and one from the North Island (Counties Manukau DHB). Hospital policies differed for glycaemic targets and testing of capillary blood glucose (CBG). During the study, Canterbury DHB moved from initially less tight glycaemic targets (fasting blood glucose < 5.5 mmol/L; 1-h postprandial < 8.0 mmol/L; and 2-h postprandial < 7.0 mmol/L) to tighter targets (fasting blood glucose ≤5.0 mmol/L; 1-h postprandial ≤7.4 mmol/

Table 1 Refined Theoretical Domains Framework adapted from Cane et al. 2012 [19] and Atkins et al. 2017 [20]

Theoretical Domains	Generic Definitions	Constructs
Knowledge	An awareness of the existence of something	- Knowledge (including knowledge of condition/ scientific rationale) - Procedural knowledge - Knowledge of task environment
Skills	An ability or proficiency acquired through practice	- Skills - Skills development - Competence - Ability - Interpersonal skills - Practice - Skill assessment
Social/Professional Role & Identity	A coherent set of behaviours and displayed personal qualities of an individual in a social or work setting	- Professional identity - Professional role - Social identity - Identity - Professional boundaries - Professional confidence - Group identity - Leadership - Organisational commitment
Beliefs about capabilities	Acceptance of the truth, reality or validity about an ability, talent, or facility that a person can put to constructive use	- Self-confidence - Perceived competence - Self-efficacy - Perceived behavioural control - Beliefs - Self-esteem - Empowerment - Professional confidence
Optimism	The confidence that things will happen for the best or that desired goals will be attained	- Optimism - Pessimism - Unrealistic optimism - Identity
Beliefs about consequences	Acceptance of the truth, reality, or validity about outcomes of a behaviour in a given situation	- Beliefs - Outcome expectancies - Characteristics of outcome expectancies - Anticipated regret - Consequents
Reinforcement	Increasing the probability of a response by arranging a dependent relationship, or contingency, between the response and a given stimulus	- Rewards (proximal/distal, valued/not valued, probable/improbable) - Incentives - Punishment - Consequents - Reinforcement - Contingencies - Sanctions
Intentions	A conscious decision to perform a behavior or a resolve to act in a certain way	- Stability of intentions - Stages of change model - Transtheoretical model and stages of change
Goals	Mental representations of outcomes or end states that an individual wants to achieve	- Goals (distal/proximal) - Goal priority - Goal/target setting - Goals (autonomous/controlled) - Action planning - Implementation intention
Memory, attention, and decision processes	The ability to retain information, focus selectively on aspects of the environment and choose between two or more alternatives	- Memory - Attention - Attention control - Decision making - Cognitive overload/tiredness
Environmental context and resources	Any circumstance of a person's situation or environment that discourages or encourages the development of skills	- Environmental stressors - Resources/material resources - Organisational culture/climate

Table 1 Refined Theoretical Domains Framework adapted from Cane et al. 2012 [19] and Atkins et al. 2017 [20] *(Continued)*

Theoretical Domains	Generic Definitions	Constructs
	and abilities, independence, social competence, and adaptive behaviour	- Salient events/critical incidents - Person × environment interaction - Barriers and facilitators
Social influences	Those interpersonal processes that can cause individuals to change their thoughts, feelings or behaviours	- Social pressure - Social norms - Group conformity - Social comparisons - Group norms - Social support - Power - Intergroup conflict - Alienation - Group identity - Modelling
Emotion	A complex reaction pattern, involving experiential, behavioural and physiological elements, by which the individual attempts to deal with a personally significant matter or event	- Fear - Anxiety - Affect - Stress - Depression - Positive/negative affect - Burn-out
Behavioural regulation	Anything aimed at managing or changing objectively observed or measured actions	- Self-monitoring - Breaking habit - Action planning

L; and 2-h postprandial ≤6.7 mmol/L). Women were asked to test their CBG at one-hour postprandial. Counties Manukau DHB used tighter glycaemic targets during the study (fasting blood glucose ≤5.0 mmol/L; 1-h postprandial ≤7.4 mmol/L; and 2-h postprandial ≤6.7 mmol/L) and women were asked to test their CBG two-hours postprandial.

Study participants

Women with GDM were eligible to participate if they had not yet given birth, had a singleton pregnancy, were able to communicate in English and had been self-monitoring their CBG concentrations for at least two weeks. All women with GDM recruited between August 2016 to February 2017 for the TARGET Trial at Canterbury and Counties Manukau DHB were sent an email invitation to consider participation in this nested study with a participant information sheet and consent form attached. Eligible women who wished to participate signed a consent form for this study.

Study materials

A question guide to facilitate the semi-structured interview was developed and pilot tested with three women who had GDM. This resulted in the addition of one question about hunger and adding the request for a pseudonym for identification rather than only a number to identify the data of participants. The data from these three women involved in piloting the question guide were included in the analyses. If women needed further guidance to share their thoughts, the question guide listed prompts and sub-questions for each broad question.

The semi-structured interview

One researcher (RM), with facilitating skills, conducted all the interviews over a six months' time period (August 2016 to February 2017). The woman's choice directed the place and timing of the interview. Consequently, face-to-face interviews were conducted at a variety of settings including a woman's home, work place, botanical gardens, cafés, on farms and hospital sites. No time constraints were applied for the interviews with most lasting about 40 min.

Data collection and analysis

All interviews were recorded using a digital recorder and were transcribed verbatim using Microsoft 2010 by independent transcribers, who had signed a confidentiality agreement. The transcripts were verified by the researcher (RM) and entered NVivo11 for windows [31] for data management and analysis. Thematic content analysis was conducted initially using an inductive approach [28] where transcripts were read and re-read in full for familiarisation with the data and analysed using open coding techniques assigning a code to each meaningful segment of text. As the open codes became saturated, a list of specific themes was generated, compared and categorised to broader overarching themes, following Braun's steps 1–5 [28] (Table 2). This was followed by a deductive approach assigning the themes with meaningful text to one or more of the 14

Table 2 Braun's (2006) Thematic Analysis Approach adapted from Braun et al. 2006 [28]

Steps	Content
1. Familiarisation with the data	Reading and re-reading the data, to become immersed and intimately familiar with its content
2. Coding	Generating succinct labels (codes) that identify important features of the data that might be relevant to answering the research question. It involves coding the entire dataset, and after that, collating all the codes and all relevant data extracts, together for later stages of analysis.
3. Searching for themes	Examining the codes and collated data to identify significant broader patterns of meaning (potential themes). It then involves collating data relevant to each candidate theme, so that you can work with the data and review the viability of each candidate theme.
4. Reviewing themes	Checking the candidate themes against the dataset, to determine that they tell a convincing story of the data, and one that answers the research question. In this phase, themes are typically refined, which sometimes involves them being split, combined, or discarded.
5. Defining and naming themes	Developing a detailed analysis of each theme, working out the scope and focus of each theme, determining the 'story' of each. It also involves deciding on an informative name for each theme.
6. Writing up	Weaving together the analytic narrative and data extracts and contextualising the analysis in relation to existing literature.

theoretical domains reflected in the Theoretical Domain's Framework [16, 20] (Table 1).

Two researchers (RM and JB) coded and classified the data and consulted with the other authors (JMC and CAC) to discuss and revise synthesising the text into the final behavioural domains with enablers and barriers identification for aspects of optimal glycaemic control. Where text fitted into multiple domains, two researchers (RM and JB) discussed and decided which text should be coded into the domain that best reflects the key theme [19] and whether a statement represented a barrier or enabler to achieving optimal glycaemic control. Reporting of this study was based on the COREQ (**Co**nsolidated Criteria for **Re**porting **Q**ualitative Research) checklist [32].

Results

During the study period, sixty-six eligible women with GDM consecutively recruited to the TARGET Trial were approached. Six women declined to be part of this study because they were too busy, having a family crisis or did not respond to the email invitation (Fig. 1). Twenty women with GDM were recruited from the Counties Manukau DHB site and 40 women with GDM from Canterbury DHB site, giving a total of 60 participants. The sociodemographic characteristics of the women who participated are reflective of a cross section of the demographics of New Zealand's pregnant population [33–35] (Table 3). Data were analysed and coded from 858 transcribed pages (249,692 words).

Women were diagnosed with GDM at a mean gestational age of 27.8 weeks (standard deviation (SD) ± 2.0. Ten women (16.7%) reported having GDM in a previous pregnancy and twenty-seven (45%) women reported a family history of diabetes (Table 3). When interviewed, the women had been checking their daily CBG for an average of 6.8 ± 2.3 weeks (Table 3). Twenty-eight women (47%) were checking their daily CBG concentration six times (before and after breakfast, lunch and dinner) and thirty-two women (53%) were checking CBG concentrations four times a day (before breakfast and after breakfast, lunch and dinner) (Table 3). Almost a third of women (18, 30%) were treated with diet alone. Thirteen (21.7%) women were treated with subcutaneous insulin for their GDM, 17 (28.3%) women with metformin and 12 (20%) women were treated with insulin and metformin (Table 3). For the interview 34 (57%) women chose to be interviewed face-to-face and 26 (43%) women by telephone (Table 3).

Women's initial response to being diagnosed with GDM

As an introduction to the interview, women were asked how they responded when diagnosed with GDM and if that response changed over time. This enabled women to share their emotions and thoughts about GDM, to recognise how far they had come on their journey with GDM and provided an effective platform for discussing enablers and barriers to achieving optimal glycaemic control [36]. Over a third of the women described their initial response as being shocked (21, 35%).

> *"Shocked, I don't feel like I have diabetes, as I feel normal and okay" (Belle 19A).*

Seven (11.7%) women described it as unexpected, while five (8.3%) women felt okay about the diagnosis.

> *"The initial gut reaction is like, oh my God, I did not expect this and what does this mean for my baby?" (Karen 09A).*

> *"I felt okay, because I know lots of Asian people, my friends around, they are pregnant. And a lot of Asian women they very, very easily get diabetes, pregnancy diabetes. So, I am prepared. I am okay" (Casey 01A).*

The remainder of women described their initial response as being disappointed (4, 6.7%), gutted (3, 5%),

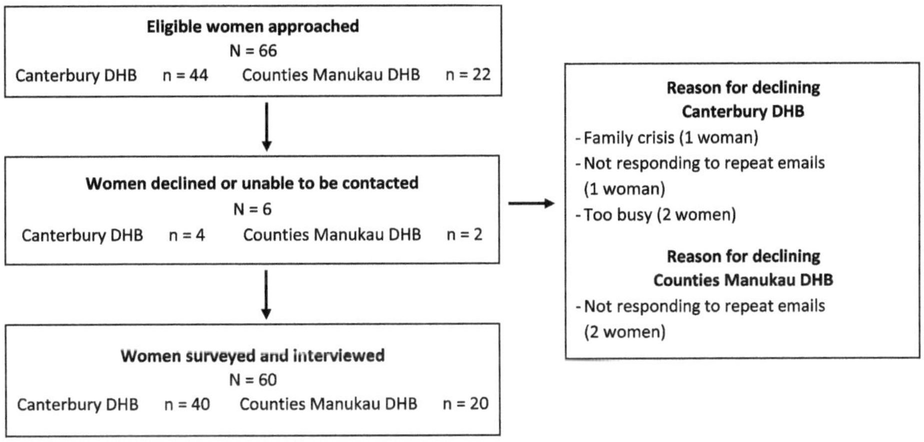

Fig. 1 Flowchart of recruitment

annoyed (3, 5%), upset (3, 5%), guilty (3, 5%), devastated (3, 5%), defeated (2, 3.3%), freaked out (2, 3.3%), angry (2, 3.3%) miffed (1, 1.7%) and heart-broken (1, 1.7%).

> *"I think disappointing, because my diet's pretty clean anyway. In that sense, it was disappointing" (Sian 11A).*

> *"Can't be true, gutted, made them do another test, otherwise I would not do the treatment" (Larissa 01B).*

Women's response to living with GDM at the time of the interview

Women at the time of the interview had been living with GDM for an average of 6.8 ± 2.3 weeks (Table 3). Most of the women commented that they had moved on from their initial response (49, 81.7%). They accepted the diagnosis as 'okay' because it would only last a finite time, but did not like the focus on the numbers of their glycaemic targets, their CBG results, weight gain and 90th percentile of fetal growth.

> *"It's hard because we have to change our routine, we have to change our food patterns and all those sort of things, changing our life to be frank, but when it comes to the reality, that makes you know, a huge difference, in our life, so it's a big change, a big challenge but we have to accept it, even though the numbers run my life but we have to do the things. The other good thing after my delivery, it will go away" (Anna 07).*

> *"It's quite overwhelming in the beginning you kind of realise now that it's not as big it kind of first seems. You just kind of adjust to it I guess and then its ok, always have to keep a look out for the numbers though" (Collette 09B).*

Theoretical domains framework – Enablers and barriers

Following Braun's [28] (Table 2) thematic content analysis, the emerging themes were categorised into the TDF domains assigning the themes with meaningful text to one or more of the 14 theoretical domains [16, 20] (Table 1) for enablers and barriers identification. The results are reported for each of the study questions. The 10 categorised domains, their definitions and identified enablers and barriers from women with GDM are listed in Tables 4, 5 and 6.

What is it like for a woman to monitor her CBG concentrations?

The themes emerging from the interviews from women with GDM for the first research question 'What is it like for a woman to monitor her CBG concentrations?' were categorised within nine out of the possible fourteen TDF domains. These were: Knowledge, Skills, Beliefs about capabilities, Beliefs about consequences, Memory, attention and decision process, Environmental context and resources, Social influences, Emotion and Behavioural regulation (Table 4). The domains represented most strongly in the interviews in the context of this question were: Beliefs about capabilities, Social influences and Emotions.

Knowledge

The domain 'Knowledge' in the context of monitoring optimal CBG control refers to a woman knowing her glycaemic targets and procedural knowledge of how to test accurately. Nearly all women knew their glycaemic targets and most understood the importance of adhering to them, enabling the process of performing routinely CBG testing. Enablers to assist this knowledge were identified as having information aids, such as stickers at the front of the recording booklet displaying the

Table 3 Demographic characteristics of women who participated in the survey

Characteristics	Women total $n = 60$ (%)
Age (years)[a]	33 (±4.5)
Primigravida (G_1P_0)	27 (45)
BMI category[b]	
- Normal	21 (35)
- Overweight	11 (18.3)
- Obese (Class I)	11 (18.3)
- Obese (Class II)	8 (13.3)
- Obese (Class II)	9 (15)
- Total obese	28 (46.6)
Ethnicity[c]	
- European	24 (40)
- Māori	6 (10)
- Asian	22 (36.7)
- Pacific Peoples	7 (11.6)
- MELAA	1 (1.7)
Highest educational qualifications after leaving school[d]	
1. No qualification	3 (5)
2. Level 1 certificate	2 (3.3)
3. Level 2 certificate	4 (6.7)
4. Level 3 certificate	6 (10)
5. Level 4 certificate	4 (6.7)
6. Level 5 and level 6 Diploma	13 (21.7)
7. Bachelor degree and level 7 qualification	25 (41.6)
8. Post-graduate and honours degree	1 (1.7)
9. Master degree	2 (3.3)
New Zealand Deprivation index[e]	
- 1 (least deprived)	8 (13.5)
- 2	5 (8.4)
- 3	5 (8.4)
- 4	10 (16.7)
- 5	7 (11.8)
- 6	2 (3.4)
- 7	5 (8.5)
- 8	6 (10)
- 9	5 (8.7)
- 10 (most deprived)	6 (10)
Lead Maternity Carer (LMC)[f]	
- Midwife	55 (91.7)
- Obstetrician	1 (1.7)
- Hospital Team	4 (6.7)
Health history	
Gestational age at GDM diagnosis (weeks)[a]	27.8 (±2.0)

Table 3 Demographic characteristics of women who participated in the survey *(Continued)*

Characteristics	Women total $n = 60$ (%)
Previous GDM	10 (16.7)
Previous hypertension	2 (3.3)
Current hypertension	3 (5)
Family history of hypertension	24 (40)
Family history of diabetes	27 (45)
Current smoker	3 (15)
Capillary blood glucose testing (CBG)	
Weeks of self-testing capillary blood glucose at interview[a]	6.8 (±2.3)
Daily self-testing CBG: four times (Before breakfast, after breakfast, after lunch and after dinner)	32 (53)
Daily self-testing CBG: six times (Before and after breakfast, lunch and dinner)	28 (47)
Current treatment	
- Diet only	18 (30)
- Insulin and diet	13 (21.7)
- Metformin and diet	17 (28.3)
- Insulin, Metformin and diet	12 (20)
Interview type	
Face-to-face interview	34 (57)
Phone interview	26 (43)

Figures are numbers and percentages
[a]Mean and standard deviation
[b]BMI categories: Underweight < 18.50; Normal range: ≥ 18.55–24.99; Overweight: ≥ 25.00–29.99; Obese (Class I) ≥ 30.00–34.99; Obese (Class II): Severe obese ≥35.00–39.99; Obese (Class II): Morbid obese: ≥ 40.00 (according to WHO and Ministry of Health categories) [44, 45]
[c]as categorised by New Zealand government statistics groups for major ethnic groups. MELAA is an acronym for Middle Eastern/Latin American/African. http://www.stats.govt.nz/Census/2013-census/profile-and-summary-reports/infographic-culture-identity.aspx
[d]as categorised by New Zealand government statistics groups. http://archive.stats.govt.nz/?_ga=2.86002648.1123263351.1521524783-1632759419.1521524783
[e]as categorised by New Zealand 2013 Deprivation Index, University of Otago, Department of Public Health. *Deprivation score was unknown for one woman, as her address had no meshblock listed* Http://www.otago.ac.nz/wellington/departments/publichealth/research/hirp/otago020194.html
[f]A Lead Maternity Carer (LMC) in New Zealand provides lead maternity care (is in charge). This can be either a Midwife, Obstetrician, or GP. https://www.midwife.org.nz/in-new-zealand/contexts-for-practice

glycaemic targets, post-it notes for a work computer and glycaemic targets recorded on their mobile phone. Using a visual step-by-step pamphlet to ensure correctly obtaining capillary blood for glucose testing enabled procedural knowledge retention.

> *"I actually understood why I had to do this air tight control, so I do it. The sticker on the booklet reminds me of my numbers and the booklet in glucometer with pictures reminds me what to know" (Erin 04B).*

Table 4 Enablers and Barriers for women with GDM to monitor their CBG concentration

Domains and Definitions	Enablers	Barriers
Knowledge Refers to a woman knowing her glycaemic targets and procedural knowledge of how to test accurately	Glycaemic targets on: - sticker on the recording booklet - post-it notes on work computer - mobile phone notebook - visual step-by-step pamphlet - list how to perform CBG testing	- different glycaemic targets to previous pregnancy - unable to read the 'how to do it list' in first language - no visual images of how to perform CBG testing
Skills Refers to a woman's ability to perform the CBG testing, working the glucometer correctly and documenting results and completing a food diary	Techniques for CBG flow: - alternating warm fingers & hands - not using soap - pricking on side of finger pads Food diary documenting	- no apps available for recording CBG results - food diary writing space too small - food diary not in first language - not knowing how to go back on glucometer
Beliefs about capabilities Refers to a woman's beliefs about her capability to perform, control and monitor her CBG concentration	- can-do attitude - perceived control of GDM - in control of CBG testing - capable of interpreting CBG results and adjusting food intake	- can't-do it attitude, too difficult - belief that it is not necessary to test regularly - perceived lack of control
Beliefs about consequences Refers to a woman's expectations about optimal CBG control	Anticipated positive consequences: - adhering to glycaemic targets will control GDM - secure healthy future for the baby - baby will be a normal size - belief future health will be better - belief family health will be better	Anticipated negative consequences: - fingerpicks damage finger pads, too difficult to play the piano or guitar - testing and controlling CBG did not work last time
Memory, attention, and decision process Refers to a woman's ability to remember when and decide where, to perform CBG testing	- mobile phone alarm reminder - setting timer on microwave - dedicated bag ready access to glucose testing equipment - able to decide where to do CBG testing	- forgetful - no reminder plan in place - unable to think outside the square - concern for doing CBG testing outside the home
Environmental context and resources Refers to a woman's access to equipment and to a health professional when unsure about results	- free resources for CBG testing - phone access to diabetes midwife - booklet fits into glucometer bag - pharmacist teaching CBG testing - group teaching sessions for learning CBG testing	- costs of resources needed for CBG testing - no phone access to diabetes health professionals - booklet too big for glucometer bag - health professional not believing results
Social influences Refers to a woman's social interactions for CBG monitoring and maintaining optimal CBG control	- supportive and engaged social interactions - do it wherever, no concern - work colleagues remind them - provide healthy food at work	- social pressure and loss of choice - worried about performing CBG testing in public, being judged - being told to leave restaurant for CBG testing - work demands, meetings, unable to stop work for CBG testing
Emotion Refers to a woman's reaction/feelings to monitoring and maintaining her CBG concentrations	- privilege to have been diagnosed - enabled learning a new skill that directed positive lifestyle changes - fun doing everyone's CBG level - not as painful as anticipated	- anxiety, scared, needle phobia - stress to remember doing CBG testing, - feeling guilty when forgotten - focus on numbers not the woman - not enjoying reading
Behavioural regulation Refers to a woman's focus on self-monitoring effectively and planning how to incorporate this into her daily life	- action plan to monitor CBG - motivated by the baby to monitor CBG regularly - documenting honestly - sharing on social media glycaemic target achievements	

Women reported barriers as being confused by different glycaemic targets compared to their last pregnancy with GDM and information that would have aided their procedural knowledge not being provided in enough visual detail or the information was not in their first language.

"The consultant gave me something that I haven't looked at, but it was 'I quit sugar' and I wouldn't recommend that, as it sounded like sugar is poison and all this kind of stuff. Pictures would be so much better" (Alice 10A).

Table 5 Enablers and barriers for women with GDM understanding what effects their CBG concentrations

Domains and Definitions	Enablers	Barriers
Knowledge Refers to a woman's understanding of what affects her CBG concentrations	- understanding the difference between carbohydrates, proteins, and fats - ability to read and comprehend food labels - able to understand how physical activity or inactivity affects their CBG concentrations	- lack of understanding which foods and exercises raise the CBG concentrations - not knowing how to read food labels - knowing how to increase insulin to eat favourite sweets
Belief about consequences Refers to a woman's expectations about what affects her CBG concentration	- eating the same food every day for optimal glycaemic control - using commercially available, pre-assembled ready for cooking, health food bags for optimal glycaemic control - hearing other women's stories encourages anticipated regret - regular activities easy to incorporate into daily life and ensures healthy baby	- belief only medication controls CBG concentrations - belief that exercises have no effect on CBG concentrations - belief that physical activity can cause pre-term labour
Environmental context and resources Refers to a woman's access to food, exercise equipment and health professionals	- access to dietitian and group sessions - food diary and discussion - food costs are less (no fast foods) - vegetable garden - recipes on social media - identifying food in pantry which are suitable with stickers - being organised - appropriate food available when not at home - access to exercise equipment (home bicycle, tread mill) - family and children creating motivating resources	- dietetic service unavailable - transport and time issues - not documenting a food diary or not knowing about it - health professionals do not discuss content of food diary - food is more expensive (fruit, special bread) - no ethnic food options included - unavailable professional assessment for exercise/physical activities - easy access to sugary food and drinks
Emotions Refers to a woman's reaction/feelings to what affects her CBG concentrations	- excited to understand the link between food and exercise and CBG concentrations	- stressed about trying hard but not able to achieve optimal CBG concentrations - feeling hungry most of the time
Behavioural regulation Refers to a woman's focus on self-monitoring effective food intake and exercise and planning how to incorporate this into daily life	- self-monitoring with food diary - developing an activity diary - calling exercise physical activity - calling diet food intake, or what to eat - action plan for physical activities - creatively incorporating family exercises affecting CBG concentrations - family and children creating motivating resources together	- dislike of exercises - medication and food is enough to maintain CBG levels - stress or excitement increases CBG concentrations, too hard to control

"I think it's important to give us something to take away, and some bullet points or pictures, now that you are diagnosed, these things you need to do, why we are doing it and in the right language" (Christina 15A).

Skills

The domain 'Skills' refers to a woman's ability to perform the CBG testing, working the glucometer correctly and documenting results and completing a food diary. Women identified various effective techniques to enable good capillary blood flow and reducing discomfort. This included not using soap for washing hands (as a belief that soap contains sugar), pricking on the edge of the finger pads, placing sufficient pressure on finger pads, wiping the first blood spot off and alternating of warm fingers and hands. Keeping a food diary helped women to make a connection between what they ate and what the test results meant, encouraging the up-keep of both regular accurate testing and recording in the food diary.

"Just pressing your fingers firmly against the end of the pricky thing on the side, because no one wants to do it twice. Next time either side of the next finger and then keep going to the next finger, all makes it less painful and better blood drops" (Toni 03B).

Barriers included having a needle phobia and women feeling frustrated that a phone app for recording CBG results was not available or not being able to document into an electronically food diary. Over half of the women wanted instructions for CBG testing in their first

Table 6 Enablers and barriers of support for women with GDM about maintaining optimal CBG control?

Domains and Definitions	Enablers	Barriers
Beliefs about consequences Refers to a woman's expectation to sharing her diagnosis of GDM with others	- telling others about GDM diagnosis gains valuable support	Not telling others about GDM diagnosis because: - concern for other family members - being judged by family, friends and work colleagues - being told what and what not to eat
Reinforcement Refers to a woman's ability to reinforce skills and coping strategies for self-support in maintaining optimal glycaemic control	- continuing with food diary, feeling better - photos of food eaten instead of written food dairy - self-rewards with non-food items - documenting CBG results - activities connected with family fun	
Environmental context and resources Refers to a woman's ability to have access to learning resources and professional services for optimal glycaemic control	- written information in first language - visual information - informative websites - partner and extended family able to attend teaching or clinic sessions - work colleagues enquiring and providing healthy food options - efficient clinic appointment system - health professional phone support - free health shuttle for appointments - hospital crèche - stickers with healthy GDM messages encourages adherence to healthy food and exercises	- health professional impatient - health professionals inconsistent with advice - not seeing the same health professional twice - long waiting times at clinic - not taught in first language - unable to write the food dairy in first language - no visual information available - website information random and scary - poor parking facilities - no transport available - unable to pay for petrol - no child care support - restaurants unable provide an ingredients list for meals - partner and extended family provide unhealthy meals
Social influences Refers to a woman's access to social interaction to learning/reinforcing optimal glycaemic control	- social media (Facebook) - sharing recipes - group teaching - meeting other women with GDM - partner, family, and friend's interest - work colleagues support	- unsupportive family members and workplaces - no social media groups or support groups in NZ - not knowing anyone with GDM - unable to perform testing in public - told what to eat by family members

language, the opportunity to record their food diary in their first language and more writing space in the hard copy food diary. Some women did not know how to go back on the glucometer to check their previous results. All these barriers prevented women from either mastering or performing regular glucose testing and recording their food intake.

> *"To be honest, the diabetes books are quite small to write in what you are eating and that can be off putting, for me I found anyway. It would so much better to have everything on my phone, like a phone app for the blood sugars and like a kind of electronic diary, everything else is on my phone, then I would do it more regularly I think" (Janet 07A).*

> *"I think they give you a lot of information that.... I mean it's good to have. But then again, yeah, I'm probably not much of a reader. I just like to speak to thing, maybe give me a YouTube clip [link], and have picture that remind me how to, that would definitely help especially if it's your first language" (Larissa 01B).*

Beliefs about capabilities

'Belief about capabilities' refers to a woman's belief about her capability to perform, control and monitor her CBG concentration. The most common reported constructs were self-confidence and having control to help women to do their CBG testing without concerns, alter their food intake accordingly and developed a 'can-do attitude'. Barriers were identified as having a 'can't-do' attitude, believing that it is not necessary to test their CBG concentrations regularly and a feeling of not being in control.

> *"The dietician and the doctor were very impressed with my numbers, and that made me feel amazing*

and proud, and chuffed with myself. I can do this" (Anneri 14B).

"It's too hard, I can't do it" (Yoko 15B).

Women who had firm beliefs about their capability reported how they were not concerned to do the CBG testing in public or at work and were highly motivated to do the testing at the appropriate times, even if it meant interrupting what they were doing.

"I am good at this, do it always on time. I do it when I am commuting on the bus or when I am attending mass. Even though I am in the middle of kneeling and everyone is quiet, I will just quickly get out my kit and quickly prick myself even though it may make some noise" (Karroll 05B).

Women with uncertain beliefs about their capabilities became increasingly scared to do their CBG testing. They had to repeat tests more often, as there was either not enough blood for the test or the glucometer would show error messages, which led them to test less often than recommended, or not at all. Women's feelings voiced of not being in control, as the CBG concentrations directed their food, exercise and/or medication intake, contributed to low self-belief in their capabilities.

"Yes, I get frustrated with it and then the glucometer does not work. Yes, I have my days where I'm tired and I'm sick of it, and belief I can't do it. I don't do my blood tests then, and I don't manage my food. It just runs my life" (Karrena 17B).

Beliefs about consequences

This domain refers to a woman's expectations about optimal CBG control. Participating women reported that anticipated positive or negative consequences strongly influenced their actions; whether they tested their CBG concentrations, adhered to the glycaemic targets, changed their food intake and physical activities, or took their medication. This domain was represented strongly throughout the interviews.

"They did tell us like that if mums are not taking care, there may be a chance for the baby to have the diabetes when the baby is a teenager or when it is little, that was a good thing, that is the one reason which I'm more careful, which I don't want to give anything to my kids which is from me you know, whatever the life brings to them that's their luck you know, but I don't want to give anything from me to my next generation, so you know, if I can be more careful about that then I have to, totally changed everything and never forget to do blood sugars"(Anna 07).

"Well, can I play the guitar with so many holes in my fingers? Who wants that? So, pricking only alternative days and not on my left hand is sort of ok, but if I have to play in church, I don't do it the week before" (Yasmin 01).

Memory, attention, and decision process

This domain refers to a woman's ability to remember when, and decide where, to perform CBG testing. Women identified memory aids, such as alarms on mobile phones, setting a timer and having a dedicated bag for all the CBG testing equipment to aid their memory and the decision process of performing the test, regardless of where they were. Forgetfulness was identified as a perceived barrier for doing regular CBG testing, in particular when away from their home, causing considerable frustration and anger for some women.

"Yeah husband reminds me at night most of the time (Amali 16). I get my partner to ring me and then do it. A couple of times when I've been driving I did it while I was driving" (Angela 15). "I keep my alarm on the phone, as otherwise you know, I can't remember the particular time" (Hana 11B). "Just put an alarm in my head and watch my clock every couple of hours" (Neethu 02).

"I do it anywhere... And they will ask me what are you doing? And that is the time I start talking to them about gestational diabetes and I say, 'you know I have gestational diabetes and I have to do this'. And then about at the same time I am like a tool for everybody to find out about diabetes and they learn about it" (Karroll 05B).

I tend to stress about it for the first half an hour after a meal, that I've got to remember, and then it just slips your mind some days, so frustrating (Erin 18B).

Environmental context and resources

'Environmental context and resources' refers to a woman's access to equipment and to a health professional when unsure about results. The most commonly reported barrier was the cost of resources, no phone access to a health professional when the woman was unsure about results and health professionals not believing the women's documented CBG results. Different sizes of CBG recording booklets were either experienced as enablers or barriers. Some women found it frustrating that their CBG recording booklet did not fit into the glucometer bag, which meant it had to be carried separately. This meant for some women CBG results were not recorded when outside their homes.

In New Zealand women receive a free glucometer, blood lancets, and testing strips from the diabetes in pregnancy services at their local hospital or they are given a prescription for these resources to be picked up from their local pharmacy. While some women could pay the costs of the prescription fee, some women found it too difficult over time and then did not continue CBG testing.

> *"It's definitely more expensive ... and then prescriptions fees for the testing bits. It all adds up and you want to be sure it's worth it. Some weeks it is not" (Jean 16B).*

> *"Yeah, like insinuating that I eat overnight, because my levels are high in the morning, like no, I am busy sleeping actually, but yeah that I struggled with, not being believed by the diabetes consultant. Why should I continue testing then?" (Alice 10A).*

Social influences

In the context of this study the domain 'social influences' refers to a woman's social interactions for CBG monitoring and maintaining optimal CBG control. Engaged social interactions, such as work colleagues asking after CBG concentrations and reminding women to do their testing, as well as providing healthy food choices and stopping meetings to provide opportunity for the women to do their testing were enablers. Barriers were being told to leave the restaurant (or other public places) when performing CBG testing and being unable to stop work for the testing. Women working as managers, bus drivers, factory workers, nurses and doctors found it difficult to adhere to the post-prandial timeframes for CBG testing, as there was often little opportunity to stop their work.

> *"Well, at work they gave me private corner to do it [CBG testing] and they are really interested what my levels are. My colleagues remind me. So helpful" (Yoko 15B).*

> *"I feel bad if I don't do it, but yeah it's usually as I've just been somewhere where I feel I couldn't do it, or I can't stop at work, especially now that I had the experience of being told to leave the restaurant and they think you are a druggie scum bag" (J.M.T.J.M.P. 14).*

Emotion

The domain 'Emotion' in this study refers to a woman's reaction and feelings to monitoring and maintaining her CBG concentrations. Some women felt it was a privilege to have been diagnosed with GDM as it meant they learnt new skills that directed positive lifestyle changes. The sense of achievements in mastering CBG collection and staying within recommended glycaemic targets enabled optimal glucose monitoring. This led to testing family and friends without understanding that this would be recorded on the glucometer as their results.

> *"It's been a good adjustment, kind of a joy, I learnt how to test blood sugars and I am living healthy, it's kind of like a good stepping stone to continue that healthy life. It's kind of giving you this mirror glass into the future that you could have diabetes in the future (Esther 07B). I'm brave, I never forget to do the pricks" (Raynia 09).*

Barriers included emotions of stress and being scared to do the capillary testing at the appropriate times, especially where a needle phobia existed. The constant focus on the numbers discouraged some women from performing regular CBG testing.

> *"Ah yes, I am scared, first of all 'cause I hate needles. One thing, it should be different that putting like, when we test our diabetes, the needle we put in our fingers, it's very painful, like all my fingers have holes, because every day I prick and then I stop. So, there should be different type of thing we can measure the diabetes" (Shairin 11).*

> *"Um, I guess, having had that experience before as part of my medical training, I kinda knew what it was like [being a doctor], but I think it's the repetitiveness, focusing on numbers and having to do it so many times a day, I mean I wince at the lancet, when it goes off as its getting to the point where it's actually getting, you know, traumatised by the pain that comes from the pricked fingers" (Christina 15A).*

Behavioural regulation

'Behavioural regulation' refers to a woman's focus on self-monitoring effectively and planning how to incorporate this into her daily life. Women who decided to have all their testing and documentation equipment in a dedicated bag and leaving it at dedicated place at home indicated how helpful this was to undertake the testing regularly. Sharing their glycaemic target achievements on social media, with overseas GDM Facebook groups, and thinking of the health of their baby were identified as motivators to regulate behaviour.

> *"You just put yourself into a routine. You just have to, for the baby, and have all your gear in a bag, ready to be used anytime and anywhere" (Sabrina 05).*

> *"Yes, having it all planned helps. Every morning at 10.30 I have 30 minutes' walk. And also after afternoon tea and dinner I have 30 minutes walking. It's very good, and I feel I have more energy" (Casey 01A).*

What affects a woman's CBG concentration and how does she maintain optimal glycaemic control with this knowledge?

The themes emerging from the interviews from women with GDM relating to the second research question 'What affects a woman's CBG concentration and how does she maintain optimal CBG control with this knowledge?'were categorised into five of the theoretical domains. These were: Knowledge, Beliefs about consequences, Environmental context and resources, Emotion, and Behavioural regulation (Table 5). The domains: Belief about consequences, Environmental context and resources and Behavioural regulation were represented most strongly in the context of this question.

Knowledge

In the context of the second research question the domain 'knowledge' refers to a woman's understanding of what affects her CBG concentrations. Women who knew the differences between carbohydrates, proteins, and fats, could read food labels and understood how exercises affected their blood glucose concentrations were more likely to embrace dietary and exercise changes and continue with regular blood glucose monitoring.

> *"You just fill it up with other stuff, like veggies, depends on what you eat regularly, it you eat KFC all the time then your buggered" (Danielle 06).*

> *"Yeah, so whenever I do my walking after meal, my blood sugar gets low right away, but if I snuggle in the bed after a meal, the blood sugar is high, that's what I notice" (Belle 19A).*

Barriers identified included not knowing how to read food labels or how food intake and activity levels impact on glycaemic control or unable to read the information provided, as it was not in the woman's first language. Two women knew how to increase their subcutaneous insulin, so they could continue eating their favourite sweets and carbohydrates and not be concerned about any behavioural lifestyle changes.

> *"I don't really understand what these food labels mean. I eat the same stuff anyway, not much use knowing it" (Jisha 04).*

> *"So, I ask them, can I just have some insulin, and they say, "Okay". They give me the long-term insulin and now I can have sweets but my levels are ok" (Casey 01A).*

Belief about consequences

The 'Belief about consequences' domain refers to a woman's expectations about what affects her CBG concentration. Several women started eating the same food every day. Some women ordered weekly commercially available, pre-assembled ready for cooking, health food bags, as this enabled women to keep their CBG concentrations within the recommended glycaemic targets. While this method of food intake was identified as an enabler by the women, it is unclear how effective long-term lifestyle changes would be sustained, as the women were not planning to eat in a similar way after the baby was born. Further enablers were identified as hearing other women's stories about GDM, which encouraged anticipated regret ('I know if I do this I will regret it, therefore I will not do it'). This meant women were diligent about routinely exercising and following their diabetic diet.

> *"I focused on it's a short period of time, eating the same every day, you can get through it, and after pregnancy it's going to be so awesome that you can eat what you want to eat, you focus on the fact that it's not forever, I always think of trying to push a baby out that is too big, that's an incentive, they can dislocate if it's too wide, so I just focus on every little bit, makes a difference, that's what I picked up from the obstetrician, you might go "oh this biscuit won't hurt" but yeah it makes a difference, no option but do it consistently. I know of women who so regretted that they did not do it properly" (Annie 16A).*

Women in the study who believed that exercises had no effect on CBG concentration were not likely to engage in any physical activity. Women who believed that too much physical activity may cause pre-term labour would do occasionally a short walk. The belief that the diabetes medication would control CBG concentrations prevented women from engaging in understanding the effects of food intake and glycaemic control.

"I've never tested after doing exercise, yeah, so I couldn't say, I don't belief it makes a difference, so don't do it really" (Alice 10A).

"I don't want my baby to come before 35 weeks, you know, I'm scared it comes early, more exercise makes it too early, but I will walk or swim after that time if it makes a difference" (Anna 07).

"I feel better now that I'm on the right medication. My sugars are well controlled and I don't need to worry about eating and walking" (Erin 04B).

"I didn't read it, because it's easier for him to read in English about what types of food you need to eat, it should be in colour and pictures. He doesn't like to read either, but when you give me a colour picture, these are the things you need to eat a lot, and these are things you need to not eat in colour, that would make a difference, then I would understand" (Zeinab 12A).

"I don't do much exercise because I am working all the time. Don't know how to fit it in. Maybe someone needs sit down with me and show me how and when?" [to exercise] (Fiona 02A).

Environmental context and resources

In the context of this research question this domain refers to a woman's access to food, exercise equipment and health professionals. Women in this study, who had access to group or individual sessions with a dietitian, could understand and alter their food intake and keep a food diary. Being taught CBG testing by a pharmacist or by a diabetes midwife in a group session was experienced as an enabler by most women interviewed. Having easy access to exercise equipment, such as a tread-mill or stationary bicycle, enabled women to exercise if they were unable to leave the house. Other enablers were identified as ensuring 'right' food in the pantry, having access to a vegetable garden, lower food costs, less fast food meals, and easy phone access to a diabetes dietitian.

"Walking through a personalised diet is really helpful, and not just a mass-produced 'try these things' and straight access to the dietitian via phone or email. I know what I can and can't eat now. Keeping a food diary has been good" (Anneri 14B).

"I bought a walker machine [treadmill] after being diagnosed with GDM to exercise. Every time I eat I do it. It is working well" (Belle 19A).

Barriers were identified as lack of or limited access to, resources and health professionals. This included lack of access to transport to attend group or individual sessions with a dietitian, no considerations for ethnic food options, not being able to discuss the effects on glycaemic control in the woman's first language, health professionals not looking at the food diary, higher food costs and unclear or no guidance about physical activities/exercises and its effect on CBG concentrations.

"Not sure if some food puts it up, it's possible, if I did a food diary I guess I could look it up, but that's a bit tedious" (Toni 03).

Emotions

The domain 'Emotion' refers to a woman's reaction and feelings as to what affects her CBG concentrations. Enablers most commonly reported for were positive emotions, such as being happy and excited to understand the link between food intake and exercises and glycaemic control. Barriers most commonly reported related to negative emotions, such as being stressed about not seeing any difference in glycaemic control despite trying hard to follow the dietary guidelines and feeling hungry most of the time when trying to achieve optimal glycaemic control.

"There are days when I am so worried that I am eating the wrong food and might hurt my baby, where I have checked myself 12 times just to see where I am staying at because the strict diet does not make a difference [to CBG concentrations], maybe I should just stop altogether? If you don't know, you don't know" (Aroha 10B).

"...but if I'm too hungry then I don't care, which is quite often" (Elizabeth 08B).

"I was kind of worried about what the dietician was going to say because I did have a few highs like in my first week of trying and I remember just feeling so overwhelmed and walking in she said, 'are you OK?' and I just burst into tears, it was just one of those things. She said: Oh my goodness, I'm not going to tell you off or anything, we'll work through it" (Collette 09B).

Behavioural regulation

The domain 'Behavioural regulation' refers to a woman's focus on self-monitoring effective food intake and exercise and planning how to incorporate this into daily life. Women who had action plans in place for physical activity and food intake, for example to do 20-min exercise after each main meal, bathing the toddler after the evening meal, playing ball games with the family, and starting a food and activity diary, found it easy to incorporate the changes into their daily life. Renaming exercise as physical activity and diet as food intake made a significant difference for women's confidence level to self-monitor these.

> *"Oh, you will laugh, but I don't try to vacuum the floor, I brush the floor every night time on my knees with a brush and shovel, because I can't go out and I get cold. My levels are good when I do this. No good levels when I do not do it" (Jisha 04A).*

Barriers to changing and regulating behaviour were mainly the dislike of having to exercise or to focus constantly on what to eat. Women noted that both stress and excitement would increase CBG concentrations and this discouraged effective self-monitoring.

> *"For the baby shower, I was so good with the food but my levels were still high, it's not just stress but also excitement that puts it up. So, what use is that then not to feel happy. May as well not do the testing" (Raman 17B).*

What support have women found helpful/not helpful in learning about and maintaining CBG control?

The key themes emerging from the interviews for women with GDM relating to the third research question 'What support have women found helpful/not helpful in learning about and maintaining CBG control?' were categorised into four of the theoretical domains. These are: Beliefs about consequences, Reinforcement, Environmental context and resources and social influences (Table 6). The domains Environmental context and resources and Social influences were represented most strongly in the context of this question.

Beliefs about consequences

The domain 'Beliefs about consequences' refers to a woman's expectation to sharing her diagnosis of GDM with others. Women shared their diagnosis and management of GDM with significant others and work colleagues when they believed this would gain them support for learning more about and maintaining optimal glycaemic control. Interestingly, when women perceived that sharing their diagnosis would generate a judgement and/or unhelpful advice they would not 'tell'. Some women did not 'tell' because they felt protective towards their family members and did not want to worry them unnecessarily. This created a lonely place for some women.

> *"It helps them to be more supportive if they know. I told them all. I don't want them to bring sugary items when they visit" (Collette 09B).*

> *"Did not tell, as I am big and people will say, ah, yes, you are fat, that did it" (Jean 16B).*

> *"Did not tell parents and friends, as they get too worried, but a bit lonely and hard doing it without them" (Aliisa 02B).*

Reinforcement

'Reinforcement' here refers to a woman's ability to reinforce skills and coping strategies for self-support in maintaining optimal CBG control. Continuing with a written or creating a pictorial food diary (taking photos with a mobile phone camera), honestly and diligently documenting CBG results and rewarding glycaemic achievements with non-food items or activities (for example, going to the movies) were identified as enabling reinforcement of skills and coping strategies. Family activities such as family members guessing around the dinner table what the CBG levels will be before and after the meal, creating a graph for the fridge for charting CBG levels for all to view and using stickers to identify in the pantry/fridge which foods are healthy options for women with GDM to consume were further reinforcing enablers.

> *"It's kind of a fun time. My husband and my daughter guess what the number should be after I have done the pricking. If we are all right we reward us with going to the playground park with my daughter, she loves it and so do we" (BC 17A).*

Environmental context and resources

The domain 'Environmental context and resources' refers to a woman's ability to have access to learning resources and health professional services for optimal glycaemic control. Visual information, such as a food plate with portion sizes and access to informative websites about GDM were identified as enablers. Provision of a free health shuttle for clinic appointments, a hospital crèche for child care, an efficient appointment system reducing waiting times and partner and extended family welcomed at teaching sessions and clinic appointments contributed to women's ability to perform CBG testing confidently and of feeling supported. Telephone access to discuss CBG results was available for most women and while only a few women used it, telephone access was considered a reassuring support. Provision of healthy food options by family and work colleagues was reported as a significant support.

> *"Yeah husband attending info sessions was good but next time not during office time, evenings or weekends would be better. The food plate was very helpful, but maybe more Asian food on it would help too" (Amali 16).*

Several women had experienced barriers to accessing learning resources and health professional services for optimal glycaemic control. These included health professionals being impatient and inconsistent in their advice; not seeing the same health professional twice; not being taught how to check the glucometer; long waiting times at clinic appointments; not being taught in their first language, being unable to write into their food diaries in their first language; having no transport to attend teaching sessions or clinic appointments and poor parking facilities. Of the women who searched for information through Google, some became scared and would have preferred guidance to visit a website with clear and supportive information. Restaurants being unable to provide an ingredients list for meals on the menu was identified as another inaccessible resource. Provision of unhealthy food by family and work colleagues was reported as a significant barrier.

> *"Google was a bit scary. So, it's better just to stay away from it and get your questions answered at the clinic. But that google information was in Russian, and that was good. Yeah, they need to tell me where to look on the internet. Same with menus from restaurants, their ingredients could be listed on-line" (Lilly 18A).*

> *"I saw a registrar who seemed very junior and gave me quite conflicting information to what everybody else had given me. So, I actually went back yesterday and saw a consultant, because I wasn't happy. That improved things, but it took more time and to find a carpark is nearly impossible" (Erin 18B).*

> *"He says, "Just eat whatever you want", because he likes sweet stuff. Hard not to give in" (Tara 19B).*

Social influences

The domain 'Social influences' refers to a woman's access to social interaction to learning/reinforcing optimal blood glucose control. Some women joined an American Facebook group for women with GDM. While the glycaemic targets were different for the American counterparts, women in this study enjoyed swapping recipes, sharing tips about CBG testing, celebrating successes of achieving and maintaining glycaemic control and providing encouragement when glycaemic challenges were shared. Family and friend's interest in all aspect of glycaemic control and meeting other women with GDM contributed to feeling supported and reinforcement for optimal glycaemic control.

> *"So, I soon realised, after joining a [American] Facebook group, that most people struggle with cereals. So, I removed the cereal and just went to a two-egg breakfast, and that just evened it out. So, then I felt a bit better again" (Anneri 14B).*

> *"Yes, in the morning, if I want to sleep in then he will do for me the fingerpicks" (Shairin 11).*

Participating women identified social disconnections as barriers for learning and reinforcing optimal glycaemic control. This included unsupportive family members and workplaces, unavailability of a support group for women with GDM in New Zealand, on-line or face-to-face, being judged in public and being constantly' told what to eat and what not to eat by family members.

> *"...I guess that's why I eat my chocolate with my yoghurt. I like chocolate, I'm going to have chocolate. You tell me I can't, then I'm not going to listen. And I'm going to want it more and I'm going to binge eat it and don't worry about my levels" (Aroha 10B).*

The results from the three questions explored in this study identified enablers and barriers for women with GDM representing their experiences of monitoring CBG concentrations, what affects this monitoring and what supports have been helpful for them to achieve optimal glycaemic control. As a summary, Table 7 outlines some considerations for practice and research that may be useful for health professionals and diabetes in pregnancy services providing care for women with GDM.

Discussion

Our results highlight the complex interactions between women with GDM monitoring their CBG concentrations, their understanding of the link between dietary intake, exercise and glycaemic control, having stress-free access to health care providers and resources, and their social context and support. The study used interviews and the validated TDF to determine the enablers and barriers women with GDM experience to achieve optimal CBG control. We categorised emerging enablers and barriers into a total of nine domains across three study questions. These were: Knowledge, Skills, Beliefs about capabilities,

Table 7 Considerations for practice and research

Practice considerations	Research considerations
Monitoring for optimal glycaemic control	Monitoring for optimal glycaemic control
• Enable women with GDM to attend group teaching for CBG testing and interpretation and include women who have had GDM to share their stories. • Discuss individual strategies for regular CBG monitoring, food intake and physical activity. • Encourage partner and family attendance at any clinic or teaching sessions (may need to be offered at evenings or weekends). • Provide information relating to GDM in a woman's first language and/or more visually, including ethnic food suggestions. • Investigate the possibility of community pharmacists' involvement in teaching CBG testing.	• Explore opportunities for companies to create phone Apps, e.g. for electronic food and activity diaries, recording of CBG results and medication intake. • Do phone apps have an impact on optimal glycaemic control for women with GDM? • Does a name change for GDM reduce anxiety in pregnant women?
Dietary intake and exercise for glycaemic control	Dietary intake and exercise for glycaemic control
• Enable easy access to a diabetes dietitian with diet recommendations tailored to an individual woman's context (cultural, financial, and emotional). • Engage in meaningful discussions about the content in a food diary and provide multi-modal opportunity for the woman to record the food diary in her first language or enable mobile phone photo collection of food intake. • Regularly address hunger for women with GDM. • Encourage a physical activity diary alongside the food diary. • Consider engaging a physical (activity) therapist for clear in-depth assessment and guidance of exercise that women can incorporate into their daily life.	• Does keeping a physical activity diary impact on glycaemic control? • Does engaging a physical activity therapist contributes to the understanding and up-take of physical activity for women with GDM? • Why do women with GDM seem to be hungry despite quality dietary recommendations? • What affect has self-imposed dietary practices by women with GDM during their pregnancy on long term lifestyle behaviour?
Support for optimal glycaemic control	Support for optimal glycaemic control
• Provide free CBG monitoring equipment, health shuttles and child care when attending clinic appointments and reduce clinic waiting times. • Consider face-to-face support groups for women with GDM. • Consider setting up a social media group for women. With current GDM (e.g. Facebook). • Include regular mental health assessment for women with GDM. • Provide direct phone access to multi-disciplinary health professionals.	• Limited research available for regular mental health assessment for women with GDM. • Limited research about the effect of a GDM diagnosis on partners and family members. • Limited research on how partners and families can best support a woman with GDM in their context. • Does social media or face-face group support make a difference for women with GDM for maintaining optimal glycaemic control?

Beliefs about consequences, Reinforcement, Memory, attention and decision processes, Environmental context and resources, Social influences, Emotion and Behaviour regulation (Tables 4, 5 and 6). Through our iterative process we identified when no new themes were emerging within the TDF domains, thus ensuring that data saturation had been achieved [37, 38]. Transcript analysis revealed a range of enablers and barriers that impact on a woman's ability to achieve optimal glycaemic control.

The initial response of women being diagnosed with GDM was predominantly of being shocked. At the time of the interview the women had generally accepted the diagnosis, knowing it would only last a finite time and were motivated by making a difference for the baby. Maternal shock, fear and anxiety associated with a diagnosis of GDM have been reported in the literature with a trend towards acceptance as the pregnancy progressed [39–44]. Kalra and colleagues [45] suggest that these findings support an onomastic (re-naming) opportunity, arguing that the phrase gestational diabetes can cause significant psychosocial morbidity. Alternative names suggested for GDM were Gestational Dysglycemia of Nutritional Origin (GDNO) or Pregnancy Related Intolerance to Glucose (PRIG). This indicates further research is needed to determine if an onomastic change would achieve less maternal psychosocial morbidity. Some women in our study, once they overcame the initial shock, thought that it was a 'privilege 'and a 'good thing' to have been diagnosed with GDM, as this supported change to a healthier lifestyle and provided them with skills such as being able to read and understand food labels. This advocates for an opportunity for promoting lasting lifestyle changes during the remainder of the pregnancy. Other studies reiterate these findings, and found that for some women with GDM, the knowledge gained enhanced the motivation and self-efficacy to initiate lasting lifestyle changes [40, 46, 47].

While most women accepted that they had GDM and adapted to the change, many women disliked the change of focus for their pregnancy to numbers of CBG concentrations, glycaemic targets, 90th percentile for fetal growth and maternal weight. This contributed to a feeling of reduced control, which exacerbated emotions and created barriers for some women. This meant a few women in the study did not continue with or reduced their self-monitoring of CBG concentrations, decided they were too busy to attend some of the clinic appointments, refused referrals for serial growth scans and were less committed to adhere to diet recommendations. Negative feelings acting as a deterrent to intervention up-take has been reported for women with GDM by some studies [41, 48, 49]. This suggests that emotional support and mental health assessments need to be an imperative part of heath care for women with GDM.

Monitoring for optimal glycaemic control

Nearly all women in our study knew their optimal glycaemic targets and the importance to adhere to them. Despite this knowledge, participating women reported that this did not necessarily mean they would self-monitor their glycaemic control as advised. Responses varied on how they felt about their self-monitoring skills, if they had access to equipment, and their context, evident through the most strongly represented domains of Belief about capabilities, Emotions and Social influences. Women were less likely to do the CBG testing or stopped altogether for a variety of reasons. These included being scared and unsure about pricking their finger for CBG testing, playing a musical instrument, believing high CBG concentrations would harm their baby, being asked to leave a restaurant when testing, not being able to take a break to perform the test because of the nature of their work, and not being believed that their recorded CBG results were correct. Women were more likely to continue with regular CBG testing if they thought it was less painful than anticipated, attended a group session to learn how to perform CBG testing, took family members to teaching sessions, were shown by a community pharmacist how do to the testing, had the belief they knew how to do it, were praised by health professionals for their efforts, and had fun 'pricking' friends and family. There is a need for health professionals to provide clear and meaningful information about CBG testing, discuss strategies for overcoming barriers particularly in work situations, enable family members to be part of this process and to believe a woman's CBG recordings (Table 7). These findings are echoed in other literature [41, 50]. The notion for a community pharmacist to initially teach women diagnosed with GDM how to perform CBG testing may be a valuable option to consider when time, cost and distance are a barrier. Some studies involving patients (pre-diabetic or with T2DM) self-monitoring their CBG concentration have found community pharmacies specialised in diabetes care can provide this service effectively [51, 52]. An extensive literature search did not identify any studies involving women with GDM and the effects of being taught CBG testing by a local community pharmacist. Clearly this is an area where further research is required (Table 7).

Dietary intake and exercise for optimal glycaemic control

Our study demonstrated that the domains Belief about consequences, Environmental context and resources and Behavioural regulation were represented most strongly in the context of dietary intake and exercise for enabler and barrier identification. Studies have reported that women with GDM who were treated with dietary advice and were self-monitoring CBG concentrations had fewer macrosomic babies, less maternal weight gain and less birth trauma [8, 53]. A Cochrane systematic review assessed evidence from 19 trials for ten different dietary interventions and concluded that while dietary advice is the main strategy for managing GDM it remains unclear which type of diet is best [54]. Dietary self-management guided by CBG concentrations alone without a particular diet may be difficult for women with GDM. In our study, participants who understood the benefits and consequences of dietary self-management and regular exercise for controlling their CBG concentrations had access to professional dietetic advice and could incorporate effective physical activities into their daily life achieved optimal glycaemic control most of the time. This is consistent with other studies [44, 50, 55, 56]. Women in our study saw self-imposed dietary restrictions such as eating the same meal every day or ordering commercially pre-packed health food options as enablers, and for them these were solutions to their current hyperglycaemia, as GDM was understood to be transitory. This self-imposed practice resulted in a woman's CBG concentrations staying within her recommended glycaemic targets most of the time. It is questionable if this approach would achieve long-term lifestyle changes. It is possible that the women in our study may not have understood the link between GDM and the risk for subsequent development of T2DM, and the importance of health behaviour regulation for reducing future diabetes risk [42, 57, 58]. Health professionals need to ascertain from women the reasons for any self-imposed dietary practices and ensure future health implications are understood. Further research is needed to explore in depth if self-imposed dietary practices by women with GDM during their pregnancy affect long term lifestyle behaviour (Table 7).

Over half of the women in this study identified a barrier to written information, as it was only provided in English. They wanted the health information in either their first language or for it to be more visually presented to better understand their GDM diagnosis, what optimal blood glucose control meant and to include ethnic food options (Table 7). These are similar findings reported by qualitative studies for women with GDM in Vietnam [42], Italy [59] and South Tamil Nadu [60]. Women in our study identified Google as a helpful tool, especially if they could access websites in their first language through Google. Health professionals need to be aware that women will access information beyond the clinic environment and that the quality of this information may vary. Health literacy providing clear and relevant health messages for women with GDM or other types of diabetes has been identified as an effective way to help people manage their own health care [61–63].

Most women commented on being hungry, but felt they could endure this for their babies' health, if it kept their CBG concentrations within the recommended glycaemic targets. Dietetic advice needs to include how to address hunger for women with GDM (Table 7).

Regular aerobic exercises involving large muscle groups such as walking, swimming and stationary cycling have been reported to be beneficial in pregnancy and are not associated with harms to the baby [64, 65]. The prevalence of exercise for women with GDM during their pregnancy appeared to be related to their understanding of what type of exercise they could do and its duration. This was further compounded by their inability to incorporate exercises into their busy daily life and the fact that it was called exercise. The lack of specific recommendation on type, intensity, and duration of exercises from health professionals and women's beliefs that exercises could cause pre-term labour or that rest is required when pregnant has been reported in the literature [48, 55, 66, 67]. Participating women, who approached exercises as meaning to be physical activity, were more likely to think outside the (exercise) square, and welcomed discovering which physical activity, such as bathing the toddler after the evening meal, had an impact on their glycaemic control. A Cochrane systematic review on exercise for pregnant women with GDM for improving maternal and fetal outcomes summarised evidence from 11 randomised controlled trials and found while exercises appeared to lower fasting and post-prandial CBG concentrations, they did not find any differences in other outcomes for pregnant women with GDM [68]. However, even if exercise does not provide any benefit during pregnancy, this change in lifestyle may persist after birth, and may help prevent the onset of type 2 diabetes and its long-term complications. A prospective study of 4554 women with previous GDM, who were followed for 16 years showed that increased physical activity levels lowered T2DM development and its risks [69]. This may mean that for women with GDM it could be worthwhile to record physical activities alongside or as part of their food diary for them to understand the effect physical activities have on their CBG concentrations (Table 7). It is common practice for the dietitian or the Lead Maternity Carer (LMC) midwife to recommended daily walking but without further in-depth guidance. Meeting with a physical activity professional or therapist who assesses where and what physical activities could be adapted to a woman's daily context, alongside other health professionals at the diabetes in pregnancy clinic, may be an option to consider and would benefit from further research (Table 7).

Support for glycaemic optimal control

Women reported that support from partners, family, friends, work colleagues and health professionals made a significant difference for them to accept their diagnosis, adhere to prescribed treatment and maintain optimal glycaemic control. This support facilitated self-management and healthy lifestyle behaviours. Partners and extended family support was reported as valuable in particular for increasing exercise and the provision of healthy meals. Similar findings have been reported in the literature [39, 41, 46, 50]. The key domains identified for this section of social influences and belief about consequences reflect this. Other suggestions for support included joining a social media network for women with current GDM, for example on Facebook, and/or attend a local support group for women with GDM. Neither of these are currently available in New Zealand and support organisations for Diabetes or DHB's may want to consider this (Table 7).

Some women in this study found their family's excessive concerns or providing unhealthy meals a challenge and reported that this contributed to them feeling stressed and unable to perform CBG monitoring. A qualitative study of perceived needs in women with GDM found similar findings and indicates the importance for health professionals to increase their awareness for the need of social support for women with GDM [70]. Other studies including women with borderline GDM and T2DM reiterate this [54, 71–73] and recommend, that health professionals as part of clinic appointments need to include discussions about effective strategies to cope with situations that are challenging for women with GDM. Research about the effect of a GDM diagnosis on partners and family members and how they can best support a woman with GDM in their context is limited (Table 7). Complexities of social determinants of health is often studied with ethnographic research [74] and it may be appropriate to encourage this type of research for partner and family experience who are living and supporting women with GDM.

Within the identified key domain of belief about consequences, a surprise finding was that several women reported not sharing their GDM diagnosis with anyone other than their partners. The main reasons for this decision was fear of being judged, not wanting to be scrutinised for daily activities including food intake, or not wanting to worry extended family members. This created social isolation, and contributed to a woman's feeling of shame, guilt, and reduced her ability to achieve optimal glycaemic control. Qualitative studies support these findings [43, 75–77]. The women in our study had not shared this decision with their respective health professionals. This suggests the need for greater awareness among health professionals that some women with GDM 'do not tell' and on-going assessment of a woman's mental well-being should be included in the health services provision [40].

This study adds to the body of knowledge about enabling women with GDM to achieve optimal glycaemic control. While some studies have explored the GDM experience from the woman's point of view, none have specifically studied the enablers and barriers to achieving optimal glycaemic control using the validated Theoretical Domains Framework. The sample size was reflective of a cross section of the demographics of New Zealand's pregnant population and reached data saturation.

Limitations of our study were that participating women were not from rural or remote areas in New Zealand and only women who were fluent in English were eligible. Women from different cultural backgrounds were well represented in this study (Table 3). It is unclear if the interviews with women in their first language would have elicited different enablers and barriers for optimal glycaemic control. Women interviewed often asked for information in their first language. Future research should consider conducting interviews in a participant's first language.

Conclusions

This qualitative study categorised identified enablers and barriers for women with GDM to achieve optimal glycaemic control into 10 theoretical domains across three main areas. This provided insights to how women adapt to regular CBG self-monitoring, adhere to recommended treatments, undertake necessary lifestyle changes and can be supported.

Barriers included: lack of health information, teaching sessions, consultations, and food diaries in a woman's first language; long waiting times at clinic appointments; seeing a different health professional every clinic visit; inconsistent advice; no tailored physical activities assessments; not knowing where to access appropriate information on the internet; unsupportive partners, families, and workplaces; and unavailability of social media or support groups for women with GDM. Perceived judgment by others led some women only to share their GDM diagnosis with their partners. This created social isolation.

Enablers included: the ability to attend group teaching sessions with family and hear from women who have had GDM; easy access to a diabetes dietitian with diet recommendations tailored to a woman's context including ethnic food and financial considerations; free CBG monitoring equipment, health shuttles to take women to appointments; child care when attending clinic appointments; and being taught CBG testing by a community pharmacist.

The enablers and barriers identified are multidimensional and may assist health professionals and diabetes in pregnancy services on how best to meet the needs of this diverse group of women and their families to achieve optimal CBG control and so reduce adverse outcomes for women with GDM and their babies.

Abbreviations

BMI: Body Mass Index; CBG: Capillary Blood Glucose; DHB: District Health Board; GDM: Gestational Diabetes Mellitus; LMC: Lead Maternity Carer; T2DM: Type 2 Diabetes Mellitus; TDF: Theoretical Domains Framework; WHO: World Health Organisation.

Acknowledgements

The authors would like to express their sincere thanks to all the women who participated. A special thank you to the four independent transcribers and their speedy transcribing and Jane Yates, research assistant, who helped compile the demographic information. We thank the Liggins Institute, at the University of Auckland, for Institutional support.

Funding

Ruth Martis, PhD candidate, is the recipient of a University of Auckland Senior Health Research Scholarship. The TARGET Trial is supported by a grant from the Health Research Council of New Zealand (14/499).

Authors' contributions

RM designed the qualitative study, recruited the women, conducted the interviews, led the analysis, and prepared the first draft of the manuscript and subsequent drafts. RM and JB coded and classified the data, revised and synthesised text into final domains and consulted with the other authors CAC and JMC during the process. CAC and JB contributed to the study design, project administration, thematic interpretation, and commented on drafts of the manuscript. All authors read and approved the final version.

Competing interests

None of the authors have any financial conflict of interests associated with this publication. CAC and JB are lead investigators for the TARGET Trial.

Author details

[1]Liggins Institute, The University of Auckland, Private Bag 92019, Auckland 1142, New Zealand. [2]Faculty of Health & Environmental Sciences, AUT, Auckland University of Technology, Private Bag 92006, Auckland 1142, New Zealand.

References

1. ADHB, Auckland District Health Board. National women's annual clinical report 2015. Auckland: Auckland District Health Board; 2016.
2. Garrison A. Screening, diagnosis and management of gestational diabetes mellitus. Am Fam Physician. 2015;91(7):460–7.

3. Wu CS, Nohr EA, Bech BH, Vestergaard M, Olsen J. Long-term health outcomes in children born to mothers with diabeetes: a population-based cohort study. PLoS One. 2012;7:e36727. https://doi.org/10.1371/journal.pone.0036727.
4. McCance DR. Pregnancy and diabetes. Best Pract Res Clin Endocrinol Metab. 2011;25:945–58.
5. Bellamy L, Casas J, Hingorani AD, Williams D. Type 2 diabetes mellitus after gestational diabetes: a systematic review and meta-analysis. Lancet. 2009; 373:1773–9.
6. Tieu J, Middleton P, Crowther CA. Preconception care for diabetic women for improving maternal and infant health. Cochrane Database Syst Rev. 2010;12 https://doi.org/10.1002/14651858.CD007776.pub2.
7. Landon MB, Spong CY, Thom E, Carpenter MW, Ramin SM, Casey B, et al. A multicenter, randomized trial of treatment for mild gestational diabetes. N Engl J Med. 2009;361(14):1339–48.
8. Crowther CA, Hiller JE, Moss JR, McPhee AJ, Jeffries WS, Robinson JS. Effect of treatment of gestational diabetes mellitus on pregnancy outcomes. N Engl J Med. 2005;352(24):2477–86.
9. Lawrence J. Women with diabetes in pregnancy: different perceptions and expectations. Best Practice & Research Clinical Obstetrics & Gynaecology. 2011;25(1):15–24.
10. Coney S. For the New Zealand guideline group (NZGG). Effective consumer voice and participation for New Zealand. A systematic review of the evidence. Auckland: New Zealand Guideline Group; 2004.
11. Health and disability commissioners Act 1994. Wellington: Ministry of Health. Reprinted as at 1 December 2014. http://legislation.govt.nz/act/public/1994/0088/latest/whole.html.
12. Health and disability services Consumers' rights regulation 1996. Wellington: Ministry of Health. Reprinted as at October 2015. http://www.hdc.org.nz/your-rights/about-the-code/code-of-health-and-disability-services-consumers-rights/.
13. Morley RF, Norman G, Golder S, Griffith P. A systematic scoping review of the evidence for consumer involvement in organisations undertaking systematic reviews: focus on Cochrane. Research Involvement and Engagement. 2016;2:36. https://doi.org/10.1186/s40900-016-0049-4.
14. Boote JD, Twiddy M, Baird W, Birks Y, Clarke C, Beever D. Supporting public involvement in research design and grant development: a case study of a public involvement award scheme managed by a National Institute for Health Research (NIHR) research design service (RDS). Health Expect. 2013; 18:1481–93. https://doi.org/10.1111/hex.12130.
15. NICE. National Institute for health and clinical excellence. Diabetes in pregnancy: management of diabetes and its complications from preconception to the postnatal period. NICE guideline NG3. National Institute for Health and Care Excellence: London; 2015.
16. Michie S, van Stralen MM, West R. The behaviour change wheel: a new method for characterising and designing behaviour change interventions. Implement Sci. 2011;6:42. https://doi.org/10.1186/1748-5908-6-42.
17. Michie S, Johnston M, Francis J, Hardeman W, Eccles M. From theory to intervention: mapping theoretically derived behavioural determinants to behaviour change techniques. Appl Psychol. 2008;57(4):660–80.
18. Michie S, Johnston M, Abraham C, Lawton R, Parker D, Walker A. Making psychological theory useful for implementing evidence based practice: a consensus approach. Quality and Safety in Health Care. 2005;14(1):26–33.
19. Atkins L, Francis J, Islam R, O'Connor D, Patey A, Ivers N, et al. A guide to using theoretical domains framework of behavioural change to investigate implementation problems. Implement Sci. 2017;12(1):77. https://doi.org/10.1186/s13012-017-0605-9.
20. Cane JOCD, Michie S. Validation of the theoretical domains framework for use in behaviour change and implementation research. Implement Sci. 2012;7:37. https://doi.org/10.1186/1748-5908-7-37.
21. French SD, Green SE, O'Connor DA, McKenzie JE, Francis JJ, Michie S, et al. Developing theory- informed behaviour change interventions to implement evidence into practice: a systematic approach using the theoretical domains framework. Implement Sci. 2012;7:38. https://doi.org/10.1186/1748-5908-7-38.
22. Davies P, Walker AE, Grimshaw JM. A systematic review of the use of theory in the design of guideline dissemination and implementation strategies and interpretation of the results of rigorous evaluations. Implement Sci. 2010;5:14.
23. McGoldrick EL, Crawford T, Brown JA, Groom KM, Crowther CA. Consumers attitudes and beliefs towards the receipt of antenatal corticosteroids and use of clinical practice guidelines. 2016;16:259. https://doi.org/10.1186/s12884-016-1043-4
24. Burgess C, Wright AJ, Forster AS, Dodhia H, Miller J, Fuller F, et al. Influences on individuals' decisions to take up the offer of a health check: a qualitative study. Health Expect. 2014;18(6):2437–48.
25. Penn L, Dombrowski SU, Sniehotta FF, White M. Perspectives of UK Pakistani women on their behaviour change to prevent type 2 diabetes: qualitative study using the theory domain framework. BMJ Open. 2014;4:e004530. https://doi.org/10.1136/bmjopen-2013-004530.
26. Nicholson SL, Donaghy M, Johnston M, Sniehotta FF, van Wijck F, Johnston D, et al. A qualitative theory guided analysis of stroke survivors' perceived barriers and facilitators to physical activity. Disabil Rehabil. 2014;36(22):1857–68.
27. Kim H, Sefcik JS, Bradway C. Characteristics of qualitative descriptive studies: a systematic review. Res Nurs Health. 2017;40:23–42.
28. Braun V, Clarke V. Using thematic analysis in psychology. Qual Res Psychol. 2006;3(2):77–101.
29. Sandelowski M. What's in a name? Qualitative description revisited. Res Nurs Health J. 2010;33:77–84.
30. Glanz K. Health behavior and health education: theory, research, and practice. 4th ed. San Francisco: Jossey-Bass; 2008.
31. QSR 2011 International Pty Ltd. NVivo11 qualitative research software. 2011. http://www.qsrinternational.com/nvivo-product/nvivo11-for-windows.
32. Tong A, Sainsbury P, Craig J. Consolidated criteria for reporting qualitative research (COREQ): 32-item checklist for interviews and focus groups. Int J Qual Health Care. 2007;19(6):349–57.
33. New Zealand Census 2013. http://www.stats.govt.nz/browse_for_stats/population/census_counts/2013CensusUsuallyResidentPopulationCounts_HOTP2013Census.aspx. Accessed 31 July 2017.
34. Counties Manakau Population Count. http://www.health.govt.nz/new-zealand-health-system/my-dhb/counties-manukau-dhb/population-counties-manukau-dhb. Accessed 31 July 2017.
35. Canterbury Population Count. http://www.health.govt.nz/new-zealand-health-system/my-dhb/canterbury-dhb/population-canterbury-dhb. Accessed 31 July 2017.
36. Edwards R, Holland J. What is qualitative interviewing? London: Bloomsbury Publishing Plc; 2013.
37. Wright A, Maloney FL, Feblowitz JC. Clinician attitudes toward and use of electronic problem lists: a thematic analysis. BMC Med Info Decis Making. 2011;11:36. https://doi.org/10.1186/1472-6947-11-36.
38. Sanders LD. Discovering research methods in psychology. London: John Wiley & Sons Ltd.; 2010.
39. Kaptein S, Evans M, McTavish S, Banerjee AT, Feig DS, Lowe J, et al. The subjective impact of a diagnosis of gestational diabetes among ethnically diverse pregnant women: a qualitative study. Can J Diabetes. 2015;39(2): 117–22. https://doi.org/10.1016/j.jcjd.2014.09.005.
40. Morrison MK, Lowe JM, Collins CE. Australian women's experiences of living with gestational diabetes. Women Birth. 2014;27(1):52–7. https://doi.org/10.1016/j.wombi.2013.10.001.
41. Parsons J, Ismail K, Amiel S, Forbes A. Perceptions among women with gestational diabetes. Qual Health Res. 2014;24(4):575–85.
42. Hirst JE, Thach ST, My An TD, Forsyth R, Morris JM, Jeffery HE. Women with gestational diabetes in Vietnam: a qualitative study to determine attitudes and health behaviours. BMC Pregnancy & Childbirth. 2012;12(1):81.
43. Collier SA, Mulholland C, Williams J, Mersereau P, Turay K, Prue C. A qualitative study of perceived barriers to management of diabetes among women with a history of diabetes during pregnancy. J Women Health. 2011;20:1333–9.
44. Persson M, Winkvist A, Mogren I. From stun to gradual balance'-women's experiences of living with gestational diabetes mellitus. Scand J Caring Sci. 2010;24(3):454–62. https://doi.org/10.1111/j.1471-6712.2009.00735.x.
45. Kalra S, Baruah MP, Gupta Y, Kalra B. Gestational diabetes: an onomastic opportunity. Lancet Diabetes Endocrinology. 2013;1(2):91. https://doi.org/10.1016/S2213-8587(13)70104-9.
46. Devsam BU, Bogossian FE, Peacock AS. An interpretive review of women's experiences of gestational diabetes mellitus: proposing a framework to enhance midwifery assessment. Women and Birth. 2013;26(2):e69–76.
47. Evans MK, O'Brien B. Gestational diabetes: the meaning of an at-risk pregnancy. Qual Health Res. 2005;15(1):66–81.
48. Carolan-Olah MC. Educational and intervention programmes for gestational diabetes mellitus (GDM) management: an integrative review. Collegian. 2016;23(1):103–14.
49. Razee H, van der Ploeg HP, Blignault I, Smith BJ, Bauman AE, McLean M,

et al. Beliefs, barriers, social support, and environmental influences related to diabetes risk behaviours among women with a history of gestational diabetes. Health Promo J Aust. 2010;21(2):130–7.
50. Carolan M, Gill GK, Steele C. Women's experiences of factors that facilitate or inhibit gestational diabetes self-management. BMC Pregnancy and Childbirth. 2012;12:99. doi.org/10.1186/1471-2393-12-99
51. Müller U, Hämmerlein A, Casper A, Schulz M. Community pharmacy-based intervention to improve self-monitoring of blood glucose in type 2 diabetic patients. Pharm Pract. 2006;4(4):195–203.
52. Mansell K, Evans C, Tran D, Sevany S. The association between self-monitoring of blood glucose, hemoglobin A1C and testing patterns in community pharmacies: results of a pilot study. Cana Pharm J (Ott). 2016; 149(1):28–37. https://doi.org/10.1177/1715163515618420.
53. Hawkins JS, Casey BM, Lo JY, Moss K, DD MI, Leveno KJ. Weekly compared with daily blood glucose monitoring in women with diet-treated gestational diabetes. Obstet Gynecol. 2009;113(6):1307–12. https://doi.org/10.1097/AOG.0b013e3181a45a93.
54. Han S, Middleton P, Shepherd E, Van Ryswyk E, Crowther CA. Different types of dietary advice for women with gestational diabetes mellitus. Cochrane Database Syst Rev. 2017;2 https://doi.org/10.1002/14651858.CD009275.pub3.
55. Wang C, Guelfi KJ, Yang H. Exercise and its role in gestational diabetes mellitus. Chronic DisTrans Med. 2016;2:208–14.
56. Hui AL, Sevenhuysen G, Harvey D, Salamon E. Barriers and coping strategies of women with gestational diabetes to follow dietary advice. Women Birth. 2014;27:292–7.
57. Balas-Nakash M, Rodríguez-Cano A, Muñoz-Manrique C, Vásquez-Peña P, Perichart-Perera O. Adherence to a medical nutrition therapy program in pregnant women with diabetes, measured by three methods, and its association with glycemic control. Clin Trans Invest. 2010;62(3):235–43.
58. Kapur K, Kapur A, Ramachandran S, Mohan V, Aravind SR, Badgandi M, et al. Barriers to changing dietary behavior. J Assoc Physic India. 2008;56:27–32.
59. Lapolla A, Di Cianni G, Di Benedetto A, Franzetti I, Napoli A, Sciacca L, et al. Quality of life, wishes, and needs in women with gestational diabetes: Italian DAWN pregnancy study. Int J Endocrinol. 2012; https://doi.org/10.1155/2012/784726.
60. Bhavadharini B, Deepa M, Nallaperumal S, Anjana RM, Mohan V. Knowledge about gestational diabetes mellitus amongst pregnant women in South Tamil Nadu. J Diabetol. 2017;8(1):22–6.
61. Hussain Z, Yusoff ZM, Sulaiman SA. Evaluation of knowledge regarding gestational diabetes mellitus and its association with glycaemic level: a Malaysian study. Prim Care Diab. 2015;9(3):184–90. https://doi.org/10.1016/j.pcd.2014.07.007.
62. Work base Education Trust. Māori health literacy research: gestational diabetes mellitus. Wellington: Ministry of Health; 2014.
63. Al Sayah F, Majumdar SR, Williams B, Robertson S, Johnson JA. Health literacy and health outcomes in diabetes: a systematic review. J Gen Intern Med. 2013;28(3):444–52. https://doi.org/10.1007/s11606-012-2241-z.
64. ACOG (American College of Obstetricians and Gynecologists). Physical activity and exercise during pregnancy and the postpartum period. Committee opinion no. 650. Obstet Gynecol. 2015;126:e135–42. https://doi.org/10.1097/AOG.0000000000001214.
65. Russo LM, Nobles C, Ertel KA, Chasan-Taber L, Whitcomb BW. Physical activity interventions in pregnancy and risk of gestational diabetes mellitus: a systematic review and meta-analysis. Obstet Gynecol. 2015;125(3):576–82. https://doi.org/10.1097/AOG.0000000000000691.
66. Momeni Javid F, Simbar M, Dolatian M, Alavi Majd H, Mahmoodi Z. A comparative study on dietary style and physical activity of women with and without gestational diabetes. Acta Medica Iranica. 2016;54(10):651–6.
67. Mudd LM, Owe KM, Mottola MF, Pivarnik JM. Health benefits of physical activity during pregnancy: an international perspective. Med Sci Sports Exer. 2013;45(2):268–77.
68. Brown J, Ceysens G, Boulvain M. Exercise for pregnant women with gestational diabetes for improving maternal and fetal outcomes. Cochrane Database Syst Rev. 2017;6 https://doi.org/10.1002/14651858.CD012202.pub2.
69. Bao W, Tobias DK, Bowers K, Chavarro J, Vaag A, Grunnet LG, et al. Physical activity and sedentary behaviors associated with risk of progression from gestational diabetes mellitus to type 2 diabetes mellitus: a prospective cohort study. JAMA Intern Med. 2014;174(7):1047–55.
70. Khooshehchin TE, Keshavarz Z, Afrakhteh M, Shakibazadeh E, Faghihzadeh S. Perceived needs in women with gestational diabetes: a qualitative study. Elect Physic. 2016;8(12):3412–20. https://doi.org/10.19082/3412.
71. Greenhalgh T, Clinch M, Afsar N, Choudhury Y, Sudra R, Campbell-Richards D, et al. Socio-cultural influences on the behaviour of south Asian women with diabetes in pregnancy: qualitative study using a multi-level theoretical approach. BMC Med. 2015;13:120. https://doi.org/10.1186/s12916-015-0360-1.
72. Miller TA, DiMatteo MR. Importance of family/social support and impact on adherence to diabetic therapy. Diab Metabol Syndrome Obes Targets Therapy. 2013;6:421–6.
73. Mayberry LS, Osborn CY. Family support, medication adherence and glycemic control among adults with type 2 diabetes. Diabetes Care. 2012; 35:1239–45.
74. Bandyopadhyay M. Tackling complexities in understanding the social determinants of health: the contribution of ethnographic research. BMC Public Health. 2011,11(Suppl 5):S6. https://doi.org/10.1186/1471-2458-11-S5-S6.
75. Ghaffari F, Salsali M, Rahnavard Z, Parvizy S. Compliance with treatment regimen in women with gestational diabetes: living with fear. Iran J Nurs Midwifery Res. 2014;19(7Suppl1):S103–11.
76. Schabert J, Browne JL, Mosely K, Speight J. Social stigma in diabetes: a framework to understand a growing problem for an increasing epidemic. Patient-Patient-Centered Outcomes Res. 2013;6(1):1–10. https://doi.org/10.1007/s40271-012-0001-0.
77. Abdoli S, Mardanian L, Mirzaei M. How public perceives diabetes: a qualitative study. Iran J Nurs Midwifery Res. 2012;17(5):370–4.

6

Lower vitamin D levels in Saudi pregnant women are associated with higher risk of developing GDM

Abdulrahman Al-Ajlan[1], Sara Al-Musharaf[2], Mona A. Fouda[8], Soundararajan Krishnaswamy[3], Kaiser Wani[3], Naji J. Aljohani[4], Amal Al-Serehi[5], Eman Sheshah[7], Naemah M. Alshingetti[8], Iqbah Z. Turkistani[9], A. Afrah Alharbi[3,4], Buthaynah A. Alraqebah[3,4], Aisha Mansoor Ali[6], Gawaher Al-Saeed[9] and Nasser M. Al-Daghri[3,4*]

Abstract

Background: Gestational diabetes mellitus (GDM) has serious consequences such as increased risks of preeclampsia, macrosomia and cesarean delivery. Even though the mechanistic basis of GDM has not been completely understood, several risk factors have been identified and one of these is vitamin D. However, the link between vitamin D deficiency and development of GDM is yet to be proven with certainty.

Methods: This study aimed to investigate the link between the incidence of GDM and serum vitamin D level in pregnant women of Saudi Arabia. 515 Saudi women (ages 18–46) in their 24-28th week of pregnancy, visiting various hospitals of Riyadh, participated in this study. Serum vitamin D and various biochemical and anthropometric parameters were determined in the first trimester and the recruits were screened for GDM by OGTT according to IADPSG criteria in their 2nd trimester. The association between vitamin D deficiency and development of GDM was calculated based on odds ratio of the incidence of GDM among vitamin D deficient and normal women.

Results: In this study cohort of 515 pregnant women, in the first trimester vitamin D deficiency (< 50 nmol/l) was detected in 425 (82.5%). On their 2nd visit (2nd trimester), 116 (27.7%) were diagnosed with GDM out of 419 with OGTT, according to IADPSG criteria. GDM risk was significantly higher among vitamin D deficient than non-deficient women (Odds Ratio: 2.87; Confidence Interval: 1.32–6.25; $P = 0.008$) even after adjusting for season, sun exposure and vitamin D intake (OR: 2.9; CI: 1.07–7.89). Of the various anthropometric and biochemical parameters, the GDM women differed significantly from non-GDM women with respect to serum levels of triglycerides (in mmol/l) (1.3 ± 0.6; 1.5 ± 0.6, $p = 0.018$) and fasting glucose (in mmol/l) [4.7 (4.3–5.2); 5.1 (4.6–5.6), $p < 0.01$]. Also, fasting glucose level in the 2nd trimester correlated inversely to serum vitamin D level determined during the 1st trimester ($r = -0.121$; $p = 0.014$).

Conclusions: Results of our study reveal a significantly higher risk of development of GDM among pregnant women having deficient vitamin D status.

Keywords: 25(OH) D, Gestational diabetes mellitus, Oral glucose tolerance test, Type 2 diabetes mellitus, Insulin resistance

* Correspondence: aldaghri2011@gmail.com
[3]Prince Mutaib Chair for Biomarkers of Osteoporosis, Department of Biochemistry, College of Science, King Saud University, PO Box, 2455, Riyadh 11451, Saudi Arabia
[4]Obesity, Endocrine and Metabolism Center, King Fahad Medical City, Faculty of Medicine, King Saud bin Abdulaziz University for Health Sciences, Riyadh 11525, Saudi Arabia
Full list of author information is available at the end of the article

Background

Gestational diabetes mellitus (GDM) is increasing in prevalence in parallel with the dramatic increase in the prevalence of overweight and obesity in women of child-bearing age [1]. GDM has a serious short- and long-term adverse health outcomes for both mothers and offspring. Factors which cause GDM have not been completely elucidated although several risk factors have been identified.

On the other hand, vitamin D deficiency, which was initially considered only to influence bone metabolism, is now known to exert a wide spectrum of extra-skeletal effects, including impairment of immune system [2], increased risk in cardiovascular disease and hypertension [3], disturbances in neuropsychiatric function [4] and even increased mortality [5]. The detection of vitamin D receptor expressed ubiquitously in almost all body cells suggests an involvement of vitamin D-mediated effects on critical metabolic pathways [6]. Recent epidemiological studies have found an association between 25(OH)D levels and risk of type 2 diabetes mellitus (T2DM) [7–9]. In vivo, vitamin D deficiency causes dysregulation of glucose metabolism by increasing insulin resistance through deteriorating β-cell function and mass [10, 11]. Vitamin D deficiency was also identified as a risk factor for obesity and T2DM in women at late reproductive age [12]. Furthermore, in pregnant women, vitamin D deficiency has important implications for the mother and lifelong health of the child, as it has been linked to maternal and child infections, small for gestational age (SGA), preterm delivery, preeclampsia, GDM, as well as DNA imprinting in the infant for lifelong chronic diseases [13]. Recent vitamin D supplementation (up to 4000 IU/d) studies involving pregnant women have suggested risk reduction in infection, preterm labor, and preterm birth [14]. However, observational studies about maternal vitamin D status and risk of GDM are conflicting, mostly due to differences in population characteristics such as ethnicity, geographic location, age of gestation at sampling and diagnostic criteria for GDM [15].

Vitamin D deficiency (< 50 nmol/L) which is found to be common globally and in various ethnicities, has a prevalence of 26–98% in pregnancy [16–18]. It has been reported to be high among women of child-bearing age in Saudi Arabia with approximately one third of reproductive-age Saudi women being vitamin D deficient [19] and a recent report showing < 5% having sufficient levels [20]. High rates of GDM incidence have been reported from Saudi Arabia, considered to be among the highest in the world [21].

Despite several studies, the link between GDM and maternal vitamin D status is yet to be fully understood. We aimed to investigate the effect of serum vitamin D level in the incidence of GDM along with its consequences on various biochemical parameters in pregnant women in Saudi Arabia, a country with a high prevalence of obesity, vitamin D deficiency and GDM.

Methods

Subjects

A total of 515 Saudi women identified to be at high risk of GDM (personal history of GDM or polycystic ovarian syndrome, glycosuria, family history of T2DM, severe obesity, macrosomia), recruited at various hospitals in Riyadh, Saudi Arabia were included in this study. In brief, only pregnant Saudi women aged 18–35 were included and non-Saudis were excluded to have a relatively homogenous cohort. Additional criteria for inclusion/exclusion have been described previously [20]. Sample size was determined using a level of confidence is at 0.05 and study power at 80% with the ratio of unexposed to exposed group 1:1 and the frequency of the outcome = 10%. The required sample is 438 pregnant women. To adjust for non-response rates, an extra 10% of the calculated sample will be added to sum up with 515 pregnant women.

Written informed consent was obtained from each subject before inclusion in the study. The study was approved by the Ethics Committee of the College of Science, King Saud University, Riyadh, Kingdom of Saudi Arabia (KSA).

Anthropometry and blood collection

Pregnant women in their first trimester pre-natal visit were subjected to anthropometric and blood withdrawal procedures as described previously [20].

Sample analyses

Blood samples collected from the subjects during their first visit were analyzed for 25(OH)D and various biochemical parameters. Serum 25(OH)D was determined as described before [20] with a Roche Elecsys modular analytics (Cobas e411) using an electrochemiluminescence immunoassay (Roche Diagnostics, GmbH, Mannheim, Germany) and commercially available IDS kits (IDS Ltd., Boldon Colliery, Tyne & Wear, UK). Variation for the 25(OH)D ELISA were 5.3% and 4.6%, respectively, with 100% cross-reactivity to 25(OH)D3 and 75% cross-reactivity to 25(OH)D2. It should be noted that the laboratory where samples were analyzed (Biomarkers Research Program, BRP) is a participating entity in the Vitamin D External Quality Assessment Scheme (DEQAS), and Quality Assurance (QA) standards are maintained by ISO 9000 and 17,025. The QA department audits the BRP laboratory at regular intervals. Serum glucose, lipid profile, calcium, and phosphorous were measured using a chemical analyzer (Konelab, Espoo, Finland). Serum-free insulin concentration was determined by electro-chemiluminescence method (Cobas e411; Roche Diagnostics, Mannheim, Germany).

Oral glucose tolerance test (OGTT)

Out of 515 pregnant women recruited for the study, only 419 visited the hospitals during their 2nd trimester and consented for OGTT. Dropout rate was 19.2%. OGTT was conducted with ingestion of seventy-five gram glucose and GDM was diagnosed according to International Association for Diabetes in Pregnancy Society Group (IADPSG) guidelines [22], if one of the following applies: fasting glucose ≥5.1 mmol/l, 1 h glucose ≥10 mmol/l or 2 h glucose ≥8.5 mmol/l.

Data analysis

Data was analyzed using the SPSS statistical Package (22.0 Version). The Kolmogorov-Smirnov test was used to analyze the normal distribution of the variables. The continuous normal variables are presented as mean ± standard deviations, while non-normal continuous variables are presented as medians and percentiles. Frequencies and percentages were used to present categorical variables. Hypothesis testing for significant differences was performed using independent Student t-test and Mann-Whitney U test for both normal and non-normal variables, respectively. Hypothesis testing for significant association was performed using chi-square test of independence. Logistic regression was performed taking GDM status as a dependent variable and vitamin D deficiency status as an independent variable. The statistical analysis was conducted at 95% confidence level and a P-value < 0.05 was considered statistically significant.

Results

Prevalence of vitamin D deficiency

Based on the recently recognized vitamin D cut-off [23], we classified pregnant women having < 50 nmol/l as deficient and those having > 50 nmol/l as non-deficient/normal. According to this criteria, out of 515 subjects of our study, 425 (82.5%) had deficient levels of vitamin D while the rest 90 (17.5%) were vitamin D sufficient. Severe vitamin D deficiency (< 25 nmol/l) was observed in 198 (38.4%) subjects.

Prevalence of GDM

Out of the 419 subjects subjected to OGTT on the second visit, 116 (27.7%) were diagnosed as positive for GDM.

Comparison of maternal and biochemical parameters of GDM women with non-GDM women

The non-GDM and GDM groups differed significantly with respect to serum vitamin D deficiency: 249 (82.5%) and 108 (93.1%), ($p = 0.006$); glucose (in mmol/l): [4.7 (4.3–5.2)], [5.1 (4.6–5.6)], ($p < 0.01$); age (years): (28.6 ± 5.1), (30.3 ± 5.6), ($p = 0.03$); HbA1c: (5 ± 0.4), (5.2 ± 0.5) ($p < 0.01$); triglycerides (mmol/l): (1.3 ± 0.6), (1.5 ± 0.6), ($p = 0.018$) and insulin (in uU/ml) [8.7 (4.4–19.5)], [11.5 (6.2–19.8)], ($p = 0.048$). Lastly, all obesity indices (pre-pregnancy BMI, BMI, waist size, hip size and WHR) were significantly higher among the GDM women compared to non-GDM women (all p-values < 0.05) (Table 1).

Analysis of association between vitamin D deficiency and GDM

Analysis of vitamin D status vs GDM incidence, as given in methods, indicated significantly higher risk for GDM among women who were deficient for vitamin D [OR: 2.87 (1.32–6.25) ($p = 0.008$)] (Table 2). The risk of development of GDM associated with vitamin D deficiency was also analyzed after adjusting the data for three sets of variables, which are known to influence carbohydrate metabolism or serum vitamin D levels. The risk of GDM among women with deficient vitamin D was sustained or increased significantly after adjusting the data for: 1) season of blood sampling, sun exposure and vitamin D intake (OR: 2.90, CI: 1.07–7.89, $p = 0.037$), 2) season of blood sampling, sun exposure and vitamin D intake, BMI at visit 1, maternal age, physical activity, family history of GDM, parity, HbA1c, WHR, triglycerides (OR: 4.41, CI: 1.19–16.42, $p = 0.027$), and adjustment 1 + adjustment 2 + gestational weight gain (OR = 6.05, CI: 1.16–31.42, $p = 0.033$).

For all the subjects ($n = 419$), serum vitamin D level measured at visit 1 was negatively correlated to fasting glucose determined at the time of 2nd visit ($r = -0.121$; $p = 0.014$) and the results are represented as a scatter plot (Fig. 1).

Discussion

Recent literature indicates a high level of incidence of GDM as well as vitamin D deficiency in Saudi Arabia and in this study we aimed to investigate the link, if any, between the two by determining the vitamin D level in the 1st trimester and assessing its association with GDM, determined by performing OGTT in the second semester. In a cohort of 515 pregnant women visiting different hospitals of Riyadh, Saudi Arabia, vitamin D deficiency was detected in 82.5% in the first trimester. On their 2nd visit, during the 2nd trimester of pregnancy, 27.7% of the 419 women who participated in OGTT were diagnosed with GDM. Analysis of the association between vitamin D status and incidence of GDM indicated a 2.87 fold increased risk of development of GDM among vitamin D deficient compared to vitamin D non-deficient women and this risk was sustained or substantially increased when the data was analyzed after adjusting for sunlight exposure, physical activity, calcium and vitamin D intake and other factors that are known to influence vitamin D levels. Of the various anthropometric and biochemical parameters, the GDM women differed significantly from non-GDM women with

Table 1 Subject characteristics at baseline (visit 1) defined according to GDM status (visit 2)

Parameters	Non-GDM	GDM	*P*-values
N	303	116	–
Vitamin D deficiency	249 (82.5%)	108 (93.1%)	0.006
Age (years)	28.6 ± 5.1	30.3 ± 5.6	0.003
Age at menarche (years)	12.5 ± 1.5	12.7 ± 1.8	0.39
Age at 1st pregnancy (years)	24.3 ± 4.4	24.9 ± 5	0.35
Parity	2 (1.0–3.0)	2 (1.0–4.0)	0.03
Gestational age (weeks)	11.4 ± 2.6	11.4 ± 2.9	0.98
Pre-BMI (kg/m^2)	26.4 ± 6.1	28.8 ± 6.3	0.003
BMI (kg/m^2)	28.1 ± 6.7	31.2 ± 7.2	< 0.001
Waist (cm)	89.3 ± 12.6	94.8 ± 13.8	0.001
Hips (cm)	107.1 ± 11.9	110.9 ± 11.6	0.011
WHR	0.8 ± 0.1	0.9 ± 0.1	0.03
Systolic blood pressure (mmHg)	113.8 ± 13.6	111.7 ± 12.5	0.23
Diastolic blood pressure (mmHg)	66.9 ± 8.7	67.7 ± 10.2	0.63
Glucose (mmol/l)	4.7 (4.3–5.2)	5.1 (4.6–5.6)	< 0.001
Insulin (μU/mL)	8.7 (4.4–19.5)	11.5 (6.2–19.8)	0.05
HbA1c (%)	5 ± 0.4	5.2 ± 0.5	< 0.001
Triglycerides (mmol/l)	1.3 ± 0.6	1.5 ± 0.6	0.02
Total cholesterol (mmol/l)	4.9 ± 1.0	5.1 ± 1.0	0.06
HDL-cholesterol (mmol/l)	1.3 ± 0.3	1.3 ± 0.3	0.22
LDL-cholesterol (mmol/l)	3 ± 0.8	3.1 ± 0.9	0.10
Calcium (mmol/l)	2.2 ± 0.2	2.1 ± 0.1	0.66
Corrected calcium (mmol/l)	2.2 ± 0.2	2.2 ± 0.1	0.94
Albumin (g/l)	35.8 ± 4.2	35.6 ± 4	0.64
Alkaline phosphatase (mmol/l)	8.3 ± 3.1	9.6 ± 3.6	0.09
PTH (pg/ml) #	10.9 (2.1–13.3)	10.9 (2.3–12.2)	0.56
Creatinine # (μmol/l)	45.1 (27.4–55.8)	45.5 (24.0–60.6)	0.93
Vitamin D (nmol/l) at visit 1 #	25.5 (17.3–41.9)	24.4 (17.4–37.1)	0.49

Data presented as Mean ± SD for continuous normal variables and medians (25th percentile – 75th percentile) for continuous non-normal variables; # indicates non-normal variables; categorical variables are presented as frequency (%). Independent sample t-test and Mann-Whitney U test are used for significance testing for Gaussian and non-Gaussian variables, respectively, while chi-square test of independence was used for categorical variable(s). Serum vitamin D level < 50 nmol/l was considered as deficient. GDM was diagnosed according to IADPSG guidelines [22]

respect to serum levels of triglyceride, fasting glucose and insulin, among others. Furthermore, all the obesity indices, pre-pregnancy BMI, BMI, waist size, hip size and WHR were significantly higher in the GDM women compared to non-GDM women suggesting a strong confounder effect from obesity. Also, overall, fasting glucose levels determined in the 2nd trimester showed an inverse association with vitamin D levels determined in the 1st semester and while this association was statistically significant it was weak, which may be due to the analysis being performed at different time points. A recent Australian study involving 3393 adults (ages 18–75 years) indicated a direct, protective effect of higher 25(OH)D on fasting plasma glucose and

Table 2 Association between GDM and vitamin D deficiency in Saudi pregnant women

Vitamin D Status	Unadjusted	Adjustment 1	Adjustment 2	Adjustment 3
< 50 nmol/l	2.87 (1.32–6.25)	2.90 (1.07–7.89)	4.41 (1.19–16.42)	6.05 (1.16–31.42)
P value	0.008	0.04	0.03	0.03

Data presented as Odd Ratios (95% CI); Logistic regression was used taking GDM status as dependent variables and vitamin D Deficiency status as independent variable. Adjustment 1: season of blood sampling, sun exposure and vitamin D intake (IU/day). Adjustment 2: adjustment 1 + pre-pregnancy BMI, maternal age, physical activity, Family history of GDM, parity, HbA1c, WHR, triglycerides; Adjustment 3: adjustment 1 + adjustment 2 and gestational weight gain

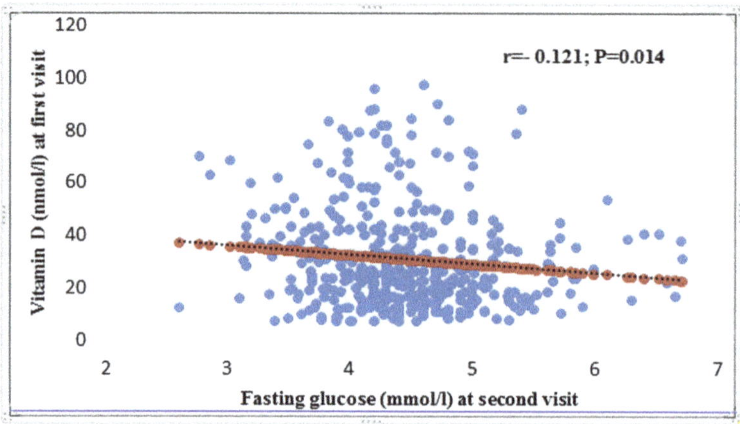

Fig. 1 Correlational analysis of baseline serum 25(OH) D with 2nd trimester fasting glucose in pregnant women

HbA1c, two criteria for assessment of risk of T2DM. Overall, results of our study indicate a significant association between vitamin D deficiency and increased risk of GDM development during the course of pregnancy.

Vitamin D deficiency is common in healthy Saudi adults and is more pronounced in females and especially in the younger age groups [24]. In a recent study performed in Riyadh, the prevalence of vitamin D deficiency (25(OH)D < 50 nmol/l) was high in both premenopausal and postmenopausal groups (80% and 68%, respectively) during the summer, as well as during the winter (85% and 76%, respectively) [25]. Vitamin D deficiency has been reported to be common among pregnant Saudi women living in Riyadh as observed by Al-Farris, recently [26].

The prevalence of GDM varies from 1 to 20%, and is rising worldwide, and the amount of GDM varies in direct proportion to the prevalence of T2DM in a given population, or ethnic group. In a recent retrospective cohort study (2013) involving 3041 women who delivered at King Khalid University Hospital, 569 (18.7%) had GDM [21]. Another study in Saudi Arabia (2015), adopting IADPSG criteria, identified 183 out of a total of 445 women (22.1%) as having GDM [26]. In a prospective cohort study (2015) involving 277 Saudi women who underwent OGTT, 47 (16.9%) were diagnosed by the former American Diabetes Association (ADA) criteria and 115 (41.5%) by the IADPSG criteria, indicating wide difference on the rates of incidence GDM depending on the method adopted. The IADPSG criteria identified all women with GDM by the former ADA criteria and an additional 68 cases [27]. In this context, our results indicating a 30.5% GDM, adopting the IADPSG criteria, may be representative of the current levels of GDM in this region.

The influence of vitamin D on the development of GDM during the course of pregnancy appears uncertain as revealed by the analysis of several individual as well as meta-analysis reports. A meta-analysis of 20 Observational studies that comprised 9209 participants showed that women with vitamin D deficiency experienced a significantly increased risk for developing GDM with a little heterogeneity [28]. A systematic review and meta-analysis of 24 observational studies (2013) found that women with circulating 25(OH)D level < 50 nmol/l in pregnancy experienced an increased risk of preeclampsia and GDM [29]. Also, a systematic review and meta-analysis to study the link between vitamin D and gestational diabetes (2012) indicated a significant inverse relation between serum 25(OH)D and the incidence of GDM and vitamin D deficiency (25(OH)D < 50 nmol/l) in pregnancy was significantly related to the incidence of GDM [30]. However, in a prospective cohort study (Spain, 2015) involving 2382 pregnant women, overall, 31.8% and 19.7% vitamin D insufficiency [25(OH)D3 20–29.99 ng/ml] and deficiency [25(OH)D3 < 20 ng/ml], respectively, showed no association between maternal 25(OH)D3 concentration and risk of GDM [31].

A similar level of uncertainty is suggested by results available from a large number of vitamin D supplementation studies. Meta-analysis (2015) performed on 13 randomized controlled trials (RCTs) ($n = 2299$) performed to study the effect of vitamin D supplementation during pregnancy on maternal and neonatal outcomes concluded that incidence of GDM was not influenced by vitamin D supplementation [32]. This was, despite the increase in circulating 25(OH)D levels that was associated with vitamin D supplementation. However, across RCTs, the doses and types of vitamin D supplements, gestational age at first administration, and outcomes were heterogeneous. A systematic review of seventy-six studies (2014) involving vitamin D supplementation in pregnancy, sponsored by The National Institute for Health (NIH) Research, found considerable heterogeneity between the studies and for most outcomes, including GDM, there was conflicting evidence [33].

High-parity and older age have previously been found to be important risk factors for GDM in the Saudi population [34], where multiparous women were found to be > 8 times increased risk of GDM than nulliparous women. The same study also reported a 2% to 21% increase in GDM incidence when age increased from 20 to 40 years. In addition to high-parity and older age, higher maternal weight was shown to be associated with higher rates of GDM by an earlier study on Saudi women conducted in the 90s [35].

The susceptibility of Saudi women to high rates of GDM may be related to the cultural restrictions on female physical activities that may lead to physical inactivity and increased access to fast foods, both causing obesity. A recent review has shown high prevalence among Saudi women of smoking (up to 9%), hypertension (22%), diabetes (up to 27.6%), overweight (27%), and obesity (40%), and physical inactivity (53.2% to 98. 1%), hypercholesterolemia (24.5%) and metabolic syndrome (MetS) (up to 40.3%) [36]. MetS is a cluster of established risk factors that together increase predisposition to major chronic diseases such as heart diseases and diabetes mellitus and a recent study (2014) on adults from several regions of Saudi Arabia confirmed > 28% incidence of MetS [37]. Vitamin D deficiency, a widely prevalent condition in Saudi Arabia, has been cited to be associated with MetS in several cross-sectional studies involving middle-aged East Asians and Europeans, but not in multicultural populations of United States and New Zealand [38]. Our results may mean that MetS is a converging point of vitamin D deficiency and obesity related issues eventually leading to increased rates of GDM in Saudi Arabian women.

A consistent association between the obesity levels, as determined from BMI and other indices, and GDM observed in this study suggests a confounding role from obesity. Altogether, results from our study performed on women living in a region which is reported to have high rates of obesity and T2DM, in general, clearly indicate a 2.8-fold increased risk among women who are vitamin D deficient.

Conclusions

Conflicting reports currently exist on the association between maternal serum vitamin D status and GDM. Our assessment of GDM status and serum vitamin D levels in pregnant women of Saudi Arabia, a population known to suffer from high incidence of both GDM and vitamin D deficiency, suggests an increased risk of development of GDM in women who are deficient for vitamin D when compared to their non-GDM counterparts. Further studies such as a robust randomized controlled trial involving dietary supplementation of vitamin D during pregnancy may clearly define the role of vitamin D in development of GDM in Saudi women.

Abbreviations

25(OH)D: 25 hydroxy Vitamin D; BMI: Body mass index; GDM: Gestational diabetes mellitus; IADPSG: The International Association of the Diabetes and Pregnancy Study Groups; OGTT: Oral glucose tolerance test; T2DM: Type 2 Diabetes Mellitus; WHR: Waist to height ratio

Acknowledgements

The authors would like to acknowledge Malak Nawaz Khan Khattak and Syed Danish Hussain for the statistical analyses.

Funding

The project was funded by funded by the National Plan for Science, Technology and Innovation (NPSTI MAARIFAH), King Abdulaziz City for Science and Technology (KACST), Kingdom of Saudi Arabia (Award Number 12-MED2504-02).

Authors' contributions

AA, SK, NJA, SA and NMA contributed to the study design; subject selection and data collection was performed by KW, ES, AAS, NA and MF; data interpretation was done by MF and IZT; manuscript was prepared by SK and reviewed by SA, NJA, MF, IZT, AAS, ES, AAA, BAA, AMA, GA and NMA. All authors read and approved the final manuscript for publication.

Consent for publication

Not Applicable

Competing interests

The authors declare no competing interests.

Author details

[1]Department of Clinical Lab Sciences, College of Applied Medical Sciences, King Saud University, Riyadh 11451, Kingdom of Saudi Arabia. [2]Division of Metabolic and Vascular Health, University of Warwick, CV47AL, Coventry, UK. [3]Prince Mutaib Chair for Biomarkers of Osteoporosis, Department of Biochemistry, College of Science, King Saud University, PO Box, 2455, Riyadh 11451, Saudi Arabia. [4]Obesity, Endocrine and Metabolism Center, King Fahad Medical City, Faculty of Medicine, King Saud bin Abdulaziz University for Health Sciences, Riyadh 11525, Saudi Arabia. [5]Maternal-Fetal Medicine Department, King Fahad Medical City, Riyadh 59406, Saudi Arabia. [6]Diabetes Care Center, King Salman Bin Abdulaziz Hospital, Riyadh, Saudi Arabia. [7]Obstetrics and Gynaecology Department, King Salman Bin Abdulaziz Hospital, Riyadh 11564, Saudi Arabia. [8]Department of Medicine, Endocrinology Division, College of Medicine, King Saud University, Riyadh 11461, Saudi Arabia. [9]Department of Obstetrics and Gynecology, College of Medicine, King Saud University, Riyadh 11461, Saudi Arabia.

References

1. Kampmann U, Madsen LR, Skajaa GO, Iversen DS, Moeller N, Ovesen P. Gestational diabetes: A clinical update. World J Diabetes. 2015;6(8):1065–72.
2. Szymczak I, Pawliczak R. The active metabolite of vitamin D3 as a potential Immunomodulator. Scand J Immunol. 2016;83(2):83–91.
3. Pilz S, Verheyen N, Grubler MR, Tomaschitz A, Marz W. Vitamin D and cardiovascular disease prevention. Nat Rev Cardiol. 2016;13(7):404–17.
4. Balion C, Griffith LE, Strifler L, Henderson M, Patterson C, Heckman G, Llewellyn DJ, Raina P. Vitamin D, cognition, and dementia: a systematic review and meta-analysis. Neurology. 2012;79(13):1397–405.
5. Schottker B, Ball D, Gellert C, Brenner H. Serum 25-hydroxyvitamin D levels and overall mortality. A systematic review and meta-analysis of prospective cohort studies. Ageing Res Rev. 2013;12(2):708–18.
6. Prasad P, Kochhar A. Interplay of vitamin D and metabolic syndrome: a review. Diabetes & Metabolic Syndrome. 2015;10(2):105–12.
7. Stadlmayr A, Aigner E, Huber-Schonauer U, Niederseer D, Zwerina J, Husar-Memmer E, Hohla F, Schett G, Patsch W, Datz C. Relations of vitamin D status, gender and type 2 diabetes in middle-aged Caucasians. Acta Diabetol. 2015;52(1):39–46.

8. Pittas AG, Nelson J, Mitri J, Hillmann W, Garganta C, Nathan DM, Hu FB, Dawson-Hughes B. Plasma 25-hydroxyvitamin D and progression to diabetes in patients at risk for diabetes: an ancillary analysis in the diabetes prevention program. Diabetes Care. 2012;35(3):565–73.
9. Afzal S, Bojesen SE, Nordestgaard BG. Low 25-hydroxyvitamin D and risk of type 2 diabetes: a prospective cohort study and metaanalysis. Clin Chem. 2013;59(2):381–91.
10. Park S, Kim da S, Kang S. Vitamin D deficiency impairs glucose-stimulated insulin secretion and increases insulin resistance by reducing PPAR-gamma expression in nonobese type 2 diabetic rats. J Nutr Biochem. 2016;27:257–65.
11. Esteghamati A, Aryan Z, Nakhjavani M. Vitamin D deficiency is associated with insulin resistance in nondiabetics and reduced insulin production in type 2 diabetics. Horm Metab Res. 2015;47(4):273–9.
12. Grineva EN, Karonova T, Micheeva E, Belyaeva O, Nikitina IL. Vitamin D deficiency is a risk factor for obesity and diabetes type 2 in women at late reproductive age. Aging (Albany NY). 2013;5(7):575–81.
13. Olmos-Ortiz A, Avila E, Surand-Carbajal M, Diaz L. Regulation of calcitriol biosynthesis and activity: focus on gestational vitamin D deficiency and adverse pregnancy outcomes. Nutrients. 2015;7(1):443–80.
14. Hollis BW, Wagner CL. Clinical review: the role of the parent compound vitamin D with respect to metabolism and function: why clinical dose intervals can affect clinical outcomes. J Clin Endocrinol Metab. 2013;98(12):4619–28.
15. Joergensen JS, Lamont RF, Torloni MR. Vitamin D and gestational diabetes: an update. Curr Opin Clin Nutr Metab Care. 2014;17(4):360–7.
16. Hamilton SA, McNeil R, Hollis BW, Davis DJ, Winkler J, Cook C, Warner G, Bivens B, McShane P, Wagner CL. Profound vitamin D deficiency in a diverse Group of Women during pregnancy living in a sun-rich environment at latitude 32 degrees N. Int J Endocrinol. 2010;2010:917428.
17. Johnson DD, Wagner CL, Hulsey TC, McNeil RB, Ebeling M, Hollis BW. Vitamin D deficiency and insufficiency is common during pregnancy. Am J Perinatol. 2011;28(1):7–12.
18. Al-Daghri NM. Vitamin D in Saudi Arabia: prevalence, distribution and disease associations. J Steroid Biochem Mol Biol. 2018;175:102-107.
19. Al-Turki HA, Sadat-Ali M, Al-Elq AH, Al-Mulhim FA, Al-Ali AK. 25-Hydoxyvitamin D levels among healthy Saudi Arabian women. Saudi Med J. 2008;29(12):1765–8.
20. Al-Ajlan A, Krishnaswamy S, Alokail MS, Aljohani NJ, Al-Serehi A, Sheshah E, Alshingetti NM, Fouda M, Turkistani IZ, Al-Daghri NM. Vitamin D deficiency and dyslipidemia in early pregnancy. BMC Pregnancy Childbirth. 2015;15:314.
21. Wahabi HA, Esmaeil SA, Fayed A, Alzeidan RA. Gestational diabetes mellitus: maternal and perinatal outcomes in King Khalid University Hospital, Saudi Arabia. J Egypt Public Health Assoc. 2013;88(2):104–8.
22. Gupta Y, Kaira B, Baruah MP, Singla R, Kalra S. Updated guidelines on screening for gestational diabetes. Int J Women's Health. 2015;7:539–50.
23. Al-Daghri NM, Al-Saleh Y, Aljohani N, Sulimani R, Al-Othman AM, Alfawaz H, Fouda M, Al-Amri F, Shahrani A, Alharbi M, Alshahrani F, Tamimi W, Sabico S, Rizzoli R, Reginster JY. Vitamin D status correction in Saudi Arabia: an experts' consensus under the auspices of the European Society for Clinical and Economic Aspects of osteoporosis, osteoarthritis, and musculoskeletal diseases (ESCEO). Arch Osteoporos. 2017;12(1):1.
24. Alsuwadia AO, Farag YM, Al Sayyari AA, Mousa DH, Alhejaili FF, Al-Harbi AS, Housawi AA, Mittal BV, Singh AK. Prevalence of vitamin D deficiency in Saudi adults. Saudi Med J. 2013;34(8):814–8.
25. Kanan RM, Al Saleh YM, Fakhoury HM, Adham M, Aljaser S, Tamimi W. Year-round vitamin D deficiency among Saudi female out-patients. Public Health Nutr. 2013;16(3):544–8.
26. Al-Faris NA. High prevalence of vitamin D deficiency among pregnant Saudi women. Nutrients. 2016;8(2):77.
27. Alfadhli E. Gestational diabetes in Saudi women identified by the International Association of Diabetes and Pregnancy Study Group versus the former American Diabetes Association criteria: a prospective cohort study. Annals Saudi Med. 2015;35(6):428–34.
28. Zhang MX, Pan GT, Guo JF, Li BY, Qin LQ, Zhang ZL. Vitamin D deficiency increases the risk of gestational diabetes mellitus: a meta-analysis of observational studies. Nutrients. 2015;7(10):8366–75.
29. Wei SQ, Qi HP, Luo ZC, Fraser WD. Maternal vitamin D status and adverse pregnancy outcomes: a systematic review and meta-analysis. J Matern Fetal Neonatal Med. 2013;26(9):889–99.
30. Poel YH, Hummel P, Lips P, Stam F, van der Ploeg T, Simsek S. Vitamin D and gestational diabetes: a systematic review and meta-analysis. Euro J Int Med. 2012;23(5):465–9.
31. Rodriguez A, Garcia-Esteban R, Basterretxea M, Lertxundi A, Rodriguez-Bernal C, Iniguez C, Rodriguez-Dehli C, Tardon A, Espada M, Sunyer J, Morales E. Associations of maternal circulating 25-hydroxyvitamin D3 concentration with pregnancy and birth outcomes. BJOG Int J Obstetr Gynaecol. 2015; 122(12):1695–704.
32. Perez-Lopez FR, Pasupuleti V, Mezones-Holguin E, Benites-Zapata VA, Thota P, Deshpande A, Hernandez AV. Effect of vitamin D supplementation during pregnancy on maternal and neonatal outcomes: a systematic review and meta-analysis of randomized controlled trials. Fertil Steril. 2015;103(5):1278–88.
33. Harvey NC, Holroyd C, Ntani G, Javaid K, Cooper P, Moon R, Cole Z, Tinati T, Godfrey K, Dennison E, et al. Vitamin D supplementation in pregnancy: a systematic review. Health Technol Assess. 2014;18(45):1–190.
34. Al-Rowaily MA, Abolfotouh MA. Predictors of gestational diabetes mellitus in a high-parity community in Saudi Arabia. East Mediterr Health J. 2010; 16(6):636–41.
35. Nasrat H, Fageeh W, Abalkhail B, Yamani T, Ardawi MS. Determinants of pregnancy outcome in patients with gestational diabetes. Int J Gynaecol Obstet. 1996;53(2):117–23.
36. Alshaikh MK, Filippidis FT, Baldove JP, Majeed A, Rawaf S. Women in Saudi Arabia and the prevalence of cardiovascular risk factors: a systematic review. J Environ Public Health. 2016;2016:7479357.
37. Aljohani NJ. Metabolic syndrome: risk factors among adults in Kingdom of Saudi Arabia. J Family Commun Med. 2014;21(3):170–5.
38. Al-Daghri NM, Alkharfy KM, Al-Saleh Y, Al-Attas OS, Alokail MS, Al-Othman A, Moharram O, El-Kholie E, Sabico S, Kumar S, Chrousos G. Modest reversal of metabolic syndrome manifestations with vitamin D status correction: a 12-month prospective study. Metab Clin Exp. 2012;61(5):661–6.

7

Maternal overweight is not an independent risk factor for increased birth weight, leptin and insulin in newborns of gestational diabetic women: observations from the prospective *'EaCH'* cohort study

Raffael Ott[1,2], Jens H. Stupin[1], Andrea Loui[3], Elisabeth Eilers[3], Kerstin Melchior[1,2], Rebecca C. Rancourt[1,2], Karen Schellong[1,2], Thomas Ziska[1,2], Joachim W. Dudenhausen[1], Wolfgang Henrich[1] and Andreas Plagemann[1,2*]

Abstract

Background: Both gestational diabetes mellitus (GDM) as well as overweight/obesity during pregnancy are risk factors for detrimental anthropometric and hormonal neonatal outcomes, identified to 'program' adverse health predispositions later on. While overweight/obesity are major determinants of GDM, independent effects on critical birth outcomes remain unclear. Thus, the aim of the present study was to evaluate, in women with GDM, the relative/independent impact of overweight/obesity vs. altered glucose metabolism on newborn parameters.

Methods: The prospective observational 'Early CHARITÉ (*EaCH*)' cohort study primarily focuses on early developmental origins of unfavorable health outcomes through pre- and/or early postnatal exposure to a 'diabetogenic/adipogenic' environment. It includes 205 mother-child dyads, recruited between 2007 and 2010, from women with treated GDM and delivery at the Clinic of Obstetrics, Charité – Universitätsmedizin Berlin, Germany. Recruitment, therapy, metabolite/hormone analyses, and data evaluation were performed according to standardized guidelines and protocols. This report specifically aimed to identify maternal anthropometric and metabolic determinants of anthropometric and critical hormonal birth outcomes in *'EaCH'*.

Results: Group comparisons, Spearman's correlations and unadjusted linear regression analyses initially confirmed that increased maternal prepregnancy body-mass-index (BMI) is a significant factor for elevated birth weight, cord-blood insulin and leptin (all $P < 0.05$). However, consideration of and adjustment for maternal glucose during late pregnancy showed that no maternal anthropometric parameter (weight, BMI, gestational weight gain) remained significant (all n.s.). In contrast, even after adjustment for maternal anthropometrics, third trimester glucose values (fasting and postprandial glucose at 32nd and 36th weeks' gestation, HbA1c in 3rd trimester and at delivery), were clearly positively associated with critical birth outcomes (all $P < 0.05$).

(Continued on next page)

* Correspondence: andreas.plagemann@charite.de
[1]Clinic of Obstetrics, Charité – Universitätsmedizin Berlin, corporate member of Freie Universität Berlin, Humboldt-Universität zu Berlin, and Berlin Institute of Health, Campus Virchow-Klinikum, Berlin, Germany
[2]Division of 'Experimental Obstetrics, Charité – Universitätsmedizin Berlin, corporate member of Freie Universität Berlin, Humboldt-Universität zu Berlin, and Berlin Institute of Health, Campus Virchow-Klinikum, Berlin, Germany
Full list of author information is available at the end of the article

(Continued from previous page)

Conclusions: Neither overweight/obesity nor gestational weight gain appear to be *independent* determinants of increased birth weight, insulin and leptin. Rather, 3rd trimester glycemia seems to be crucial for respective neonatal outcomes. Thus, gestational care and future research studies should greatly consider late pregnancy glucose in overweight/obese women with or without GDM, for evaluation of critical causes and interventional strategies against 'perinatal programming of diabesity' in the offspring.

Keywords: Gestational diabetes mellitus, Maternal overweight/obesity, Gestational weight gain, Maternal glucose, Birth weight, Cord-blood insulin, Cord-blood leptin, Newborn outcomes, Perinatal programming,

Background

Gestational diabetes mellitus (GDM) and maternal overweight/obesity are the most prevalent disorders/diseases during gestation, affecting > 10 and > 30% of pregnant women in westernized countries, respectively [1–4]. Both GDM as well as maternal overweight/obesity are causally linked to adverse birth and long-term outcomes in the offspring [5, 6]. Especially GDM, often a consequence of overweight/obesity, has manifold been identified epidemiologically, clinically and experimentally as risk condition in terms of critical birth outcomes related to long-term health adversity [7, 8]. In general, altered birth weight was recognized as an important surrogate marker for later disorders and diseases [9–11]. More precisely, altered humoral and hormonal parameters, e.g. increased glucose, insulin, leptin etc., in utero and at birth were identified as causal, mechanistic factors for 'perinatal programming' of increased susceptibility to develop disorders/diseases later in life [8, 12–14]. Similar 'programming' effects may also occur in offspring of overweight/obese mothers. Accordingly, during recent years overweight/obesity has been suggested, beyond GDM, as independent and additive risk condition for adverse short- and long-term outcomes [5, 15].

Fortunately, regular GDM screening and optimized treatment has become widely distributed since the past few years due to rapid progress in the GDM field. Moreover, greater emphasis worldwide has been placed on optimal management of glucose levels after a positive GDM screening test, especially as the HAPO study and large randomized controlled trials have strongly shown beneficial influences of treating GDM for birth outcomes [16–18]. However, similar convincing data are so far missing regarding the role of overweight during pregnancy. A major challenge here is the tight link between overweight/obesity and glycemia, which complicates the evaluation of the relative contribution of maternal anthropometry vs. glucose metabolism for birth outcomes. Moreover, most studies have solely relied on glucose values at GDM screening, typically performed at 24-28th weeks' gestation, while maternal glycemia in later pregnancy is hardly considered. Thus, it remains open whether maternal overweight per se is an independent factor for respective adversity or if rather accompanied, undetected and/or not considered maternal (hyper-) glycemia, especially in 3rd trimester, is ultimately responsible. This needs further investigation since it would have far ranging implications for better understanding of pathophysiology, general risk estimation and optimal gestational care.

The 3rd trimester plays a major role for fetal growth, differentiation and maturation, in particular for growth of insulin-sensitive tissues, e.g. fat tissue [19]. Treatment of GDM, i.e., achieving good glycemic control, has been shown to effectively reduce in utero overgrowth and increased birth weight risk [17, 18]. Similarly, adequate glucose management has been observed to prevent perinatal hyperinsulinism and, consequently, related long-term risk of developing impaired glucose tolerance [20]. Interestingly, offspring of women with treated GDM may remain more likely to become overweight or exhibit features of the metabolic syndrome even with 'normalized' birth weight [21]. This indicates that 'programming' effects, which could similarly occur in offspring of overweight/obese mothers, are also apparent below adverse birth weight cut-offs, e.g. macrosomia. Exact mechanisms remain unknown but could be attributable to altered hormones during perinatal development, e.g. hyperinsulinism and hyperleptinism, even in newborns with 'normal' birth weight [8, 14]. Therefore, consideration of hormonal birth outcomes appears important in respective study interpretations.

In order to contribute to a clearer understanding of such important perinatal risk factors, the 'Early CHARITÉ (*EaCH*)' cohort was created to explore unreflected/unknown factors associated with the pre- and neonatal development in offspring of mothers with diabetes/overweight during pregnancy, and to characterize potential mechanisms and pathophysiological factors from the clinical to the molecular level. We initially focused on characterization of relations of maternal anthropometry, especially body-mass-index (BMI) and gestational weight gain (GWG), and maternal glucose metabolism on critical anthropometric and cord-blood hormone outcomes at birth.

Methods

Study aims and design

The *'EaCH'* approach is a prospective observational cohort study in mother-child dyads with maternal GDM and/or overweight/obesity, with the primary focus on early developmental origins of unfavorable health outcomes through pre- and/or early postnatal exposure to a 'diabetogenic/adipogenic' environment. The primary aim of *'EaCH'* is to identify metabolic, hormonal, nutritional, epigenetic and other causal factors/determinants that are critically associated with pre- and neonatal acquired disease susceptibility. The overall goal is to deliver new mechanistic and/or preventive approaches and strategies to reduce disease risk in affected offspring.

The study includes a final GDM cohort of 205 mother-child dyads (75% of eligible cases, Fig. 1), from initially 562 women with GDM and delivery between June 2007 and December 2010 at the Clinic of Obstetrics, Charité – Universitätsmedizin Berlin, Campus Virchow-Klinikum, Germany (Flow chart, including exclusion criteria, shown in Fig. 1). A major exclusion criterion was non-sufficient German/English speaking, due to a relatively high proportion of immigrants attending our clinic. Research design and methods were conducted in accordance with the Declaration of Helsinki, revised in 2004 [22], and approved by the local Ethics Committee (EA2/026/04). All participants provided written informed consent before inclusion into the study.

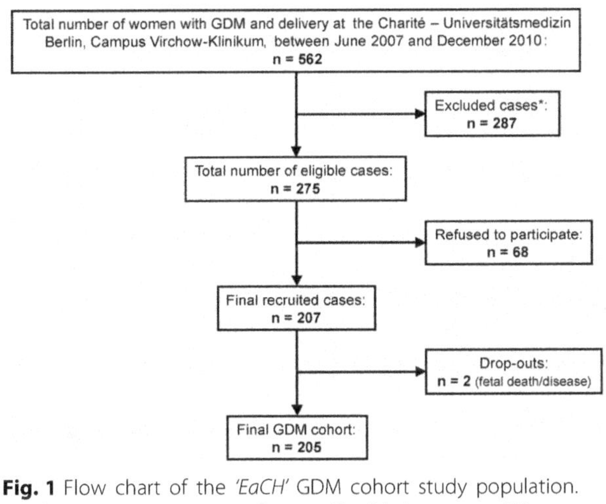

Fig. 1 Flow chart of the *'EaCH'* GDM cohort study population. *Exclusion criteria: missing German/English language skills, prepregnancy underweight (body-mass-index <18.5 kg/m^2), assisted reproductive technology, chronic diseases/infections (including type 1 and type 2 diabetes; HIV, hepatitis B/C *etc.*), multiple pregnancy, substance abuse, special nutrition (*e.g.* vegetarians), special surgical conditions (*e.g. placenta previa*), first visit at the clinic after 32nd weeks' gestation and/or fetal diseases/malformations. GDM: Gestational diabetes mellitus

Parental socio-economic, lifestyle, and anthropometric data

Respective data were collected at the woman's first visit at our clinic by personal interview via standardized questionnaire. Parental educational background, current employment status (before maternity leave) and job description were recorded and used for socio-economic status (SES) categorization, as applied previously [23, 24]. The resulting SES categories were further assigned to lower (categories: unemployed, manual worker, non-manual worker without university degree) or higher SES (category: non-manual worker with university degree).

Paternal height and weight was recorded via standardized questionnaire at enrollment and the BMI (kg/m^2) was calculated. Maternal height and weight before conception, weight change in the 1st, 2nd and 3rd trimester as well as the last weight measured within one week prior to delivery were abstracted/calculated from the 'Mutterpass'. This 'Mutterpass' is a standardized maternity record/documentation in Germany, containing essential information about pregravid health/conditions, regular screening/medical examinations throughout pregnancy as well as clinically important perinatal data [25]. Prepregnancy BMI was calculated using pregravid weight and height and then categorized according to WHO criteria (normal weight: 18.5–24.9 kg/m^2, overweight: 25.0–29.9 kg/m^2, obese: ≥30.0 kg/m^2). Total gestational weight gain (GWG) was calculated as the difference between prepregnancy weight and nearest weight to delivery and categorized in line with the Institute of Medicine (IOM) guidelines from 2009 using the labels inadequate, adequate and excessive weight gain, respectively [26]. As an indicator of the genuine maternal weight gain during pregnancy, net GWG was calculated by subtracting birth weight and placental weight from total GWG.

GDM diagnosis and treatment

Gestational diabetes screening was conducted generally between the 24th–28th week of pregnancy (mean ± SD: 25.6 ± 3.8) using 75-g oral glucose tolerance test (oGTT) according to the guidelines of the German Society of Gynecology and Obstetrics at the time of recruitment [27]. Respective guidelines were based on the Carpenter and Coustan criteria [28]. GDM was diagnosed if two values were equal to or above either capillary fasting glucose (FG) ≥90 mg/dL (5.0 mmol/L) and/or 1-h glucose ≥180 mg/dL (10.0 mmol/L) and/or 2-h glucose ≥155 mg/dL (8.6 mmol/L). Subsequent diabetic care was provided according to above mentioned guidelines, aiming especially for the following glucose targets: FG 60–90 mg/dL (3.3–5.0 mmol/L) and 1-h postprandial glucose (PPG) ≤140 mg/dL (7.8 mmol/L). Among all GDM cases, 63% ($n = 129$) were treated by diet and moderate physical activity only, while 37% ($n = 76$)

received additional insulin therapy to achieve glycemic control. Insulin-sensitizing drugs (e.g. metformin) were not applied here. Overall, women were instructed to monitor blood glucose at least 4-times daily, i.e., morning FG and three 1-h PPG values, using the Accu-Chek glucose meter (Roche Diagnostics, Mannheim, Germany). From these individual profiles, mean FG (based on three values) and mean PPG levels (based on nine values) were calculated from three days within the 32nd and 36th week of gestation, respectively. As marker for long-term glycemic status, glycated hemoglobin A1c (HbA1c) was assessed in the third trimester (mean ± SD: 33.2 ± 2.5 weeks' gestation), and, additionally, at delivery by standardized high-performance liquid chromatography (Variant II System, Bio-Rad, Hercules, CA, USA) at the clinic's central laboratory. Based on recent guidelines from the American Diabetes Association [29], an HbA1c value above 6% was used as indicator of poorer metabolic control for evaluations.

Clinical pregnancy-related characteristics

A variety of maternal parameters, including parity, history of GDM, comorbidities (e.g. gestational hypertension), mode of delivery, gestational age at birth, were abstracted from the standardized 'Mutterpass' and medical records, respectively. Gestational hypertension and preeclampsia were diagnosed according to the guidelines of the German Society of Gynecology and Obstetrics [30]. Mode of delivery was defined according to HAPO study criteria [31], i.e., spontaneous, vaginal-operative, primary or repeat Cesarean section (CS). Gestational age was estimated based on woman's last menstrual period in combination with subsequent ultrasound examinations at first trimester.

Birth outcomes

Information about infant's sex, preterm birth (< 37 weeks' gestation), placental weight, birth weight, length and head circumference was abstracted from medical records. Placental weight was measured immediately after delivery with umbilical cord attached. Additional anthropometric outcomes included relative birth weight (g/cm), ponderal index ($g/cm^3 \times 100$), and macrosomia (defined as birth weight ≥ 4000 g). Furthermore, based on sex- and ethnic-specific birth weight for gestational age percentiles [32–34], infants were categorized into small-for-gestational age (SGA, <10th percentile), appropriate-for-gestational age (AGA, 10th–90th percentile) or large-for-gestational age (LGA, > 90th percentile). Occurrence of further adverse neonatal outcomes, e.g. hypoglycemia and/or shoulder dystocia, was retrieved from medical records.

Venous umbilical cord-blood was collected immediately after delivery and plasma samples stored at − 80 °C. Commercially available radioimmunoassays were used for analyses of insulin (Cat# 10624, Radim Diagnostics, Pomezia RM, Italy), C-peptide and leptin (C-peptide: Cat# RIA-1252, leptin: Cat# RIA-1624, DRG Instruments, Marburg, Germany) according to manufacturers' instructions. The 90th percentile cut-offs in this study were the following: insulin 34.2 μU/mL, C-peptide 2.2 ng/mL, and leptin 29.6 ng/mL.

Statistical analyses

Descriptive statistics are presented as means ± standard deviations (SD) or numbers and percentages, respectively. All continuous variables were tested for normal distribution using Kolmogorov-Smirnov test and evaluation of distribution plots. Group comparisons were analyzed by one-way ANOVA followed by Tukey's post hoc test or Kruskal-Wallis test followed by Dunn's post hoc test and Fisher's exact or Chi-square tests, respectively. Spearman's correlation coefficients (r) and/or linear regression models (unstandardized B coefficients with 95% confidence intervals [95% CI]) were calculated to assess relationships between paternal and/or maternal anthropometric/metabolic parameters and neonatal anthropometric and cord-blood hormone outcomes. For regression analyses, normal distribution was achieved for respective variables by transformation using the method described by Templeton [35]. Furthermore, categorical variables were dichotomized, e.g. mode of delivery was grouped into deliveries with vs. without CS etc., if required. Overall, collinearity was controlled by bivariate correlation ($r < 0.7$) and variance inflation factor (< 2.5). The following parameters were tested as independent variables for their association with birth outcomes. Anthropometry: maternal prepregnancy weight and BMI, GWG in 1st, 2nd and 3rd trimester, total and net GWG; Metabolism: FG, 1-h and 2-h glucose, and area under the curve (AUC) of glucose at oGTT, mean FG and PPG at 32nd and 36th weeks' gestation, HbA1c in 3rd trimester and at delivery. Birth outcomes were: placental weight, birth weight, relative birth weight, cord-blood insulin and leptin. All regressions are shown as crude and adjusted models. Model I included general parameters: maternal age, SES, ethnic origin, smoking in pregnancy, parity, height (except for pre-pregnancy BMI), type of therapy (diet vs. insulin), gestational age, mode of delivery, and infant's sex. To evaluate independent associations of maternal anthropometry and metabolism with birth outcomes, further adjustment models were applied. For maternal anthropometry, model II contained all parameters of model I *plus* mean FG and PPG at 32nd and 36th weeks' gestation and HbA1c partum. Accordingly, the applied model II for maternal metabolism included all parameters of model I *plus* prepregnancy weight and net GWG. In addition, forward step-wise regression analyses were carried out to identify categorical predictors of anthropometric/hormonal birth outcomes, considering paternal and maternal parameters (max. $n = 118–153$). In line with previous studies in this research area [5, 36], adjusted semipartial correlation coefficients (Sr^2) were calculated for each individual (potential) predictor entered into the final models. These coefficients estimate the contribution of each factor to the total variability of the outcome variable. Finally, owing to small numbers of unfavorable categorical anthropometric and cord-blood hormone outcomes logistic regression analyses (odds ratio, OR) were just performed for LGA ($n = 41$ in the total cohort), using the same adjustment models as described above. Additionally, percentages of relevant maternal anthropometric and metabolic variables/exposures in newborns with unfavorable anthropometric and cord-blood hormone outcomes were compared with those in reference groups that had no respective outcomes. In general, missing data analysis according to Little's MCAR test was performed and indicated random distribution. A P-value < 0.05 was considered significant (two-tailed). All calculations were performed using SPSS v. 24.0 (IBM Co., Armonk, NY, USA).

Results

General parental characteristics

Major parameters across maternal prepregnancy BMI categories are presented in Table 1. Overall, the mean paternal BMI as well as paternal SES were in alignment with those of the mothers, with highest BMI and lowest SES in partners of obese mothers (Table 1). Moreover, there was a positive correlation between paternal and maternal BMIs ($r = 0.23$, $P < 0.01$).

Maternal data showed no difference in age across prepregnancy BMI groups (Table 1). Overall, the majority of women of the total cohort was of European origin and belonged to the lower SES category, while significantly more individuals in the overweight/obese groups were of Non-European origin and had higher frequencies of lower SES. There was no difference in smoking during pregnancy between normal weight and overweight (but not obese) women; however, smoking was much more abundant in the obese group. Similarly, parity was higher in obese individuals. Amongst multiparous women, more than one-third had a history of GDM, while a non-significant trend towards higher frequencies of prior GDM was observed in overweight/obese groups compared to normal weight mothers.

Maternal anthropometrics

The GDM cohort as a whole was overweight, in terms of mean BMI, before pregnancy. Around 40% were classified as normal weight and around 30% as obese. More than half of the women in the overweight/obese groups showed excessive GWG, according to IOM criteria, as compared to only around one-third in normal weight women. Furthermore, there was a continuous decrease in inadequate GWG across prepregnancy BMI groups. Total GWG was lowest in obese women, while normal weight and overweight mothers gained similar amounts of weight during gestation. However, the calculated net GWG, i.e., excluding placental and newborn weight, showed a decrease across all BMI categories (Table 1). Both total and net GWG correlated inversely with prepregnancy BMI (total GWG: $r = -0.30$, $P < 0.001$; net GWG: $r = -0.32$, $P < 0.001$).

Maternal metabolism

In the total cohort, GDM screening revealed that the majority of women exceeded FG and 1-h glucose cut-offs while only one-third surpassed the 2-h glucose threshold at oGTT (Table 1). Among oGTT measurements, only FG and frequencies above its cut-off showed significant increase across BMI categories. In 3rd trimester, an overall decrease of mean FG and PPG values, and, thus, a reduction of frequencies above their respective guideline cut-offs was observed. Of note, application of guideline cut-offs (FG > 90 mg/dL; PPG > 140 mg/dL) regarding 3rd trimester values revealed that to a greater extent FG rather than PPG was less controlled. In line with this, among all glucose values at oGTT, only FG correlated significantly with the respective mean glucose levels later in pregnancy (FG at 32nd weeks: $r = 0.40$, $P < 0.001$; FG at 36th weeks: $r = 0.27$, $P < 0.001$). Compared to normal weight women, insulin therapy was more abundant in the overweight and obese groups, respectively. Each glucose variable in 3rd trimester, i.e., mean glucose and HbA1c levels, increased significantly with maternal prepregnancy BMI, in contrast to oGTT variables at 24–28 weeks' gestation (Table 1).

Birth outcomes

Placental weight was significantly higher in the overweight/obese groups as compared to normal weight women (Table 1). Likewise, birth weight, relative birth weight and ponderal index were higher in overweight/obese individuals. However, instead of a further increase in the obese as compared to overweight women these anthropometric measures plateaued. Moreover, birth weight and relative birth weight were highest in the overweight group. Frequencies of adverse anthropometric outcomes were more abundant in the overweight/obese groups, with the exception of SGA as there was no significant difference across BMI categories. Overweight women had the highest rate of LGA and macrosomia. In obese, the percentage of LGA was similar to the overweight group, however, the rate of macrosomia was between the normal weight and overweight category. In contrast to these observations regarding anthropometric birth outcomes, cord-blood levels of C-peptide, insulin, and leptin continuously increased across BMI categories. Accordingly,

Table 1 General and specific cohort characteristics

Characteristics	N	Total GDM cohort	Maternal prepregnancy BMI category			P-value[a]
			Normal weight	Overweight	Obese	
n		205	89[b]	51[b]	65[b]	
Paternal						
Age (years)	204	35.7 ± 7.7	35.9 ± 7.2	36.2 ± 7.6	34.9 ± 8.4	ns
Socio-economic status – %[c]						
Lower SES category	143	69.8	54.5	68.0	93.8[d]	< 0.001
Higher SES category	60	29.3	45.5	32.0	6.2[d]	< 0.001
BMI (kg/m^2)	202	26.9 ± 5.0	25.5 ± 3.2	27.0 ± 4.7[d]	28.7 ± 6.4[d]	0.002
Maternal						
Age (years)	205	31.8 ± 5.4	32.2 ± 5.5	31.2 ± 4.9	31.7 ± 5.8	ns
Ethnic origin – %						
European	129	62.9	73.0	52.9[d]	56.9[d]	< 0.001
Non-European (e.g. Turkish, Arabic)	76	37.1	27.0	47.1[d]	43.1[d]	< 0.001
Socio-economic status – %[c]						
Lower SES category	161	78.5	62.9	86.3[d]	93.8[d]	< 0.001
Higher SES category	44	21.1	37.1	13.7[d]	6.2[d]	< 0.001
Smoking in pregnancy (any) – %	30	14.6	10.1	7.8	26.2[d]	0.009
Nulliparous – %	61	29.8	37.1	37.3	13.9[d]	0.002
History of GDM (multiparous only) – %	52	40.6	29.2	48.4	46.9	ns
Height (cm)	205	165.8 ± 6.6	166.9 ± 6.6	164.9 ± 7.0	165.1 ± 6.2	ns
Prepregnancy weight (kg)	205	76.8 ± 20.9	60.6 ± 6.7	73.8 ± 6.6[d]	101.4 ± 17.6[d]	< 0.001
Prepregnancy BMI (kg/m^2)	205	28.0 ± 7.4	21.7 ± 1.7	27.1 ± 1.4[d]	37.1 ± 5.5[d]	< 0.001
Total GWG (kg)	205	13.4 ± 6.4	14.8 ± 5.3	14.0 ± 7.1	10.8 ± 6.4[d]	< 0.001
GWG category (IOM) – %						
Inadequate	43	21.0	28.1	19.6	12.3[d]	ns
Adequate	67	32.7	37.1	23.5	33.9	ns
Excessive	95	46.3	34.8	56.9[d]	53.8[d]	0.014
Net GWG (kg)	205	9.3 ± 6.3	11.0 ± 5.2	9.7 ± 7.0	6.6 ± 6.3[d]	< 0.001
BMI at delivery (kg/m^2)	205	32.8 ± 7.1	27.1 ± 2.5	32.3 ± 2.7[d]	41.1 ± 5.5[d]	< 0.001
Blood glucose at oGTT (mg/dL)[e]						
Fasting	205	94.2 ± 19.0	88.6 ± 13.3	91.8 ± 14.3	103.7 ± 24.7[d]	< 0.001
Fasting > 90 mg/dL – %[f]	118	57.6	42.7	54.9	80.0[d]	< 0.001
1 h	203	197.0 ± 28.2	196.0 ± 26.0	192.8 ± 24.0	201.8 ± 33.4	ns
1 h > 180 mg/dL – %[f]	169	83.7	86.5	80.0	82.5	ns
2 h	193	144.5 ± 37.6	140.0 ± 27.3	143.3 ± 32.4	151.4 ± 50.6	ns
2 h > 155 mg/dL – %[f]	63	32.8	28.6	34.0	37.7	ns
Area under the curve (mg/dL*h)	193	315.6 ± 44.3	310.2 ± 32.9	306.9 ± 31.0	329.6 ± 60.6	ns
Mean glucose at 32nd weeks' gestation (mg/dL)[g]						
Fasting	195	88.0 ± 11.3	83.8 ± 7.0	87.8 ± 9.0[d]	93.8 ± 14.5[d]	< 0.001
Fasting > 90 mg/dL – %[f]	70	35.9	16.9	34.7[d]	61.9[d]	< 0.001
Postprandial	183	121.7 ± 14.3	117.6 ± 11.5	122.8 ± 13.3[d]	126.4 ± 16.8[d]	< 0.001
Postprandial > 140 mg/dL – %[f]	14	7.7	2.5	6.8	15.0[d]	0.020
Mean glucose at 36th weeks' gestation (mg/dL)[g]						
Fasting	188	84.2 ± 8.0	80.8 ± 6.0	85.2 ± 8.0[d]	87.7 ± 8.4[d]	< 0.001
Fasting > 90 mg/dL – %[f]	38	20.2	6.3	20.0[d]	37.5[d]	< 0.001
Postprandial	169	118.6 ± 12.1	114.0 ± 8.9	121.5 ± 14.0[d]	122.3 ± 12.2[d]	ns
Postprandial > 140 mg/dL – %[f]	6	3.6	0.0	4.8	7.1[d]	ns

Table 1 General and specific cohort characteristics *(Continued)*

Characteristics	Total GDM cohort		Maternal prepregnancy BMI category			
			Normal weight	Overweight	Obese	*P*-value[a]
HbA1c in 3rd trimester (%)	196	5.4 ± 0.6	5.1 ± 0.4	5.5 ± 0.6[d]	5.7 ± 0.6[d]	< 0.001
HbA1c in 3rd trimester > 6% – %	24	12.2	2.4	18.8[d]	20.3[d]	< 0.001
HbA1c partum (%)	197	5.5 ± 0.6	5.3 ± 0.5	5.6 ± 0.5[d]	5.8 ± 0.6[d]	< 0.001
HbA1c partum > 6% – %	42	21.3	6.9	23.9[d]	39.1[d]	< 0.001
Insulin therapy – %	75	36.6	16.9	41.2[d]	60.0[d]	< 0.001
Prepregnancy hypertension – %	10	4.9	2.2	2.0	10.8[d]	0.035
Gestational hypertension – %	12	5.9	2.2	5.9	10.8[d]	ns
Preeclampsia – %	9	4.4	2.2	2.0	9.2	ns
Mode of delivery – %						
Spontaneous	115	56.1	66.3	45.1[d]	50.8	0.028
Vaginal-operative	20	9.8	7.9	17.7	6.2	ns
Primary Cesarean section	31	15.1	15.7	11.8	16.9	ns
Repeat Cesarean section	39	19.0	10.1	25.5[d]	26.2[d]	0.015
Gestational age at delivery (weeks)	205	38.6 ± 1.5	38.7 ± 1.6	38.9 ± 1.3	38.3 ± 1.5[d]	ns
Newborn						
Female sex – %	88	42.9	43.8	43.1	41.5	ns
Preterm birth (< 37 weeks' gestation) – %	15	7.3	6.7	3.9	10.8	ns
Placental weight (g)	201	607.0 ± 159.9	559.4 ± 124.6	666.1 ± 172.3[d]	624.9 ± 175.1[d]	< 0.001
Birth weight (g)	205	3450 ± 506	3345 ± 496	3591 ± 481[d]	3483 ± 514	0.006
Birth length (cm)	205	51.3 ± 2.5	51.2 ± 2.5	51.7 ± 2.4	50.9 ± 2.5	ns
Relative birth weight (g/cm)	205	67.1 ± 8.1	65.1 ± 7.8	69.3 ± 7.7[d]	68.2 ± 8.4[d]	0.001
Ponderal index ($g/cm^3 \times 100$)	205	2.6 ± 0.3	2.5 ± 0.2	2.6 ± 0.3	2.6 ± 0.3[d]	0.009
Birth weight category – %						
SGA	9	4.4	4.5	2.0	6.2	ns
AGA	155	75.6	84.3	70.6	67.7[d]	0.036
LGA	41	20.0	11.2	27.5[d]	26.2[d]	0.018
Macrosomia (≥4000 g) – %	27	13.2	7.9	21.6[d]	13.8	ns
Head circumference (cm)	205	34.8 ± 2.9	34.7 ± 1.8	35.3 ± 1.4	35.0 ± 1.5	ns
Hypoglycemia – %	20	9.8	5.6	7.8	16.9[d]	ns
Shoulder dystocia – %	1	0.5	0.0	0.0	1.5	ns
Cord-blood plasma levels						
C-peptide (ng/mL)	162	1.4 ± 0.7	1.3 ± 0.6	1.4 ± 0.7	1.6 ± 0.7[d]	0.016
C-peptide > 90th percentile – %[h]	17	10.5	5.4	7.7	20.4[d]	0.034
Insulin (μU/mL)	164	17.3 ± 13.7	14.3 ± 10.6	18.5 ± 17.6	20.7 ± 13.6[d]	0.022
Insulin > 90th percentile – %[h]	15	9.2	5.4	7.9	15.7	ns
Leptin (ng/mL)	164	13.3 ± 10.7	10.6 ± 8.6	15.2 ± 11.1[d]	15.9 ± 12.3[d]	0.013
Leptin > 90th percentile – %[h]	16	9.8	6.8	10.3	13.7	ns

Data are shown as mean ± SD or %. *N*: Number of subjects with characteristic. n: Total number of subjects

Abbreviations: *GDM* Gestational diabetes mellitus, *BMI* Body-mass-index, *ns* Non-significant, *SES* Socio-economic status, *GWG* Gestational weight gain, *IOM* Institute of Medicine, *oGTT* Oral glucose tolerance test, *HbA1c* Glycated hemoglobin A1c, *SGA* Small-for-gestational age, *AGA* Appropriate-for-gestational age, *LGA* Large-for-gestational age

[a]Statistical significant differences ($P < 0.05$) across all pregestational BMI groups were assessed using one-way ANOVA with Tukey's post hoc test or Kruskal-Wallis test with Dunn's post hoc test and Fisher's exact or Chi-squared tests, as appropriate. [b]n across variables: Normal weight = 74–89, overweight = 39–51, obese = 49–65. [c]Lower (unemployed, manual and non-manual worker without university degree) or higher SES (non-manual worker with university degree) [23, 24]. [d]Statistical significant difference vs. normal weight. [e]oGTT at 25.6 ± 3.8 weeks' gestation. [f]Blood glucose values above guideline cut-offs at the time of study [27]. [g]Mean fasting and 1-h postprandial glucose values were calculated using self-monitored blood glucose data from three days at respective weeks' gestation. [h]Study 90th percentile cut-offs: C-Peptide 2.2 ng/mL, Insulin 34.2 μU/mL, Leptin 29.6 ng/mL.

the same pattern was observed for frequencies above the 90th percentile cut-offs of these hormones at birth.

Associations between parental anthropometric and maternal metabolic variables and birth outcomes

Paternal BMI showed no relation to *any* of the investigated birth outcomes, neither in step-wise regression (see below) nor correlation analyses (Spearman's r of paternal BMI: vs. birth weight, $r = -0.01$; vs. relative birth weight, $r = 0.02$; vs. cord-blood insulin, $r = 0.13$; vs. cord-blood leptin, $r = -0.02$; all not significant).

Bivariate associations between maternal anthropometry and glycemia revealed that prepregnancy BMI positively correlated only with FG among oGTT measurements ($r = 0.36$, $P < 0.001$) but clearly with 3rd trimester glucose variables (mean FG at 32nd weeks' gestation: $r = 0.40$, mean FG at 36th weeks' gestation: $r = 0.41$, HbA1c in 3rd trimester: $r = 0.50$, HbA1c at delivery: $r = 0.46$; all $P < 0.001$). In contrast, the only relationship of net GWG was an inverse correlation with AUC glucose at oGTT ($r = -0.15$, $P = 0.037$).

Furthermore, prepregnancy BMI, but not net GWG, was significantly positively associated with birth outcomes, i.e., placental weight, relative birth weight, cord-blood insulin and leptin (Table 2, Fig. 2). The relationship between prepregnancy BMI and birth weight was close to significance ($r = 0.14$, $P = 0.050$). Glucose variables at oGTT were not related to birth outcomes, with the exception of a weak positive correlation between FG and placental weight. However, mean FG at 32nd weeks' gestation and HbA1c levels in 3rd trimester and at delivery were significantly positively associated with all birth outcomes, including birth weight (Table 2). Among all anthropometric and metabolic variables, HbA1c at delivery had the strongest associations with birth outcomes, in particular with relative birth weight and cord-blood insulin (Table 2, Fig. 2). Of note, placental weight was an even stronger correlate for birth weight ($r = 0.57$, $P < 0.001$) and relative birth weight ($r = 0.58$, $P < 0.001$).

The influence of maternal anthropometry on birth outcomes was further investigated in detail by comprehensive regression analyses (Table 3). There were no relationships observed between GWG in 1st and 2nd trimester and net GWG, respectively, and anthropometric birth outcomes. In the crude models, prepregnancy weight status, i.e., body weight and/or BMI, and 3rd trimester and/or total GWG were significantly positively associated with placental weight, birth weight and relative birth weight. However, their initial relations were already diminished after adjustment to general parameters (Model I, Table 3). Further addition of maternal 3rd trimester glucose variables (Model II, Table 3) completely abolished all of these associations. With regard to cord-blood hormones, there were hardly any associations observed with maternal anthropometry. In unadjusted models, only prepregnancy weight and BMI status showed significant positive associations with insulin and leptin, however, these relations no longer persisted even after adjustment only to general variables (Model I, Table 3). Taken together, neither maternal nor paternal anthropometry showed a significant relation to investigated birth outcomes, after consideration of maternal metabolic parameters.

In order to identify potential metabolic determinants responsible for these observations, regression analyses with a variety of glucose variables were carried out (Table 4). Glucose values at oGTT showed almost no relationship with any birth outcome. There was just a positive relation between FG at oGTT and placental weight, as already observed in correlation analysis (Table 2). In contrast, even an inverse relation between 1-h glucose and birth weight was observed (Table 4). Both associations, however, were no longer present after adjustment to general variables (Model I, Table 4). On the contrary, 3rd trimester glucose variables were significantly positively associated with anthropometric outcomes at birth. Particularly consistent, mean FG and PPG at 32nd weeks' gestation as well as HbA1c levels in 3rd trimester and at delivery were

Table 2 Spearman's correlations between key maternal anthropometric and metabolic variables and neonatal outcomes

Maternal characteristics	Neonatal outcomes									
	Placental weight		Birth weight		Relative birth weight		Cord-blood insulin		Cord-blood leptin	
	r	*P*-value	r	*P*-value	r	*P*-value	r	*P*-value	r	*P*-value
Prepregnancy BMI	0.24	0.001	0.14	ns	0.18	0.009	0.19	0.015	0.20	0.009
Net GWG	0.06	ns	0.09	ns	0.09	ns	0.04	ns	− 0.06	ns
FG at oGTT	0.18	0.010	0.12	ns	0.13	ns	0.10	ns	0.15	ns
AUC glucose at oGTT	−0.02	ns	− 0.09	ns	− 0.07	ns	0.02	ns	0.15	ns
Mean FG at 32nd GW	0.24	< 0.001	0.16	0.029	0.19	0.007	0.23	0.003	0.23	0.004
Mean FG at 36th GW	0.12	ns	0.10	ns	0.15	0.041	0.21	0.010	0.21	0.011
HbA1c in 3rd trimester	0.21	0.004	0.17	0.017	0.22	0.002	0.31	< 0.001	0.32	< 0.001
HbA1c partum	0.24	< 0.001	0.25	< 0.001	0.29	< 0.001	0.39	< 0.001	0.38	< 0.001

Abbreviations: *BMI* Body-mass-index, *ns* Non-significant, *GWG* Gestational weight gain, *FG* Fasting glucose, *oGTT* Oral glucose tolerance test, *AUC* Area under the curve, *GW* Gestational week, *HbA1c* Glycated hemoglobin A1c

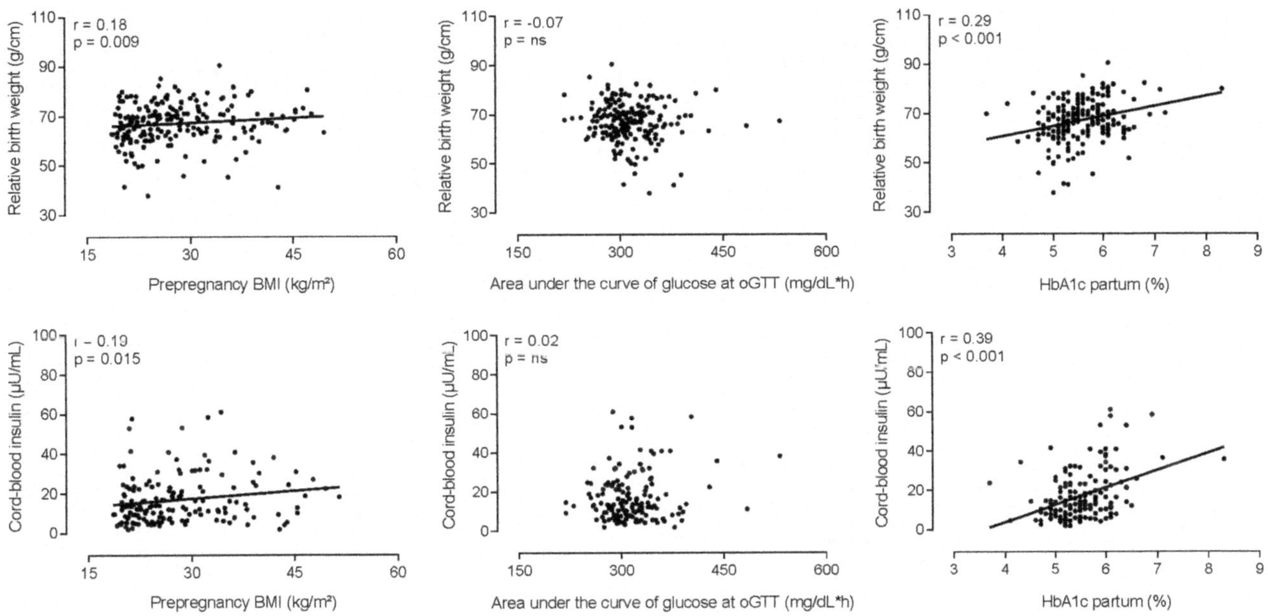

Fig. 2 Correlations between maternal parameters and birth outcomes. Maternal prepregnancy body-mass-index (BMI) and glycemia at delivery (HbA1c), but not at oral glucose tolerance test (oGTT), were significantly positively associated with relative birth weight and cord-blood insulin levels. Spearman's correlation coefficients (r) and *P*-values are shown

significantly positively associated with all anthropometric outcomes in the crude models. Importantly, most of these relations remained constant also after adjustment to general parameters (Model I, Table 4). Further inclusion of maternal anthropometric variables into the adjustment model (Model II, Table 4) abolished some initial associations. However, after adjustment to critical general as well as anthropometric variables (Model II) mean glucose values at 32nd and 36th weeks' gestation showed clear significant positive relationships with placental weight, while mean PPG at 32nd weeks' gestation and HbA1c in 3rd trimester and at delivery were significantly positively associated with birth weight and relative birth weight, respectively (Table 4). A similar pattern was observed for critical cord-blood hormones. Again, glucose variables at oGTT were hardly related to cord-blood insulin and leptin. The only association was observed between FG at oGTT and cord-blood leptin, however, this weak positive relationship was only present in the unadjusted model. In contrast, considering 3rd trimester glucose variables, in particular mean FG at 32nd and 36th weeks' gestation and HbA1c at delivery remained significantly positively associated with cord-blood insulin, even after full adjustment (Model II, Table 4). Likewise, maternal 3rd trimester glycemia, indicated by HbA1c, was significantly positively related to cord-blood leptin, and HbA1c at delivery showed the strongest effects here (Table 4). Adjustment to general and, additionally, maternal anthropometric variables only marginally altered the effect size of these associations (Model II, Table 4).

Identification of major categorical parental determinants of anthropometric birth and cord-blood hormone outcomes

Forward step-wise regression analyses with key paternal and maternal general, anthropometric, and metabolic parameters in (clinically) relevant categories were then performed to identify major predictors for critical birth outcomes (Table 5). Aside from classical birth weight determining factors, e.g. term delivery, smoking during pregnancy etc., maternal, but not paternal, anthropometric and metabolic variables, respectively, appeared as predictors. However, maternal anthropometry, i.e., prepregnant overweight/obesity and excessive GWG (according to IOM criteria), was positively related only to relative birth weight and explained around 2–3% of the variance (Table 5). On the contrary, maternal glucose during 3rd trimester showed a variety of associations. For example, mean FG at 32nd weeks' gestation > 90 mg/dL was the strongest factor for placental weight (6% of variance) and a predictor for birth weight and cord-blood insulin (Table 5). A FG value > 90 mg/dL at oGTT was a significant positive factor for cord-blood leptin at birth (3% of variance). Unexpectedly, 1-h glucose value at oGTT above the guideline cut-off (> 180 mg/dL) was associated with lower instead of higher birth weight and relative birth weight, explaining 2–4% of variances. As shown in Table 5, HbA1c at delivery was a

Table 3 Crude and adjusted linear regression analyses for maternal anthropometric variables vs. neonatal anthropometric and cord-blood outcome variables

Outcome variable	Independent variable	Crude		Adjusted[a]			
				Model I		Model II	
		B (95% CI)	*P*-value	B (95% CI)	*P*-value	B (95% CI)	*P*-value
Placental weight							
	Prepregnancy body weight	0.195 (0.06; 0.34)	0.006	0.171 (0.02; 0.33)	0.032	0.118 (− 0.09; 0.32)	ns
	Prepregnancy BMI	0.201 (0.06; 0.34)	0.005	0.164 (0.01; 0.32)	0.036	0.097 (− 0.10; 0.30)	ns
	GWG in 1. trimester	0.066 (− 0.08; 0.21)	ns	0.077 (−0.06; 0.21)	ns	0.052 (− 0.10; 0.20)	ns
	GWG in 2. trimester	0.082 (− 0.06; 0.22)	ns	0.058 (− 0.09; 0.20)	ns	0.029 (− 0.14; 0.19)	ns
	GWG in 3. trimester	0.184 (0.04; 0.32)	0.010	0.131 (−0.01; 0.27)	ns	0.057 (− 0.10; 0.22)	ns
	Total GWG	0.120 (−0.02; 0.26)	ns	0.099 (−0.04; 0.24)	ns	0.018 (− 0.14; 0.18)	ns
	Net GWG	0.054 (−0.09; 0.20)	ns	0.045 (−0.09; 0.18)	ns	−0.034 (− 0.19; 0.12)	ns
Birth weight							
	Prepregnancy body weight	0.142 (0.00; 0.28)	0.044	0.113 (− 0.03; 0.25)	ns	0.085 (−0.10; 0.27)	ns
	Prepregnancy BMI	0.103 (− 0.04; 0.24)	ns	0.102 (−0.04; 0.24)	ns	0.081 (−0.11; 0.27)	ns
	GWG in 1. trimester	0.043 (−0.10; 0.18)	ns	0.058 (−0.06; 0.18)	ns	0.025 (−0.11; 0.17)	ns
	GWG in 2. trimester	0.139 (− 0.00; 0.28)	ns	0.084 (−0.04; 0.21)	ns	0.091 (−0.06; 0.24)	ns
	GWG in 3. trimester	0.190 (0.05; 0.33)	0.007	0.146 (0.02; 0.27)	0.021	0.113 (− 0.03; 0.26)	ns
	Total GWG	0.172 (0.03; 0.31)	0.016	0.139 (0.02; 0.26)	0.028	0.108 (−0.04; 0.25)	ns
	Net GWG	0.086 (− 0.05; 0.23)	ns	0.077 (−0.05; 0.20)	ns	0.048 (−0.10; 0.19)	ns
Relative birth weight							
	Prepregnancy body weight	0.188 (0.05; 0.33)	0.007	0.133 (− 0.01; 0.28)	ns	0.069 (− 0.12; 0.26)	ns
	Prepregnancy BMI	0.150 (0.01; 0.29)	0.033	0.121 (−0.02; 0.26)	ns	0.069 (− 0.12; 0.26)	ns
	GWG in 1. trimester	0.026 (−0.12; 0.17)	ns	0.038 (− 0.09; 0.16)	ns	0.043 (− 0.10; 0.19)	ns
	GWG in 2. trimester	0.136 (−0.01; 0.28)	ns	0.105 (−0.03; 0.24)	ns	0.107 (−0.05; 0.26)	ns
	GWG in 3. trimester	0.216 (0.08; 0.35)	0.002	0.171 (0.05; 0.30)	0.008	0.105 (−0.04; 0.25)	ns
	Total GWG	0.197 (0.06; 0.33)	0.005	0.168 (0.04; 0.29)	0.009	0.131 (−0.02; 0.28)	ns
	Net GWG	0.106 (− 0.03; 0.25)	ns	0.098 (−0.03; 0.23)	ns	0.064 (−0.08; 0.21)	ns
Cord-blood insulin							
	Prepregnancy body weight	0.109 (−0.04; 0.26)	ns	0.078 (−0.09; 0.24)	ns	−0.046 (− 0.25; 0.16)	ns
	Prepregnancy BMI	0.177 (0.03; 0.33)	0.023	0.090 (−0.07; 0.25)	ns	−0.021 (− 0.23; 0.18)	ns
	GWG in 1. trimester	−0.067 (− 0.22; 0.09)	ns	− 0.059 (− 0.20; 0.08)	ns	− 0.109 (− 0.26; 0.05)	ns
	GWG in 2. trimester	0.050 (− 0.11; 0.21)	ns	0.083 (− 0.07; 0.24)	ns	0.157 (− 0.01; 0.32)	ns
	GWG in 3. trimester	0.142 (− 0.01; 0.30)	ns	0.111 (− 0.03; 0.26)	ns	0.146 (−0.02; 0.31)	ns
	Total GWG	0.107 (−0.05; 0.26)	ns	0.129 (−0.01; 0.27)	ns	0.147 (−0.01; 0.31)	ns
	Net GWG	0.069 (−0.09; 0.23)	ns	0.102 (−0.04; 0.25)	ns	0.124 (−0.04; 0.28)	ns
Cord-blood leptin							
	Prepregnancy body weight	0.159 (0.01; 0.31)	0.042	0.116 (− 0.05; 0.28)	ns	0.102 (−0.11; 0.31)	ns
	Prepregnancy BMI	0.177 (0.02; 0.33)	0.024	0.098 (− 0.06; 0.26)	ns	0.088 (− 0.12; 0.29)	ns
	GWG in 1. trimester	−0.032 (− 0.19; 0.13)	ns	− 0.018 (− 0.16; 0.12)	ns	− 0.061 (− 0.22; 0.10)	ns
	GWG in 2. trimester	−0.102 (− 0.26; 0.06)	ns	− 0.049 (− 0.20; 0.10)	ns	0.031 (− 0.14; 0.20)	ns
	GWG in 3. trimester	0.117 (− 0.04; 0.27)	ns	0.069 (−0.08; 0.22)	ns	0.103 (− 0.06; 0.27)	ns
	Total GWG	0.006 (−0.15; 0.16)	ns	0.032 (−0.11; 0.18)	ns	0.022 (− 0.14; 0.18)	ns
	Net GWG	−0.019 (− 0.18; 0.14)	ns	0.020 (− 0.12; 0.16)	ns	0.015 (− 0.15; 0.18)	ns

Abbreviations: *BMI* Body-mass-index, *ns* Non-significant, *GWG* Gestational weight gain

[a]Model I: Adjusted for maternal age, socio-economic status, ethnic origin, smoking during pregnancy, parity, height (except for BMI), type of therapy, gestational age, mode of delivery and infant's sex.

Model II: Model I adjustment plus mean fasting and postprandial glucose at 32nd and 36th weeks' gestation and HbA1c partum

Table 4 Crude and adjusted linear regression analyses for maternal metabolic variables vs. neonatal anthropometric and cord-blood outcome variables

Outcome variable	Independent variable	Crude		Adjusted[a]			
				Model I		Model II	
		B (95% CI)	*P*-value	B (95% CI)	*P*-value	B (95% CI)	*P*-value
Placental weight							
	FG at oGTT	0.170 (0.03; 0.31)	0.017	0.106 (−0.04; 0.25)	ns	0.072 (− 0.08; 0.22)	ns
	1-h glucose at oGTT	−0.084 (− 0.23; 0.06)	ns	− 0.088 (− 0.23; 0.05)	ns	−0.051 (− 0.19; 0.09)	ns
	2-h glucose at oGTT	0.046 (−0.10; 0.19)	ns	0.065 (−0.08; 0.21)	ns	0.080 (−0.07; 0.23)	ns
	AUC glucose at oGTT	−0.034 (− 0.18; 0.11)	ns	− 0.037 (− 0.19; 0.11)	ns	−0.008 (− 0.16; 0.14)	ns
	Mean FG at 32nd GW	0.250 (0.11; 0.39)	0.001	0.231 (0.07; 0.39)	0.006	0.197 (0.03; 0.36)	0.021
	Mean PPG at 32nd GW	0.300 (0.16; 0.44)	< 0.001	0.265 (0.11; 0.42)	0.001	0.234 (0.08; 0.39)	0.003
	Mean FG at 36th GW	0.145 (−0.00; 0.29)	ns	0.125 (− 0.03; 0.28)	ns	0.071 (− 0.09; 0.23)	ns
	Mean PPG at 36th GW	0.218 (0.07; 0.37)	0.005	0.215 (0.06; 0.37)	0.008	0.179 (0.02; 0.34)	0.040
	HbA1c in 3.trimester	0.220 (0.08; 0.36)	0.003	0.192 (0.04; 0.35)	0.015	0.141 (−0.02; 0.31)	ns
	HbA1c partum	0.222 (0.08; 0.37)	0.003	0.151 (−0.00; 0.30)	ns	0.106 (−0.05; 0.27)	ns
Birth weight							
	FG at oGTT	0.094 (−0.05; 0.23)	ns	0.052 (−0.08; 0.19)	ns	0.062 (− 0.08; 0.20)	ns
	1-h glucose at oGTT	−0.142 (− 0.28; − 0.00)	0.044	−0.091 (− 0.22; 0.04)	ns	−0.059 (− 0.19; 0.07)	ns
	2-h glucose at oGTT	−0.049 (− 0.19; 0.09)	ns	0.016 (− 0.12; 0.15)	ns	0.045 (− 0.09; 0.18)	ns
	AUC glucose at oGTT	−0.126 (− 0.27; 0.02)	ns	− 0.057 (− 0.19; 0.08)	ns	− 0.014 (− 0.15; 0.12)	ns
	Mean FG at 32nd GW	0.157 (0.01; 0.30)	0.032	0.147 (− 0.00; 0.30)	ns	0.120 (−0.03; 0.27)	ns
	Mean PPG at 32nd GW	0.295 (0.15; 0.44)	< 0.001	0.259 (0.12; 0.40)	< 0.001	0.233 (0.09; 0.38)	0.002
	Mean FG at 36th GW	0.125 (−0.02; 0.27)	ns	0.118 (−0.02; 0.26)	ns	0.080 (−0.06; 0.22)	ns
	Mean PPG at 36th GW	0.161 (0.01; 0.31)	0.033	0.171 (0.03; 0.32)	0.020	0.111 (−0.04; 0.26)	ns
	HbA1c in 3.trimester	0.141 (0.00; 0.28)	0.048	0.146 (0.01; 0.29)	0.040	0.112 (−0.04; 0.26)	ns
	HbA1c partum	0.218 (0.08; 0.36)	0.003	0.186 (0.05; 0.32)	0.008	0.176 (0.03; 0.32)	0.016
Relative birth weight							
	FG at oGTT	0.108 (−0.03; 0.25)	ns	0.031 (− 0.11; 0.17)	ns	0.034 (− 0.11; 0.17)	ns
	1-h glucose at oGTT	−0.108 (− 0.25; 0.03)	ns	− 0.074 (− 0.20; 0.06)	ns	−0.046 (− 0.18; 0.09)	ns
	2-h glucose at oGTT	0.005 (−0.14; 0.15)	ns	0.050 (−0.09; 0.18)	ns	0.088 (−0.05; 0.22)	ns
	AUC glucose at oGTT	−0.080 (− 0.22; 0.06)	ns	− 0.039 (− 0.18; 0.10)	ns	0.003 (− 0.14; 0.14)	ns
	Mean FG at 32nd GW	0.193 (0.05; 0.34)	0.008	0.142 (−0.01; 0.29)	ns	0.105 (−0.05; 0.26)	ns
	Mean PPG at 32nd GW	0.319 (0.18; 0.46)	< 0.001	0.285 (0.14; 0.43)	< 0.001	0.241 (0.09; 0.39)	0.002
	Mean FG at 36th GW	0.174 (0.03; 0.32)	0.017	0.139 (−0.00; 0.28)	ns	0.098 (−0.05; 0.24)	ns
	Mean PPG at 36th GW	0.175 (0.03; 0.32)	0.019	0.164 (0.02; 0.31)	0.030	0.097 (−0.06; 0.25)	ns
	HbA1c in 3.trimester	0.214 (0.08; 0.35)	0.002	0.202 (0.06; 0.34)	0.006	0.162 (0.01; 0.31)	0.037
	HbA1c partum	0.269 (0.13; 0.41)	< 0.001	0.217 (0.08; 0.35)	0.002	0.196 (0.05; 0.34)	0.008
Cord-blood insulin							
	FG at oGTT	0.114 (−0.04; 0.27)	ns	0.018 (−0.14; 0.18)	ns	0.012 (−0.15; 0.18)	ns
	1-h glucose at oGTT	0.039 (−0.12; 0.20)	ns	−0.027 (− 0.18; 0.13)	ns	0.003 (− 0.15; 0.16)	ns
	2-h glucose at oGTT	0.047 (−0.11; 0.20)	ns	0.037 (−0.11; 0.19)	ns	0.065 (−0.09; 0.22)	ns
	AUC glucose at oGTT	0.041 (−0.12; 0.20)	ns	−0.012 (− 0.17; 0.14)	ns	0.026 (− 0.14; 0.19)	ns
	Mean FG at 32nd GW	0.241 (0.08; 0.40)	0.004	0.243 (0.07; 0.41)	0.005	0.231 (0.06; 0.41)	0.010
	Mean PPG at 32nd GW	0.225 (0.07; 0.38)	0.005	0.116 (−0.04; 0.28)	ns	0.085 (−0.08; 0.25)	ns
	Mean FG at 36th GW	0.224 (0.07; 0.38)	0.006	0.194 (0.04; 0.35)	0.012	0.172 (0.01; 0.33)	0.035

Table 4 Crude and adjusted linear regression analyses for maternal metabolic variables vs. neonatal anthropometric and cord-blood outcome variables *(Continued)*

Outcome variable	Independent variable	Crude		Adjusted[a]			
				Model I		Model II	
		B (95% CI)	*P*-value	B (95% CI)	*P*-value	B (95% CI)	*P*-value
	Mean PPG at 36th GW	0.143 (−0.02; 0.31)	ns	0.080 (−0.07; 0.24)	ns	0.037 (−0.12; 0.20)	ns
	HbA1c in 3.trimester	0.315 (0.16; 0.48)	< 0.001	0.209 (0.04; 0.37)	0.014	0.180 (−0.01; 0.37)	ns
	HbA1c partum	0.386 (0.24; 0.54)	< 0.001	0.300 (0.15; 0.45)	< 0.001	0.282 (0.11; 0.45)	0.001
Cord-blood leptin							
	FG at oGTT	0.157 (0.01; 0.31)	0.042	0.065 (−0.09; 0.22)	ns	0.034 (− 0.13; 0.20)	ns
	1-h glucose at oGTT	0.084 (−0.07; 0.24)	ns	0.054 (−0.10; 0.21)	ns	0.072 (−0.09; 0.23)	ns
	2-h glucose at oGTT	0.134 (−0.02; 0.29)	ns	0.154 (0.01; 0.30)	ns	0.169 (0.02; 0.32)	0.028
	AUC glucose at oGTT	0.124 (−0.03; 0.28)	ns	0.107 (−0.05; 0.26)	ns	0.122 (−0.04; 0.28)	ns
	Mean FG at 32nd GW	0.204 (0.05; 0.36)	0.012	0.172 (0.01; 0.34)	0.043	0.149 (−0.02; 0.32)	ns
	Mean PPG at 32nd GW	0.194 (0.04; 0.35)	0.015	0.131 (−0.03; 0.29)	ns	0.122 (−0.04; 0.28)	ns
	Mean FG at 36th GW	0.188 (0.03; 0.35)	0.020	0.122 (−0.04; 0.28)	ns	0.073 (−0.10; 0.24)	ns
	Mean PPG at 36th GW	0.104 (−0.06; 0.27)	ns	0.030 (−0.13; 0.19)	ns	0.004 (−0.16; 0.17)	ns
	HbA1c in 3.trimester	0.290 (0.14; 0.44)	< 0.001	0.190 (0.03; 0.35)	0.021	0.188 (0.01; 0.37)	0.041
	HbA1c partum	0.350 (0.20; 0.50)	< 0.001	0.261 (0.11; 0.42)	0.001	0.259 (0.09; 0.43)	0.003

Abbreviations: *FG* Fasting glucose, *oGTT* Oral glucose tolerance test, *ns* Non-significant, *AUC* Area under the curve, *GW* Gestational week, *PPG* Postprandial glucose, *HbA1c* Glycated hemoglobin A1c
[a]Model I: Adjusted for maternal age, socio-economic status, ethnic origin, smoking during pregnancy, parity, height, type of therapy, gestational age, mode of delivery and infant's sex.
Model II: Model I adjustment plus prepregnancy body weight and net gestational weight gain

particular strong predictor for higher cord-blood insulin and leptin levels (7% of variance).

Finally, logistic regression analysis was performed. Because of low numbers of adverse clinical endpoints, analysis was restricted to the outcome LGA. Indeed, crude, unadjusted evaluation revealed increased prepregnancy BMI as risk factor for LGA (OR: 1.53, 95% CI: 1.06–2.20, $P = 0.023$). However, after adjustment for 3rd trimester glucose according to Model II variables (see above), neither pregravid BMI (OR: 1.39, 95% CI: 0.80–2.40) nor total GWG (OR: 1.52, 95% CI: 0.95–2.42) nor net GWG (OR: 1.34, 95% CI: 0.83–2.15) were significantly related to LGA.

Additionally, to further illustrate observations for clinically unfavorable neonatal anthropometric (LGA and macrosomia) and cord-blood outcomes (insulin and leptin > 90th percentiles), percentages of relevant anthropometric and metabolic variables/exposures, grouped according to clinical/guideline cut-offs, were compared to respective internal reference groups which did not show these adverse outcomes (Fig. 3). Following this approach, maternal prepregnancy overweight/obesity and excessive GWG only showed significantly higher relative frequencies regarding LGA (Fig. 3). In contrast, parameters of maternal hyperglycemia during 3rd trimester were associated with all unfavorable endpoints. Percentages of 3rd trimester glucose variables above cut-offs, in particular mean FG at 32nd weeks' gestation > 90 mg/dL and HbA1c > 6% in 3rd trimester as well as at delivery, were significantly higher in offspring with LGA and macrosomia, respectively. Notably, women with macrosomic offspring exceeded 2.5-times more often the cut-off for HbA1c in 3rd trimester (Fig. 3). Furthermore, both cord-blood insulin as well as leptin > 90th percentile showed strong positive associations with maternal 3rd trimester hyperglycemia, but neither with pregravid BMI nor excessive GWG. Percentages above the cut-offs of FG at oGTT and mean FG at 32nd weeks' gestation (> 90 mg/dL for both) were significantly higher in offspring with cord-blood leptin > 90th percentile. Finally, relative frequencies above the cut-off for HbA1c at both investigated time points were even increased up to 3- to 6-fold in offspring with cord-blood insulin and leptin > 90th percentile, respectively (Fig. 3).

Discussion

Maternal overweight/obesity and GDM are associated with adverse short- and long-term outcomes in the offspring [5, 7], the latter identified to be related especially to increased birth weight, insulin and leptin. In this prospective observational study of women with treated GDM the influence of maternal anthropometry on respective birth outcomes was strongly dependent on maternal glycemia in late pregnancy. After adjustment to 3rd trimester glucose metabolism, no significant effect of maternal anthropometry was observed on placental weight, birth

Table 5 Maternal categorical predictor variables affecting anthropometric birth outcomes and cord-blood hormones

Outcome variable	Predictor variable[a]	B (95% CI)	*P*-value	Adj. Sr^2
Placental weight	Mean FG at 32nd GW > 90 mg/dL	0.487 (0.18; 0.80)	0.002	0.057
	Term delivery	0.934 (0.30; 1.57)	0.004	0.040
	Cesarean section	0.424 (0.11; 0.74)	0.008	0.036
Birth weight	Term delivery	1.400 (0.80; 2.00)	< 0.001	0.118
	1-h glucose at oGTT > 180 mg/dL	−0.501 (−0.86; −0.15)	0.006	0.035
	Smoking in pregnancy	−0.561 (− 0.96; − 0.17)	0.006	0.029
	Male sex	0.333 (0.05; 0.62)	0.022	0.023
	Mean FG at 32nd GW >90 mg/dL	0.297 (0.01; 0.59)	0.044	0.017
Relative birth weight	Term delivery	1.457 (0.86; 2.06)	< 0.001	0.121
	Excessive GWG	0.332 (0.04; 0.62)	0.026	0.029
	Smoking in pregnancy	−0.565 (−0.97; −0.16)	0.007	0.025
	Prepregnancy BMI > 25 kg/m^2	0.319 (0.02; 0.61)	0.034	0.024
	1-h glucose at oGTT > 180 mg/dL	−0.375 (− 0.74; − 0.01)	0.042	0.016
	Male sex	0.295 (0.01; 0.58)	0.044	0.016
Cord-blood insulin	Cesarean section	0.679 (0.38; 0.97)	< 0.001	0.170
	HbA1c partum > 6%	0.460 (0.09; 0.83)	0.016	0.066
	Non-European ethnicity	0.438 (0.13; 0.75)	0.006	0.043
	Mean FG at 32nd GW >90 mg/dL	0.321 (0.02; 0.63)	0.038	0.020
Cord-blood leptin	HbA1c partum > 6%	0.470 (0.08; 0.86)	0.017	0.070
	Non-European ethnicity	0.519 (0.19; 0.85)	0.002	0.048
	Male sex	−0.395 (−0.71; −0.08)	0.013	0.042
	FG at oGTT >90 mg/dL	0.339 (0.03; 0.65)	0.034	0.025

Unstandardized B coefficients with 95% confidence interval and adjusted semipartial correlation coefficients (Sr^2), which estimate the contribution of each factor to the variance of the outcome variable, are shown

Abbreviations: *FG* Fasting glucose, *GW* Gestational week, *oGTT* Oral glucose tolerance test, *GWG* Gestational weight gain, *BMI* Body-mass-index, *HbA1c* Glycated hemoglobin A1c

[a]Included categorical variables: Paternal SES (lower/higher), maternal SES (lower/higher), parity (nulliparous/multiparous), ethnicity (European/Non-European), smoking in pregnancy (no/yes), type of therapy (diet/insulin), mode of delivery (Cesarean section no/yes), gestational age (preterm/term), infant's sex (female/male), paternal BMI > 25 kg/m^2 (no/yes), paternal BMI > 30 kg/m^2 (no/yes), maternal prepregnancy BMI > 25 kg/m^2 (no/yes), prepregnancy BMI > 30 kg/m^2 (no/yes), inadequate GWG (no/yes), excessive GWG (no/yes), FG at oGTT > 90 mg/dL (no/yes), 1-h glucose at oGTT > 180 mg/dL (no/yes), 2-h glucose at oGTT > 155 mg/dL (no/yes), mean FG at 32nd weeks' gestation > 90 mg/dL (no/yes), mean FG at 36th weeks' gestation > 90 mg/dL (no/yes), HbA1c in third trimester > 6% (no/yes) and partum > 6% (no/yes).

weight, relative birth weight (weight-to-length ratio), and cord-blood insulin and leptin, respectively. On the contrary, 3rd trimester glucose variables, and only marginally FG at oGTT screening, showed clear positive associations with these outcomes, even after adjustment for a variety of general as well as anthropometric parental measures. Thus, maternal (hyper-) glycemia in 3rd trimester appears to be the key target for managing and avoiding alterations of fetal growth (adiposity) and hormone levels affecting long-term health.

Our observations are in line with data from other cohort studies showing that treatment of GDM, i.e., achieving good metabolic control, can significantly reduce the potential effects of maternal (prepregnancy) BMI status on adverse anthropometric perinatal outcomes [37–39]. Beyond their focus on LGA and macrosomia, the present study additionally highlights the influence of maternal 3rd trimester glycemia on a wide birth weight and relative birth weight range. Considering, in general, a linear increase of later overweight risk with increasing birth weight [11], strict management of maternal glycemia throughout the fetal growth spectrum may therefore be beneficial for the offspring, to protect their genuine growth potential. Other studies concluded that maternal obesity per se is a major factor or even better predictor than maternal glycemia to manage fetal (over-) growth in women with treated GDM [40–42]. Similar to the present cohort, obesity was accompanied in two of these studies by higher glucose levels compared to normal weight individuals [40, 41]. However, only group comparisons [41] and no adjustments for general covariates and/or maternal glycemia in later pregnancy were performed [40, 41]. Thus, the relative contributions of maternal weight status vs. glucose may have been different after all, and might have depend lastly on the degree of 3rd trimester glycemia in these cohorts, too. Similarly, in another

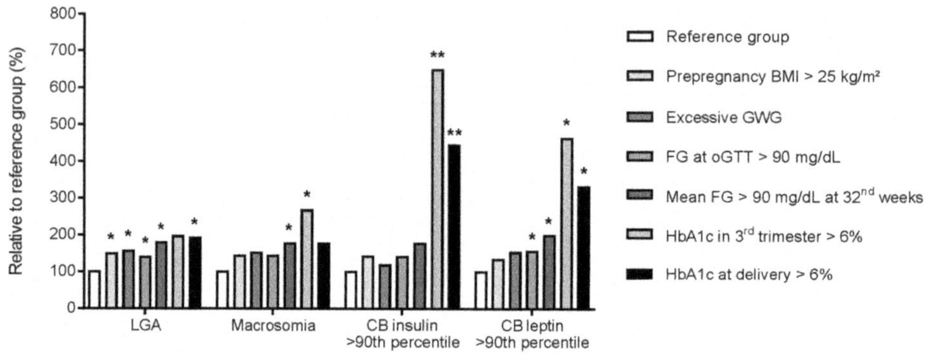

Fig. 3 Relative percentages of significant maternal anthropometric and metabolic variables/exposures in newborns with unfavorable outcomes. Frequencies of maternal key anthropometric and metabolic variables/exposures in newborns with unfavorable outcomes relative to respective reference groups (LGA/Macrosomia: Reference group consists of appropriate-for-gestational age and non-macrosomic infants; CB insulin/leptin: Reference group consists of all cases <90th percentiles) are shown. Significant differences are indicated as * $P < 0.05$, ** $P < 0.001$. Abbreviations: LGA: Large-for-gestational age, CB: Cord-blood, BMI: Body-mass-Index, GWG: Gestational weight gain, FG: Fasting glucose, oGTT: Oral glucose tolerance test, HbA1c: Glycated hemoglobin A1c

retrospective study [42] critical information about the relationship between maternal BMI and glucose was not provided and HbA1c levels in 3rd trimester and at delivery were not available. Interestingly, however, although maternal obesity was clearly associated with fetal overgrowth, it was concluded that during the period of maximum in utero growth, i.e., 3rd trimester, maternal glycemia was the predominant factor.

Furthermore, some studies reported that increased maternal GWG is an independent factor for adverse anthropometric outcomes in women with GDM [43–46]. Again, however, maternal glycemia in later pregnancy or even only at GDM screening was not considered in the final analyses, with the exception of one study [43]. Interestingly enough, here multivariable analysis revealed that total maternal weight gain during pregnancy was finally only of minor significance while increased mean blood glucose during the treatment period was associated with a 2-fold risk for LGA outcome. Hence, the effects of maternal GWG seem to decisively depend on maternal glycemia, as observed in the present study. Total and 3rd trimester GWG, both comprising fetal weight, were initially associated with birth weight and relative birth weight but no longer after adjustment to 3rd trimester glucose variables. Moreover, genuine maternal weight gain (net GWG) per se showed no relation to any outcome. Based on these observations, future studies should consider adjustment to maternal glycemia but also net GWG for clear-cut analyses and interpretation of the impact of maternal anthropometry for the outcome.

In addition to neonatal anthropometry, our study also shows that maternal glycemia in 3rd trimester, but not maternal anthropometry per se, is independently related to critical cord-blood hormones shown to promote fetal 'malprogramming'. While causal factors for adverse neonatal anthropometric outcomes are intensively studied, determinants of cord-blood insulin and leptin are less considered in clinical studies, although probably even more important mechanistically for the long-term development of metabolic disorders [8, 14, 20, 47–49]. Especially, hyperinsulinism has been shown to be crucial for long-term 'malprogramming' of the child towards 'diabesity' predisposition [20, 47, 48]. Furthermore, cord-blood leptin correlates with neonatal adiposity [50], and might act as a growth factor in utero itself [51]. There is strong evidence that maternal obesity and diabetes are associated with higher cord-blood insulin and leptin concentrations [52–55]. With regard to maternal glycemia it has been shown recently that both hormones are related to fasting and post load glucose at oGTT, adjusted for maternal BMI, in a multiethnic cohort with and without GDM [56]. Consistently, the present study indicates a strong influence of maternal glucose, but not BMI or GWG per se, on both hormones. Here, however, not glucose at the time of oGTT but in later pregnancy appeared critically linked to adverse birth outcomes. Since both clinical as well as experimental studies demonstrated the particular importance of, especially, hyperinsulinism for long-term 'diabesity programming,' this observation seems to deserve particular attention [14, 20, 57].

The HAPO study clearly showed a linear positive relationship between maternal glucose concentrations at oGTT screening, in particular FG, and critical birth outcomes, e.g. birth weight and cord-blood C-peptide > 90th percentiles, respectively [16]. Moreover, it is suggested from HAPO that maternal obesity and GDM are independent risk factors for these outcomes, while the odds are additive and higher with increasing glycemia [15]. First, this implies that maternal glycemia is generally a major factor for fetal (over-) growth and hyperinsulinemia and further that a strong interaction exists between maternal BMI and glucose metabolism, while the relative contributions are difficult to tease apart.

In HAPO, and a number of related studies addressing the influence of maternal anthropometry on neonatal outcomes, adjustment was made, however, only to oGTT glucose data [15, 58, 59], if performed at all [60, 61], while consideration of later maternal glycemia appears critical for analyses and interpretation. As indicated by the present study, the effects of maternal BMI and GWG, respectively, depend strongly on glucose metabolism not at oGTT but in later pregnancy, contributing significantly to fetal (over-) growth and critical cord-blood outcomes, respectively. Therefore, considering increasing insulin resistance in later pregnancy, regular glucose measurements in overweight/obese women appear to be recommendable even after a negative oGTT screening test. To date, however, research studies considering maternal glycemia in the 3rd trimester are very rare.

Although our data might appear to challenge the impact of maternal overweight for adverse birth outcomes, this would not be correct. Of course, maternal overweight/obesity and increased gestational weight gain play an important detrimental role, just due to tight links with glucose metabolism (insulin sensitivity). As shown here, not all initial associations of adverse birth outcomes with maternal 3rd trimester glucose withstood adjustment to maternal anthropometry. Furthermore, applying step-wise regression analyses with common categorical parameters to our dataset, pregravid overweight/obesity and excessive GWG remained predictors for relative birth weight and showed higher percentages in LGA offspring as compared to the internal reference group. However, all of these effects were rather weak and could not be confirmed using continuous variable analyses. Compared to maternal anthropometric parameters, glucose in 3rd trimester was clearly better related to birth outcomes, in particular placental weight, macrosomia and cord-blood insulin as well as leptin, the latter mainly reflecting neonatal adiposity. Taken together, our data therefore indicates that the impact of (higher) maternal weight status and GWG on critical birth outcomes is ultimately to a major extent attributable to maternal glycemia in late pregnancy, but not at the time of oGTT, i.e., potentially even independent of a negative oGTT screening test. This might have far ranging implications for clinical care.

Our study suggests, that especially maternal glucose at 32nd weeks' gestation as well as HbA1c levels, integrative characterizing 3rd trimester glycemia, are positively related to fetal (over-) growth and (adverse) cord-blood hormone outcomes, respectively. HbA1c at delivery showed particular pronounced effects. This appears plausible, as in general the 3rd trimester is the period of major fetal growth, e.g. due to accelerated fat accumulation, and intrauterine differentiation and maturation [19]. Furthermore, these observations indicate that cumulative maternal hyperglycemia during late pregnancy, characterized by HbA1c, plays a crucial role, which is in agreement with other studies [62–64]. Ensenauer and colleagues [63] reported that even non-GDM obese women with elevated HbA1c at delivery showed increased odds for LGA newborns and cord-blood C-peptide, also after adjustment for maternal prepregnancy BMI and GWG. Interestingly, in the present study, major relations between maternal glycemia and placental weight were observed especially for glucose at 32nd week' gestation. Because placental weight strongly determines/correlates with fetal weight, as shown here and in other reports [36, 65], glucose-dependent placental growth may be an important pathway by which maternal 3rd trimester glycemia influences fetal growth.

Unexpectedly, glucose values at oGTT were, with few exceptions, not significantly related to birth outcomes, which may be a consequence of GDM treatment. Even more surprising was the negative association between 1-h glucose at oGTT above the guideline cut-off (> 180 mg/dL) and birth weight/relative birth weight in step-wise regression analyses on categorical variables. While the majority of women in the total cohort exceeded this threshold, earlier and stricter treatment was applied to these women, possibly resulting in relatively lower birth weights. Moreover, relative frequencies of multiparous gestation, insulin therapy, preterm delivery and SGA outcome were non-significantly higher in women with glucose > 180 mg/dL at oGTT as compared to those below this cut-off. Possibly, all of this might cumulatively provide an explanation for this finding, which was not observed in the other analyses here.

Also worthy to note, paternal anthropometry has been suggested to be directly related to fetal growth and birth weight [66]. As no associations were found in the present study, no support can be given to this hypothesis, in line with other observations speaking clearly against relevant paternal anthropometric determination of birth weight [67]. Interestingly, however, our data indicate "assortative mating" regarding BMI and SES. This may also appear in other studies and, thus, proper adjustment to respective paternal factors should be performed.

Lastly, like all observational studies also the present one had some limitations, which may have influenced the results. First, as only women with sufficient German/English language skills were included into the study, a selection bias could be present here, which appears unavoidable. Secondly, maternal self-reported weight before pregnancy was used for data evaluation. General concordance, however, has been shown for self-reported vs. measured maternal prepregnancy weight [68]. Furthermore, GWG calculations were based on pregravid weight and the last gestational weight measured within one week prior to delivery, which is not totally accurate but common practice in such studies. In addition, due to the design of the study, only placental weight and no other placental characteristics, e.g. shape, size etc., were assessed.

Of note, in BMI group comparisons, the anthropometric outcomes birth weight, relative birth weight and LGA were similar in prepregnancy overweight and obese mothers and did not further increase in the latter, despite higher glycemia in 3rd trimester in the obese. Multiple reasons may explain these observations. For example, factors generally associated with fetal growth restriction and lower birth weight were (much) more abundant in the obese group, e.g. smoking, pregnancy-related hypertensive disorders, preterm delivery, and the mean gestational age at delivery was lower. As highlighted above, adjustment to such potential confounder variables is crucial for analyses and interpretation. Therefore, among a number of covariates, all general predictor variables, e.g. those identified in step-wise regression, were included in the adjustment models. Finally, since sex-specific differences were observed regarding determinants of the investigated fetal/ birth outcomes [36], adjustment was made to infant's sex. Interestingly, offspring's gender, indeed, appeared as potential co-predictor for birth weight and cord-blood leptin, with males more predisposed to higher weight but, remarkably, lower leptin levels at birth. Similar was already observed [54, 69] and should be further explored in future studies.

Conclusions

In summary and conclusion, in a cohort of women with treated GDM maternal BMI and GWG were not associated with birth outcomes critical for 'perinatal programming' after consideration of maternal 3rd trimester glucose metabolism. While glucose at oGTT showed almost no relationships with endpoints, glucose metabolism in later pregnancy was strongly and independently associated with anthropometric and cord-blood hormone outcomes at birth. Thus, maternal overweight does not independently contribute to the detrimental birth outcomes addressed here, while it appears mandatory to strictly manage and scientifically consider, respectively, 3rd trimester glucose in gestational care and future research studies on the short- and long-term consequences of GDM and/or overweight/ obesity during pregnancy.

Abbreviations

AGA: Appropriate-for-gestational age; AUC: Area under the curve; BMI: Body-mass-index; CB: Cord-blood; CI: Confidence interval; CS: Cesarean section; EaCH: Early CHARITÉ study; FG: Fasting glucose; GDM: Gestational diabetes mellitus; GW: Gestational week; GWG: Gestational weight gain; HAPO: Hyperglycemia and adverse pregnancy outcome study; HbA1c: Glycated hemoglobin A1c; IOM: Institute of Medicine; LGA: Large-for-gestational age; Ns: Non-significant; oGTT: oral Glucose tolerance test; OR: Odds ratio; PPG: Postprandial glucose; SD: Standard deviation; SES: Socio-economic status; SGA: Small-for-gestational age; WHO: World Health Organization

Acknowledgements

Thomas Harder, MD, (Robert-Koch Institut, Berlin, Germany) is acknowledged for initial contributions to concept, study design and preliminary analyses during the recruitment period. The authors would like to thank Sandra Schulz, M.Sc., as well as midwifes and staff of the Clinic of Obstetrics at the Charité, Campus Virchow-Klinikum, Berlin, Germany, for their support.

Funding

This study was supported in part by grants of the German Research Foundation (DFG: PL-241/5–1, GRK 1208) to Dr. Plagemann. The funders had no role in study design, data collection and analysis, decision to publish, or preparation of the manuscript.

Authors' contributions

RO contributed to design and conceptualization of the study, analyzed and interpreted the data and wrote the original draft. JHS contributed to design and conceptualization of the study and data collection and reviewed the final draft. AL was involved in study design and conceptualization of the study and data collection and reviewed the final draft. EE contributed to study design and data collection and revised the final draft. KM was involved in data collection/ management and laboratory measurements and reviewed the final draft. RCR contributed to data interpretation and revised the final manuscript. KS contributed to data collection/management and interpretation and reviewed the final manuscript. TZ performed laboratory measurements and revised the final manuscript. JWD contributed to study design, provided resources and revised the final draft. WH provided resources and reviewed the final draft. AP contributed to design and conceptualization of the study, analyzed and interpreted the data and wrote the original draft. All authors read and approved the final manuscript.

Consent for publication

Not applicable.

Competing interests

The authors declare that they have no competing interests.

Author details

[1]Clinic of Obstetrics, Charité – Universitätsmedizin Berlin, corporate member of Freie Universität Berlin, Humboldt-Universität zu Berlin, and Berlin Institute of Health, Campus Virchow-Klinikum, Berlin, Germany. [2]Division of 'Experimental Obstetrics, Charité – Universitätsmedizin Berlin, corporate member of Freie Universität Berlin, Humboldt-Universität zu Berlin, and Berlin Institute of Health, Campus Virchow-Klinikum, Berlin, Germany. [3]Department of Neonatology, Charité – Universitätsmedizin Berlin, corporate member of Freie Universität Berlin, Humboldt-Universität zu Berlin, and Berlin Institute of Health, Campus Virchow-Klinikum, Berlin, Germany.

References

1. O'Sullivan EP, Avalos G, O'Reilly M, Dennedy MC, Gaffney G, Dunne F. Atlantic diabetes in pregnancy (DIP): the prevalence and outcomes of gestational diabetes mellitus using new diagnostic criteria. Diabetologia. 2011;54:1670–5.
2. Sacks DA, Hadden DR, Maresh M, Deerochanawong C, Dyer AR, Metzger BE, et al. Frequency of gestational diabetes mellitus at collaborating centers based on IADPSG consensus panel-recommended criteria: the hyperglycemia and adverse pregnancy outcome (HAPO) study. Diabetes Care. 2012;35:526–8.

3. Melchior H, Kurch-Bek D, Mund M. Population-based analysis of a nationwide screening program. Dtsch Arztebl Int. 2017;114:412–8.
4. Flegal KM, Carroll MD, Odgen CL, Curtin LR. Prevalence and trends in obesity among US adults, 1999-2008. JAMA. 2010;303:235–41.
5. Catalano PM, Ehrenberg HM. The short- and long-term implications of maternal obesity on the mother and her offspring. BJOG. 2006;113:1126–33.
6. Metzger BE, Buchanan TA, Coustan DR, De Leiva A, Dunger DB, Hadden DR, et al. Summary and recommendations of the fifth international workshop-conference on gestational diabetes mellitus. Diabetes Care. 2007;30(Suppl 2):S251–60.
7. Reece EA. The fetal and maternal consequences of gestational diabetes mellitus. J Matern Fetal Neonatal Med. 2010;23:199–203.
8. Plagemann A. Maternal diabetes and perinatal programming. Early Hum Dev. 2011;87:743–7.
9. Barker DJP. Obesity and early life. Obes Rev. 2007;8(Suppl 1):45–9.
10. Harder T, Rodekamp E, Schellong K, Dudenhausen JW, Plagemann A. Birth weight and subsequent risk of type 2 diabetes: a meta-analysis. Am J Epidemiol. 2007;165:849–57.
11. Schellong K, Schulz S, Harder T, Plagemann A. Birth weight and long-term overweight risk: systematic review and a meta-analysis including 643,902 persons from 66 studies and 26 countries globally. PLoS One. 2012;7: e47776. https://doi.org/10.1371/journal.pone.0047776.
12. Van Assche FA, Holemans K, Aerts L. Long-term consequences for offspring of diabetes during pregnancy. Br Med Bull. 2001;60:173–82.
13. Fetita LS, Sobngwi E, Serradas P, Calvo F, Gautier JF. Consequences of fetal exposure to maternal diabetes in offspring. J Clin Endocrinol Metab. 2006;91: 3718–24.
14. Plagemann A. A matter of insulin: developmental programming of body weight regulation. J Matern Fetal Neonatal Med. 2008;21:143–8.
15. Catalano PM, McIntyre HD, Cruickshank JK, McCance DR, Dyer AR, Metzger BE, et al. The hyperglycemia and adverse pregnancy outcome study: associations of GDM and obesity with pregnancy outcomes. Diabetes Care. 2012;35:780–6.
16. HAPO Study Cooperative Research Group. Hyperglycemia and adverse pregnancy outcomes. N Engl J Med. 2008;358:1991–2002.
17. Crowther CA, Hiller JE, Moss JR, McPhee AJ, Jeffries WS, Robinson JS. Effect of treatment of gestational diabetes mellitus on pregnancy outcomes. N Engl J Med. 2005;352:2477–86.
18. Landon MB, Spong CY, Thom E, Carpenter MW, Ramin SM, Casey B, et al. A multicenter, randomized trial of treatment for mild gestational diabetes. N Engl J Med. 2009;361:1339–48.
19. Moore KL, Persaud TV, Torchia MG. The developing human. 9th ed. Philadelphia: Saunders Elsevier Inc.; 2011 Dec 19. p. 93–108.
20. Silverman BL, Metzger BE, Cho NH, Loeb CA. Impaired glucose tolerance in adolescent offspring of diabetic mothers: relationship to fetal hyperinsulinism. Diabetes Care. 1995;18:611–7.
21. Clausen TD, Mathiesen ER, Hansen T, Pedersen O, Jensen DM, Lauenborg J, et al. Overweight and the metabolic syndrome in adult offspring of women with diet-treated gestational diabetes mellitus or type 1 diabetes. J Clin Endocrinol Metab. 2009;94:2464–70.
22. World MA. World medical association declaration of Helsinki: ethical principles for medical research involving human subjects. J Int Bioethique. 2004;15:124–9.
23. Rodekamp E, Harder T, Kohlhoff R, Franke K, Dudenhausen JW, Plagemann A. Long-term impact of breast-feeding on body weight and glucose tolerance in children of diabetic mothers: role of the late neonatal period and early infancy. Diabetes Care. 2005;28:1457–62.
24. Plagemann A, Harder T, Rodekamp E, Kohlhoff R. Rapid neonatal weight gain increases risk of childhood overweight in offspring of diabetic mothers. J Perinat Med. 2012;40:557–63.
25. Gemeinsamer Bundesausschuss. Mutterpass. https://www.g-ba.de/downloads/17-98-4071/2016-02-16_Mutterpass_englisch_WEB_WZ.pdf. Accessed 12 July 2017.
26. Rasmussen KM, Yaktine AL. EdsWeight gain during pregnancy: reexamining the guidelines. Washington, DC: National Academies Press; 2009.
27. Deutsche Gesellschaft für Gynäkologie und Geburtshilfe. Diabetes und Schwangerschaft. https://www.dggg.de/fileadmin/documents/leitlinien/archiviert/beteiligt/057023_Diabetes_und_Schwangerschaft/057023_2008.pdf. Accessed 15 July 2017.
28. Carpenter MW, Coustan DR. Criteria for screening tests for gestational diabetes. Am J Obstet Gynecol. 1982;144:768–73.
29. American Diabetes Association. Standards of medical care in diabetes - 2016. Section 12. Management of diabetes in pregnancy. Diabetes Care 2016;39 Suppl 1:S94–S98.
30. Deutsche Gesellschaft für Gynäkologie und Geburtshilfe. Diagnostik und Therapie hypertensiver Schwangerschaftserkrankungen. https://www.dggg.de/fileadmin/documents/leitlinien/archiviert/federfuehrend/015018_Diagnostik_und_Therapie_hypertensiver_Schwangerschaftserkrankungen/015018_2008.pdf. Accessed 15 July 2017.
31. HAPO Study Cooperative Research Group. The hyperglycemia and adverse pregnancy outcome (HAPO) study. Int J Gynaecol Obstet. 2002;78:69–77.
32. Alshimmiri MM, Hammoud MS, Al-Saleh EA, Alsaeid KMS. Ethnic variations in birthweight percentiles in Kuwait. Paediatr Perinat Epidemiol. 2003;17:355–62.
33. Voigt M, Fusch C, Olbertz D, Hartmann K, Rochow N, Renken C, et al. Analyse des Neugeborenenkollektivs der Bundesrepublik Deutschland. Geburtshilfe Frauenheilkd. 2006;66:956–70.
34. Kurtoğlu S, Hatipoğlu N, Mazicioğlu MM, Akin MA, Çoban D, Gökoğlu S, et al. Body weight, length and head circumference at birth in a cohort of Turkish newborns. J Clin Res Pediatr Endocrinol. 2012;4:132–9.
35. Templeton GF. A two step approach for transforming continuous variables to normal: implications and recommendations for IS research. CAIS. 2011;28. 41–58. Available at: http://aisel.aisnet.org/cais/vol28/iss1/4.
36. O 'Tierney-Ginn P, Presley L, Minium J, Hauguel-de Mouzon S, Catalano PM. Sex-specific effects of maternal anthropometrics on body composition at birth. Am J Obstet Gynecol. 2014;211:292.e1–9.
37. Langer O, Yogev Y, Xenakis EMJ, Brustman L. Overweight and obese in gestational diabetes: the impact on pregnancy outcome. Am J Obstet Gynecol. 2005;192:1768–76.
38. Yogev Y, Langer O. Pregnancy outcome in obese and morbidly obese gestational diabetic women. Eur J Obstet Gynecol Reprod Biol. 2008;137:21–6.
39. Casey BM, Mele L, Landon MB, Spong CY, Ramin SM, Wapner RJ, et al. Does maternal body mass index influence treatment effect in women with mild gestational diabetes? Am J Perinatol. 2015;32:93–100.
40. Roman AS, Rebarber A, Fox NS, Klauser CK, Istwan N, Rhea D, et al. The effect of maternal obesity on pregnancy outcomes in women with gestational diabetes. J Matern Fetal Neonatal Med. 2011;24:723–7.
41. Schaefer-Graf UM, Heuer R, Kilavuz O, Pandura A, Henrich W, Vetter K. Maternal obesity not maternal glucose values correlates best with high rates of fetal macrosomia in pregnancies complicated by gestational diabetes. J Perinat Med. 2002;30:313–21.
42. Schaefer-Graf UM, Kjos SL, Kilavuz O, Plagemann A, Brauer M, Dudenhausen JW, et al. Determinants of fetal growth at different periods of pregnancies complicated by gestational diabetes mellitus or impaired glucose tolerance. Diabetes Care. 2003;26:193–8.
43. Most O, Langer O. Gestational diabetes: maternal weight gain in relation to fetal growth, treatment modality, BMI and glycemic control. J Matern Fetal Neonatal Med. 2012;25:2458–63.
44. Berggren EK, Stuebe AM, Boggess KA. Excess maternal weight gain and large for gestational age risk among women with gestational diabetes. Am J Perinatol. 2015;32:251–6.
45. Egan AM, Dennedy MC, Al-Ramli W, Heerey A, Avalos G, Dunne F. ATLANTIC-DIP: excessive gestational weight gain and pregnancy outcomes in women with gestational or pregestational diabetes mellitus. J Clin Endocrinol Metab. 2014;99:212–9.
46. Miao M, Dai M, Zhang Y, Sun F, Guo X, Sun G. Influence of maternal overweight, obesity and gestational weight gain on the perinatal outcomes in women with gestational diabetes mellitus. Sci Rep. 2017;7:305. https://doi.org/10.1038/s41598-017-00441-z.
47. Plagemann A, Harder T, Kohlhoff R, Rohde W, Dörner G. Overweight and obesity in infants of mothers with long-term insulin-dependent diabetes or gestational diabetes overweight and obesity in infants of mothers with long-term insulin-dependent diabetes or gestational diabetes. Int J Obes Relat Metab Disord. 1997;21:451–6.
48. Plagemann A, Harder T, Kohlhoff R, Rohde W, Dörner G. Glucose tolerance and insulin secretion in children of mothers with pregestational IDDM or gestational diabetes. Diabetologia. 1997;40:1094–100.
49. Freinkel N, Metzger BE. Pregnancy as a tissue culture experience: the critical implications of maternal metabolism for fetal development; in pregnancy metabolism, diabetes and the fetus. Ciba Found Symp. 1978;63:3–28.
50. Donnelly JM, Lindsay KL, Walsh JM, Horan M, Molloy EJ, McAuliffe FM. Fetal metabolic influences of neonatal anthropometry and adiposity. BMC Pediatr. 2015;15:175. https://doi.org/10.1186/s12887-015-0499-0.
51. Christou H, Connors JM, Ziotopoulou M, Hatzidakis V, Papathanassoglou E, Ringer SA, et al. Cord blood leptin and insulin-like growth factor levels are independent predictors of fetal growth. J Clin Endocrinol Metab. 2001;86:935–8.

52. Shekhawat PS, Garland JS, Shivpuri C, Mick GJ, Sasidharan P, Pelz CJ, et al. Neonatal cord blood leptin: its relationship to birth weight, body mass index, maternal diabetes, and steroids. Pediatr Res. 1998;43:338–43.
53. Tapanainen P, Leinonen E, Ruokonen A, Knip M. Leptin concentrations are elevated in newborn infants of diabetic mothers. Horm Res. 2001;55:185–90.
54. Okereke NC, Uvena-Celebrezze J, Hutson-Presley L, Amini SB, Catalano PM. The effect of gender and gestational diabetes mellitus on cord leptin concentration. Am J Obstet Gynecol. 2002;187:798–803.
55. Catalano PM, Presley L, Minium J, Hauguel-de Mouzon S. Fetuses of obese mothers develop insulin resistance in utero. Diabetes Care. 2009;32:1076–80.
56. Lawlor DA, West J, Fairley L, Nelson SM, Bhopal RS, Tuffnell D, et al. Pregnancy glycaemia and cord-blood levels of insulin and leptin in Pakistani and white British mother-offspring pairs : findings from a prospective pregnancy cohort. Diabetologia. 2014;57:2492–500.
57. Weiss PMA, Scholz HS, Haas J, Tamussino KE, Seissler J, Borkenstein MH. Long-term follow-up of infants of mothers with type 1 diabetes. Diabetes Care. 2000;23:905–11.
58. Ong KK, Diderholm B, Salzano G, Wingate D, Hughes IA, MacDougall J, et al. Pregnancy insulin, glucose, and BMI contribute to birth outcomes in nondiabetic mothers. Diabetes Care. 2008;31:2193–7.
59. Badon SE, Dyer AR, Josefson JL. Gestational weight gain and neonatal adiposity in the hyperglycemia and adverse pregnancy outcome study-north American region. Obesity (Silver Spring). 2014;22:1731–8.
60. Ehrenberg HM, Mercer BM, Catalano PM. The influence of obesity and diabetes on the prevalence of macrosomia. Am J Obstet Gynecol. 2004;191:964–8.
61. Black MH, Sacks DA, Xiang AH, Lawrence JM. The relative contribution of prepregnancy overweight and obesity, gestational weight gain, and IADPSG-defined gestational diabetes mellitus to fetal overgrowth. Diabetes Care. 2013;36:56–62.
62. Damm P, Mersebach H, Råstam J, Kaaja R, Hod M, McCance DR, et al. Poor pregnancy outcome in women with type 1 diabetes is predicted by elevated HbA1c and spikes of high glucose values in the third trimester. J Matern Fetal Neonatal Med. 2014;27:149–54.
63. Ensenauer R, Brandlhuber L, Burgmann M, Sobotzki C, Zwafink C, Anzill S, et al. Obese nondiabetic pregnancies and high maternal glycated hemoglobin at delivery as an indicator of offspring and maternal postpartum risks : the prospective PEACHES mother-child cohort. Clin Chem. 2015;61:1381–90.
64. Cyganek K, Skupien J, Katra B, Hebda-Szydlo A, Janas I, Trznadel-Morawska I, et al. Risk of macrosomia remains glucose-dependent in a cohort of women with pregestational type 1 diabetes and good glycemic control. Endocrine. 2017;55:447–55.
65. Ouyang F, Parker MG, Luo ZC, Wang X, Zhang HJ, Jiang F, et al. Maternal BMI, gestational diabetes, and weight gain in relation to childhood obesity: the mediation effect of placental weight. Obesity (Silver Spring). 2016;24:938–46.
66. Griffiths LJ, Dezateux C, Cole TJ. Differential parental weight and height contributions to offspring birthweight and weight gain in infancy. Int J Epidemiol. 2007;36:104–7.
67. Brooks AA, Johnson MR, Steer PJ, Pawson ME, Abdalla HI. Birth weight: nature or nurture? Early Hum Dev. 1995;42:29–35.
68. Lederman SA, Paxton A. Maternal reporting of prepregnancy weight and birth outcome: consistency and completeness compared with the clinical record. Matern Child Health J. 1998;2:123–6.
69. Matsuda J, Yokota I, Iida M, Murakami T, Naito E, Ito M, et al. Serum leptin concentration in cord blood: relationship to birth weight and gender. J Clin Endocrinol Metab. 1997;82:1642–4.

8

Prevalence and risk factors of gestational diabetes mellitus: findings from a universal screening feasibility program in Lima, Peru

Gloria T. Larrabure-Torrealva[1,2], Stephanie Martinez[3], Miguel Angel Luque-Fernandez[3], Sixto E. Sanchez[4,5], Pedro A. Mascaro[1,2], Hugo Ingar[1], Walter Castillo[1], Rina Zumaeta[1], Mirtha Grande[4], Vicky Motta[4], Percy Pacora[2], Bizu Gelaye[3*] and Michelle A. Williams[3]

Abstract

Background: Gestational diabetes mellitus (GDM) is a global public health concern with potential implications for the health of a mother and her offspring. However, data on the prevalence and risk factors of GDM in Latin America are scarce.
The study was designed to estimate the prevalence of GDM and identify maternal risk factors among Peruvian women.

Methods: A cross-sectional study was conducted among 1300 pregnant women attending a prenatal clinic in Lima, Peru. GDM was diagnosed using an Oral Glucose Tolerance Test (OGTT) performed between 24 and 28 gestational weeks using the International Association of Diabetes and Pregnancy Study Groups (IADPSG) criteria. Depression status was assessed using the Patient Health Questionnaire-9. Multivariate logistic regression models were used to identify risk factors of GDM.

Results: Approximately 16% of pregnant women were diagnosed with GDM. The prevalence of obesity and depression were 24.4 and 10.6%, respectively. After adjusting for confounders, mid-pregnancy obesity was associated with a 1.64-fold increased odds of GDM (OR: 1.64; 95% CI: 1.03–2.61). Participants with a family history of diabetes had a 1.5-fold increased odds of developing GDM (OR: 1.51, 95% CI: 1.10–2.07) as compared to women without this family history. Depression was associated with a 1.54-fold increased odds of GDM (OR: 1.54; 95% CI:1.09–2.17).

Conclusions: GDM is highly prevalent and was associated with maternal obesity, family history of diabetes and antepartum depression among Peruvian women. Intervention programs aimed at early diagnoses and management of GDM need to take maternal obesity, family history of diabetes and antepartum depression into account.

Keywords: Diabetes mellitus, Gestational diabetes mellitus, Obesity, Depression, Pregnancy, IADPSG criteria, Peru

Background

Gestational diabetes mellitus (GDM) is a non-communicable disease affecting pregnant women [1, 2]. Globally the median estimates of GDM range from 6 to 13% [2]. In the United States, recent estimates show up to 9% of all pregnancies are complicated by GDM [3]. In Central and South America, the recent overall prevalence of GDM is estimated at 11% [2]. There is well-established evidence showing that women with GDM are at risk for preeclampsia [4, 5], premature birth [6], increased risk of cesarean section [4, 5] and later development of type 2 diabetes [2]. GDM is also associated with increased risk of perinatal complications including malformations [7], shoulder dystocia [5], neonatal hypoglycemia [8], and perinatal mortality [8, 9].

Obesity and a family history of diabetes have been consistently identified as major risk factors for GDM in previous studies [3]. Other risk factors for GDM include

* Correspondence: belaye@hsph.harvard.edu; bgelaye@hsph.harvard.edu
[3]Department of Epidemiology, Harvard T.H. Chan School of Public Health, 677 Huntington Avenue, Kresge 505F, Boston, MA 02115, USA

advanced maternal age [10], nonwhite race [10, 11], previous unexplained stillbirth [12, 13], and obesity [10, 13]. In addition to increased GDM risk, maternal obesity increases the risk of multiple adverse maternal health outcomes including thrombosis [14], gestational hypertension [15], preeclampsia [16–18], preterm delivery [19], and cesarean section [16, 18]. Of note, significant neonatal complications have been associated with obesity and GDM. These include congenital anomalies [20, 21], macrosomia [22], and birth injury [23, 24]. An expanding body of evidence now implicates unipolar major depressive disorder as one of the major risk factors for and conditions co-occurring with GDM [25], although the evidence is inconsistent [26].

Peru, a middle-income country, is one of the countries experiencing an epidemiologic transition with increasing burden of non-communicable disease risk factors [27, 28]. A 2014 national survey in Peru of people ≥15 years old showed the prevalence of overweight is 35% and the prevalence of obesity is 18% of the population [29]. However, the prevalence of GDM and its risk factors have not been investigated in Peru. Given this gap in the literature and the increased burden of non-communicable diseases in the country, we sought to examine the prevalence of GDM and associated risk factors in a cohort of pregnant women in Lima, Peru.

Methods

Study population

The Screening Treatment and Effective Management of Gestational Diabetes Mellitus (STEM-GDM) was designed to evaluate the prevalence of GDM among Peruvian women attending perinatal care and to provide evidence to improve the local guidelines for standardized GDM screening/diagnosis, effective management, and treatment. Participants were 1300 pregnant women attending prenatal care clinic at the Instituto Nacional Materno Perinatal (INMP) in Lima, Peru (Additional file 1). Recruitment occurred between February 2013 and June 2014. The Instituto Nacional Materno Perinatal (INMP), overseen by the Peruvian Ministry of Health, is the primary referral center for maternal and perinatal care in Lima, Peru.

Women were eligible if they were at least 18 years of age, had a gestational age of 24 to 28 gestational weeks, and could speak, read and write Spanish. Participants were excluded if they planned to deliver at another hospital or location, date of last menstrual period not certain and not confirmed by ultrasound exam performed prior to 24 weeks of gestation, unable to complete an oral glucose tolerance test (OGTT), known to have a multiple pregnancy, had a previous diagnosis of overt diabetes requiring treatment with medication before the pregnancy, or were currently receiving medical treatment for chronic diseases, such as oral glucocorticoids, thiazide diuretics, β-blockers, ACE inhibitors, oral β-mimetics, Dilantin, or antiretroviral agents. All participants provided written informed consent. Study procedures were approved by institutional review boards of the INMP, Lima, Peru and the Harvard T.H. Chan School of Public Health Office of Human Research Administration, Boston, MA, USA.

Gestational Diabetes Mellitus (GDM) assessment

GDM cases were identified using the OGTT, which is considered the gold standard for this diagnosis. For the OGTT test, participants were appointed to the laboratory at INMP between 8 AM to 9 AM after 8-h overnight fasting. A trained lab technician obtained a basal venous blood sample of $15cm^3$ for measuring fasting plasma glucose (PG). Participants were administered 75 g of anhydrous oral glucose dissolved in 250 ml of water. After 1 and 2 h, new venous blood samples were obtained for measuring PG levels. Plasma glucose value was measured by the glucose oxidase-peroxidase method in duplicate using an auto-analyzer for biochemical tests. Standard clinical laboratory quality control assessment of the OGTT testing was completed to assure reliability and validity of measured plasma glucose.

Interpretation of the OGTT

According to the standard OGTT testing procedures outlined by the IADPSG recommendations [30], pregnant women were considered to have GDM if fasting plasma glucose (PG) was ≥92 mg/dl (5.1 mmol/l), 1 h-h PG ≥180 mg/dl (10 mmol/l), and/or 2-h PG ≥153 mg/dL (≥8.5 mmol/L). Overall, 205 women were diagnosed with GDM. Of the GDM diagnosed women, 186 women (90.7%) had a fasting PG ≥ 92 mg/dl, 29 women (14.1%) had a 1-h PG ≥180 mg/dl, and 24 women (11.7%) had a 2-h PG ≥153 mg/dL. Women diagnosed with GDM received glucometers, nutritional advice, and clinical care to manage their condition.

Sociodemographic characteristics

Women were interviewed using a structured questionnaire to collect detailed information on sociodemographic, lifestyle characteristics, medical and reproductive history. Sociodemographic information collected included participants' age, family history of diabetes mellitus among first degree-relatives, body weight, height, smoking status, and alcohol use. Other covariates included maternal and paternal education (≤6, 7–12, > 12 years); ethnicity (Mestizo vs. others); marital status (married/living with partner vs. others); employment status (employed vs. not employed); difficulty paying for the basics (very hard/hard, somewhat hard, not very hard); difficulty accessing medical care (very hard/hard, somewhat hard, not very hard); food insecurity (no vs. yes), and perceived health during pregnancy.

Pre-pregnancy body mass index (BMI) and mid-pregnancy BMI were calculated as weight (in kilograms) divided by the square of height (in meters and used to identify normal weight (BMI < 25 kg/m^2), overweight (BMI: 25–29.9 kg/m^2), and obese (BMI ≥ 30 kg/m^2)) women. Due to the small number of underweight women, this group was merged with normal weight women. For the purpose of our analysis, obesity was grouped into a single category of BMI of 30.0 kg/m^2 and higher. Depression status was assessed using the 9-item Spanish-language Patient Health Questionnaire-9 (PHQ-9) [31, 32], which has been validated in a population of pregnant Peruvian women [33]. The PHQ-9 score was calculated by assigning a score between 0 and 3 to the response categories of "not at all," "several days," "more than half the days," and "nearly every day." Depression was defined as a PHQ-9 score ≥ 10.

Statistical analysis

Sociodemographic characteristics were evaluated using numbers (%) for categorical variables and means (± standard deviations) for continuous variables. Chi-square tests and Student's t-tests were conducted to compare distributions between women with and without GDM. Prevalence estimates were determined for GDM in relation to socio-demographic and behavioral characteristics. Adjusting for covariates of interest, we used multivariable logistic regression procedures to calculate odds ratios (OR) and 95% confidence intervals (95% CI) to estimate associations of GDM with risk factors. Forward logistic regression modeling procedures combined with the change-in-estimate approach were used to select the final report models [34]. Variables of a priori interest (e.g., age and BMI) were forced into final models. All analyses were performed using IBM's SPSS Statistical Software for Windows (IBM SPSS Version 22, Chicago, Illinois, USA). All reported p-values are two-sided and deemed statistically significant at $\alpha = 0.05$.

Results

Maternal sociodemographic and reproductive characteristics of the study population are presented in Table 1. The average age of study participants was 28.9 years (± 6.1). A majority of participants were married or living with a partner (86.5%), Mestizo (98.1%), and unemployed (67.8%) (Table 1). The overall prevalence of GDM in our population of Peruvian pregnant women was 15.8%. The prevalence of mid-pregnancy obesity was 24.5% while 10.6% of them had depression. Compared to women without GDM, women with GDM were significantly older ($p = 0.013$), more likely to report a family history of diabetes ($p = 0.005$), have higher mid-pregnancy BMI ($p = 0.016$) and have depression ($p = 0.012$). The prevalence of GDM increased significantly with the presence of family history of diabetes mellitus (p = 0.005) and maternal mid-pregnancy obesity ($p = 0.02$) (Fig. 1).

In an unadjusted bivariate analysis, participants with a family history of diabetes had 1.53-fold increased risk of GDM (OR: 1.53, 95%CI: 1.13–2.07), and participants with mid-pregnancy obesity had 1.83-fold increased risk of GDM compared to those of normal weight (OR: 1.83, 95%CI: 1.19–2.81) (Table 2). Compared to non-depressed participants, those with depression had a 1.5-fold increased odds of GDM (OR: 1.52, 95%CI: 1.09–2.12). After adjusting for age and family history of diabetes, the association between depression status and GDM remained significant (OR: 1.53, 95%CI: 1.09–2.14). In a multivariate model, a family history of diabetes remained significantly associated with GDM (OR: 1.51, 95%CI: 1.10–2.07), mid-pregnancy obesity slightly increased the risk for GDM (OR: 1.64, 95%CI: 1.03–2.61), and depression was also significantly associated with GDM (OR: 1.54, 95%CI: 1.09–2.17) (Table 2).

Discussion

To the best of our knowledge, this is the first study to examine the prevalence of GDM in Lima, Peru using the IADPSG criteria, as well as the presence of family history of diabetes mellitus, maternal mid-pregnancy obesity, and maternal depression as independent risk factors of GDM. Approximately 16% of pregnant women were diagnosed with GDM. The prevalence of obesity was 24% and the prevalence of depression was 11%. A previous study by Sacks et al. using IADPSG criteria and a multinational cohort (n = 23,957) reported the prevalence of GDM varies from 9 to 26% and is associated with older maternal age, BMI, family history of diabetes, mean OGTT glucose values, and ethnicity [35]. Globally, the prevalence of GDM varies by study setting and diagnostic criteria. Additional influencing factors include age, obesity, and use of health services. For instance, using International Classification of Diseases (ICD) diagnostic codes (ICD-9 and ICD-10), GDM prevalence was reported as 6% in the USA [36], and 10% in Korea [37]. A meta-analysis of 22 studies in sub-Saharan Africa with a range of diagnostic criteria and study setting reported a GDM prevalence of 2–6% [13]. A study in China using a 75-g 2-h OGTT reported a GDM prevalence of 8%. A higher percentage of GDM diagnoses were made by fasting PG than 1- or 2-h glucose levels compared to previous estimates.

We found a significant association between GDM and mid-pregnancy obesity (BMI > 25). Maternal age of 30 years or older and family history of diabetes were also significantly associated with GDM. Our results are in general agreement with previous studies that have identified similar associations with GDM risk factors. For example, Kumari et al., found a GDM prevalence of 24.5%

Table 1 Maternal sociodemographic characteristics (*N* = 1300)

Characteristics	All participants (*N* = 1300)		No GDM (*N* = 1095)		GDM (*N* = 205)		*P*-value
	n	%	n	%	n	%	
Maternal age (years)[a]	28.86 ± 6.14		28.68 ± 6.06		29.83 ± 6.49		*0.013*
Maternal age (years)							
< 19	49	3.8	43	3.9	6	2.9	0.081
20–29	669	51.5	578	52.8	91	44.4	
30–34	313	24.1	258	23.6	55	26.8	
≥35	269	20.7	216	19.7	53	25.9	
Ethnicity							
Mestizo	1275	98.1	1074	98.1	201	98.0	0.974
Other	25	1.9	21	1.9	4	2.0	
Marital status							
Married or living with partner	1123	86.5	946	86.5	177	86.3	0.960
Single or living alone/divorced	176	13.5	148	13.5	28	13.7	
Educational Status (years)	12.17 ± 2.38		12.16 ± 2.39		12.25 ± 2.33		0.604
Maternal education (years)							
≤6	39	3.0	34	3.1	5	2.4	0.743
7–12	698	53.7	591	54.0	107	52.2	
> 12	563	43.3	470	42.9	93	45.4	
Paternal education (years)							
≤6	30	2.3	27	2.5	3	1.5	0.318
7–12	727	56.4	620	57.0	107	53.0	
> 12	532	41.3	440	40.5	92	45.5	
Employment							
No	881	67.8	733	66.9	148	72.2	0.140
Yes	419	32.2	362	33.1	57	27.8	
Pre-pregnancy BMI (kg/m^2)							
< 25 (normal weight)	684	53.6	580	53.8	104	52.3	0.137
25–29.9 (overweight)	446	34.9	382	35.4	64	32.2	
≥30 (obese)	147	11.5	116	10.8	31	15.6	
Mid-pregnancy BMI (kg/m^2)							
< 25 (normal weight)	324	25.0	284	26.1	40	19.5	*0.016*
25–29.9 (overweight)	653	50.5	553	50.8	100	48.8	
≥30 (obese)	317	24.5	252	23.1	65	31.7	
Family history of diabetes							
No/Don't Know	834	64.2	720	65.8	114	114	*0.005*
Yes	466	35.8	375	34.2	91	44.4	
Depression	138	10.6	106	9.7	32	15.6	*0.012*
Perceived health during pregnancy							
Excellent	18	1.4	14	1.3	4	2.0	0.696
Very Good	76	5.8	67	6.1	9	4.4	
Good	586	45.1	488	44.6	98	47.8	
Fair	568	43.7	483	44.1	85	41.5	
Poor	52	4.0	43	3.9	9	4.4	

Table 1 Maternal sociodemographic characteristics ($N = 1300$) *(Continued)*

Characteristics	All participants ($N = 1300$)		No GDM ($N = 1095$)		GDM ($N = 205$)		*P*-value
	n	%	n	%	n	%	
Difficulty paying for basics							
Very hard/hard	199	15.3	171	15.6	28	13.7	0.759
Somewhat hard	441	34.0	369	33.8	72	35.1	
Not very hard	658	50.7	553	50.6	105	51.2	
Food insecurity							
No	446	34.3	379	34.6	67	32.7	0.593
Yes	854	65.7	716	65.4	138	67.3	
Difficulties to access medical care							
Very hard/hard	248	19.1	207	18.9	41	20.0	0.728
Somewhat hard	897	69.1	760	69.5	137	66.8	
Not very hard	154	11.9	127	11.6	27	13.2	

[a]mean ± standard deviation
Italicized *p*-values are statistically significant at $\alpha = 0.05$

in obese compared to 2.2% in non-obese women ($P < 0.0001$) [38]. In a retrospective cohort study of 613 obese (BMI > 35; class II and III) and 11,313 non-obese women, there was a threefold increase of GDM for obese patients compared to non-obese women (OR: 3.2, 95%CI: 2.5–4.2) [39]. In a recent meta-analysis of published literature, Chu and colleagues reported ORs of developing GDM of 2.14 (95% CI: 1.82–2.53), 3.56 (95% CI: 3.05–4.21), and 8.56 (95% CI: 5.07–16.04) among overweight, obese, and severely obese compared with normal-weight pregnant women, respectively [40]. According to Kim et al. in a study of pregnant women from Florida, USA, the likelihood of GDM increased with increasing BMI was significant for all racial/ethnic groups investigated [41]. Additionally, the proportion of GDM cases attributable to overweight and obesity was 41.1% overall [41]. The HAPO Study Cooperative Research Group has demonstrated that

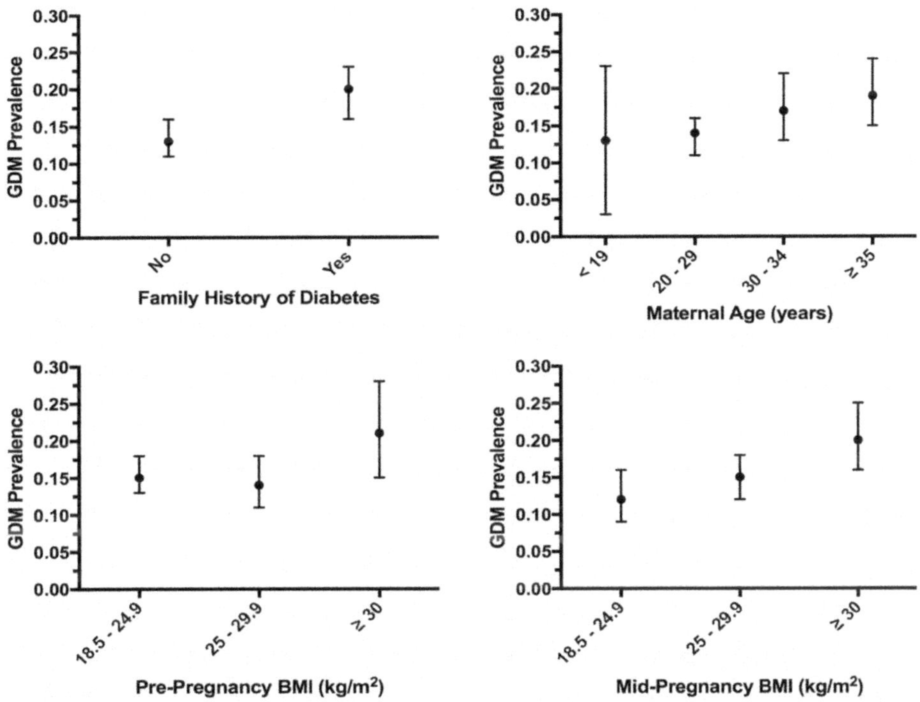

Fig. 1 Prevalence of GDM by family history of diabetes mellitus among first degree-relatives, maternal age, pre-pregnancy BMI, and mid-pregnancy BMI. Point estimates and 95%CI are reported

Table 2 Prevalence and risk factors of gestational diabetes ($N = 1300$)

Characteristics	Crude OR (95%CI)	Age and family history of diabetes adjusted OR (95%CI)[a]	Multivariate OR (95%CI)[b]
Maternal age (years)	1.03 (1.01–1.06)	–	1.03 (1.00–1.06)
Ethnicity			
Mestizo	Reference	Reference	Reference
Other	1.02 (0.35–3.00)	1.05 (0.35–3.10)	1.01 (0.34–3.02)
Marital status			
Married or living with partner	Reference	Reference	Reference
Single or living alone/divorced	1.01 (0.66–1.56)	1.10 (0.70–1.71)	1.04 (0.66–1.66)
Maternal education (years)			
≤6	Reference	Reference	Reference
7–12	1.23 (0.47–3.22)	0.79 (0.3–2.11)	1.13 (0.42–3.03)
> 12	1.35 (0.51–3.53)	0.92 (0.69–1.27)	1.13 (0.41–3.10)
Partner education (years)			
≤6	Reference	Reference	Reference
7–12	1.55 (0.46–5.21)	0.52 (0.15–1.76)	1.72 (0.50–5.88)
> 12	1.88 (0.56–6.34)	0.85 (0.63–1.16)	1.98 (0.57–6.86)
Pre-pregnancy BMI (kg/m^2)			
< 25 (normal weight)	Reference	Reference	Reference
25–29.9 (overweight)	0.93 (0.67–1.31)	0.86 (0.61–1.21)	0.90 (0.63–1.27)
≥30 (obese)	1.49 (0.95–2.33)	1.22 (0.76–1.95)	1.29 (0.80–2.07)
Mid-pregnancy BMI (kg/m^2)			
< 25 (normal weight)	Reference	Reference	Reference
25–29.9 (overweight)	1.28 (0.87–1.90)	1.18 (0.79–1.77)	1.23 (0.82–1.87)
≥30 (obese)	1.83 (1.19–2.81)	1.54 (0.98–2.41)	1.64 (1.03–2.61)
P-value for trend			0.033
Family history of diabetes			
No/Don't know	Reference	–	Reference
Yes	1.53 (1.13–2.07)	–	1.51 (1.10–2.07)
Depression			
No	Reference	Reference	Reference
Yes	1.52 (1.09–2.12)	1.53 (1.09–2.14)	1.54 (1.09–2.17)
Perceived health during pregnancy			
Excellent	Reference	Reference	Reference
Very good	0.47 (.13–1.74)	0.52 (0.14–1.93)	0.62 (0.16–2.34)
Good	0.70 (0.23–2.18)	0.75 (0.24–2.35)	0.89 (0.28–2.82)
Fair	0.62 (0.20–1.92)	0.63 (0.20–1.97)	0.69 (0.22–2.21)
Poor	0.73 (0.20–2.75)	0.73 (0.19–2.76)	0.76 (0.20–2.92)
Difficulty paying for basics			
Very hard/hard	Reference	Reference	Reference
Somewhat hard	1.19 (0.74–1.91)	1.24 (0.77–1.99)	1.18 (0.73–1.93)
Not very hard	1.16 (0.74–1.82)	1.25 (0.79–1.97)	1.19 (0.74–1.91)

[a]Adjusted for age (continuous) and family history of diabetes mellitus among first degree-relatives (yes vs. no/don't know)
[b]Main multivariate regression model adjusted for all characteristics (maternal age, ethnicity, marital status, maternal education, paternal education, mid-pregnancy BMI, family history of diabetes, depression, perceived health during pregnancy, and difficulty paying for the basics) except pre-pregnancy BMI and OR (95%CI) from this model are reported here. A second multivariate regression model adjusted for all covariates except mid-pregnancy BMI and the OR (95%CI) for pre-pregnancy BMI is reported from this model

higher maternal BMI is associated with increased likelihood of pregnancy complications, including complications related to fetal growth, adiposity, and preeclampsia [42].

There is a growing body of epidemiologic evidence that shows depression as a risk factor for GDM [43, 44]. Our study results showing a significant association between depression and GDM is in general agreement with some prior studies [25, 43] but not all [26]. Recently, a longitudinal study in the USA from Hinkle et al. found that persistently high depression scores in the 1st and 2nd trimesters were associated with three-fold increased risk of GDM (highest vs lowest quartile in both trimesters: RR: 3.21, 95% CI: 1.00–10.28) [43]. In a cross-sectional study, women with GDM were more than three times more likely to have a history of depression compared to non-depressed women (OR: 3.79, 95% CI: 1.07–13.45) [25]. However, using data from prenatal care clinics at a University of Washington Medical Center, Katon et al. found no evidence of association between GDM and antepartum depression (OR = 0.95; 95%CI: 0.68–1.33) [26]. In a addition, a 2016 meta-analysis shows there is no clear consensus on the association between depression and diabetes during pregnancy and additional studies are needed [45]. Although we do not have a clear explanation for these findings, we speculate that differences in nutrition, physical activity, and other lifestyle characteristics may have contributed to the observed differences. Pregnancy is a major life event that increases vulnerability to depression, and pregnant women who have comorbid depression and GDM with serious implications for both maternal and infant outcomes.

This study had several strengths, including the use of trained interviewers and standard laboratory procedures for measuring plasma glucose. Our relatively large sample size and the high prevalence of gestational diabetes give us statistical power to study the associations of interest. However, some limitations must be considered when interpreting the results of our study. First, a family history of diabetes was assessed based on self-report; therefore, we cannot rule out recall bias. Additionally, previous studies have shown associations between GDM and adverse pregnancy outcomes. However, information on pregnancy outcomes was not collected in our study cohort. Lastly, participants in this study were pregnant women living in Lima, and the results may not be generalizable to the whole Peruvian population. Future studies that collect objective measures potentially associated with GDM and obesity may overcome concerns about these potential errors.

Conclusion

Overweight and obesity may be prevented by implementing a healthy lifestyle that includes physical activity and nutritional counseling before pregnancy. If women are already obese when they become pregnant, O'Dwyer et al. suggests early screening for women with a body mass index > 34.9 kg/m in order to optimize maternal glycemic control during pregnancy [46]. In a retrospective cohort study, Lutsic et al. found that the proportion of women with maternal or delivery complications was highest among overweight or obese depressed pregnant women [47]. These studies provide evidence of a high prevalence of GDM in women with an elevated mid-pregnancy BMI and depression. GDM is prevalent in this population, especially in overweight/obese and depressed pregnant women. Our findings may be used to develop and implement programs aimed at supporting high-risk mothers in antenatal care.

Abbreviations

BMI: Body mass index; GDM: Gestational diabetes mellitus; IADPSG : International Association of Diabetes and Pregnancy Study Groups; INMP: Instituto Nacional Materno Perinatal; OGTT: Oral Glucose Tolerance Test; PHQ-9: Patient Health Questionnaire-9; STEM-GDM: Screening Treatment and Effective Management of Gestational Diabetes Mellitus

Acknowledgments

The authors wish to thank the dedicated staff members of Asociacion Civil Proyectos en Salud, Peru, and INMP, Peru, for their expert technical assistance with this research.

Funding

This research was supported by Roche Diagnostic Operations Inc., project number 208617-5074547 and National Institute for Minority Health and Health Disparities, National Institutes of Health (T37-MD0014490).

Authors' contributions

GLT, MALF, BG, SES, and MAW conceived and designed the study. SM, BG, SES, and MAW analyzed data and drafted the manuscript. GTL, SM, MALF, SES, PMS, JI, WC, RZ, MG, VM, PP, BG, and MAW interpreted the data, critically revised the draft for important intellectual content, and gave final approval of the manuscript to be published.

Consent for publication

Not applicable.

Competing interests

The authors declare that they have no competing interests and the content is solely the responsibility of the authors. The funding agency did not participate in the writing of the manuscript or the decision to submit it for publication.

Author details

[1]Instituto Nacional Materno Perinatal de Lima, Lima, Perú. [2]Departamentos de Medicina y Ginecología y Obstetricia, Universidad Nacional Mayor de San Marcos, Lima, Perú. [3]Department of Epidemiology, Harvard T.H. Chan School of Public Health, 677 Huntington Avenue, Kresge 505F, Boston, MA 02115,

USA. [4]Asociación Civil Proyectos en Salud, A.C. PROESA, Lima, Perú. [5]Facultad de Medicina, Universidad Particular San Martin de Porres, Lima, Peru.

References

1. Ferrara A. Increasing prevalence of gestational diabetes mellitus: a public health perspective. Diabetes Care. 2007;30(Suppl 2):S141–6.
2. Zhu Y, Zhang C. Prevalence of gestational diabetes and risk of progression to type 2 diabetes: a global perspective. Curr Diab Rep. 2016;16(1):7.
3. DeSisto CL, Kim SY, Sharma AJ. Prevalence estimates of gestational diabetes mellitus in the United States, Pregnancy Risk Assessment Monitoring System (PRAMS), 2007-2010. Prev Chronic Dis. 2014;11:E104.
4. Waters TP, Dyer AR, Scholtens DM, Dooley SL, Herer E, Lowe LP, Oats JJ, Persson B, Sacks DA, Metzger BE, et al. Maternal and neonatal morbidity for women who would be added to the diagnosis of GDM using IADPSG criteria: a secondary analysis of the hyperglycemia and adverse pregnancy outcome study. Diabetes Care. 2016;39:2204–10.
5. Fadl HE, Ostlund IK, Magnuson AF, Hanson US. Maternal and neonatal outcomes and time trends of gestational diabetes mellitus in Sweden from 1991 to 2003. Diabet Med. 2010;27(4):436–41.
6. Hedderson M. Gestational diabetes mellitus and lesser degrees of pregnancy hyperglycemia: association with increased risk of spontaneous preterm birth. Obstet Gynecol. 2003;102(4):850–6.
7. Sheffield J, Butler-Koster E, Casey B, McIntire D, Leveno K. Maternal diabetes mellitus and infant malformations. Obstet Gynecol. 2002;100(5 Pt 1):925–30.
8. Bartha JL, Martinez-Del-Fresno P, Comino-Delgado R. Gestational diabetes mellitus diagnosed during early pregnancy. Am J Obstet Gynecol. 2000; 182(2):346–50.
9. Wood S, Jick H, Sauve R. The risk of stillbirth in pregnancies before and after the onset of diabetes. Diabet Med. 2003;20(9):703–7.
10. Solomon C, Willett W, Carey V, Rich-Edwards J, Hunter D, Colditz G, Stampfer M, Speizer F, Spiegelman D, Manson J. A prospective study of pregravid determinants of gestational diabetes mellitus. JAMA. 1997;278(13): 1078–83.
11. Hunsberger M, Rosenberg KD, Donatelle RJ. Racial/ethnic disparities in gestational diabetes mellitus: findings from a population-based survey. Womens Health Issues. 2010;20(5):323–8.
12. McMahon M, Ananth C, Liston R. Gestational diabetes mellitus. Risk factors, obstetric complications and infant outcomes. J Reprod Med. 1998;43(4):372–8.
13. Mwanri AW, Kinabo J, Ramaiya K, Feskens EJ. Gestational diabetes mellitus in sub-Saharan Africa: systematic review and metaregression on prevalence and risk factors. Tropical Med Int Health. 2015;20(8):983–1002.
14. Larsen TB, Sorensen HT, Gislum M, Johnsen SP. Maternal smoking, obesity, and risk of venous thromboembolism during pregnancy and the puerperium: a population-based nested case-control study. Thromb Res. 2007;120(4):505–9.
15. Gaillard R, Steegers EA, Hofman A, Jaddoe VW. Associations of maternal obesity with blood pressure and the risks of gestational hypertensive disorders. The generation R study. J Hypertens. 2011;29(5):937–44.
16. Rahman MM, Abe SK, Kanda M, Narita S, Rahman MS, Bilano V, Ota E, Gilmour S, Shibuya K. Maternal body mass index and risk of birth and maternal health outcomes in low- and middle-income countries: a systematic review and meta-analysis. Obes Rev. 2015;16(9):758–70.
17. Young OM, Twedt R, Catov JM. Pre-pregnancy maternal obesity and the risk of preterm preeclampsia in the American primigravida. Obesity (Silver Spring). 2016;24(6):1226–9.
18. Vinturache A, Moledina N, McDonald S, Slater D, Tough S. Pre-pregnancy Body Mass Index (BMI) and delivery outcomes in a Canadian population. BMC Pregnancy Childbirth. 2014;14:422.
19. Cnattingius S, Villamor E, Johansson S, Bonamy AE, Persson M, Wikström A, Granath F. Maternal obesity and risk of preterm delivery. JAMA. 2013;309(22):2362–70.
20. Moore L, Singer M, Bradlee M, Rothman K, Milunsky A. A prospective study of the risk of congenital defects associated with maternal obesity and diabetes mellitus. Epidemiolog. 2000;11(6):689–94.
21. Martínez-Frías M, Frías J, Bermejo E, Rodríguez-Pinilla E, Prieto L, Frías J. Pre-gestational maternal body mass index predicts an increased risk of congenital malformations in infants of mothers with gestational diabetes. Diabet Med. 2005;22(6):775–81.
22. Ehrenberg HM, Mercer BM, Catalano PM. The influence of obesity and diabetes on the prevalence of macrosomia. Am J Obstet Gynecol. 2004;191(3):964–8.
23. Shoar Z, Zivot A, Nasiri S, Mandhani N, Kelly B. Maternal obesity, maternal gestational diabetes mellitus, and maternal and neonatal outcomes. J Obes Weight Loss Therapy. 2016;06(01):1-12.
24. Wendland EM, Torloni MR, Falavigna M, Trujillo J, Dode MA, Campos MA, Duncan BB, Schmidt MI. Gestational diabetes and pregnancy outcomes–a systematic review of the World Health Organization (WHO) and the International Association of Diabetes in Pregnancy Study Groups (IADPSG) diagnostic criteria. BMC Pregnancy Childbirth. 2012;12:23.
25. Byrn M, Penckofer S. The relationship between gestational diabetes and antenatal depression. J Obstet Gynecol Neonatal Nurs. 2015;44(2):246–55.
26. Katon JG, Russo J, Gavin AR, Melville JL, Katon WJ. Diabetes and depression in pregnancy: is there an association? J Women's Health (Larchmt). 2011;20(7):983–9.
27. Checkley W, Ghannem H, Irazola V, Kimaiyo S, Levitt NS, Miranda JJ, Niessen L, Prabhakaran D, Rabadan-Diehl C, Ramirez-Zea M, et al. Management of NCD in low- and middle-income countries. Glob Heart. 2014;9(4):431–43.
28. Nabel EG, Stevens S, Smith R. Combating chronic disease in developing countries. Lancet. 2009;373(9680):2004–6.
29. Informática INdEse. Peru Enfermedades No transmísibles y Transmisibles 2014. Lima: INEI; 2015. Available at: http://www.inei.gob.pe/media/MenuRecursivo/publicaciones_digitales/Est /Lib1212/Libro.pdf
30. International Association of D, Pregnancy Study Groups Consensus P, Metzger BE, Gabbe SG, Persson B, Buchanan TA, Catalano PA, Damm P, Dyer AR, Leiva A, et al. International association of diabetes and pregnancy study groups recommendations on the diagnosis and classification of hyperglycemia in pregnancy. Diabetes Care. 2010;33(3):676–82.
31. Wulsin L, Somoza E, Heck J. The feasibility of using the Spanish PHQ-9 to screen for depression in primary care in Honduras. Prim Care Companion J Clin Psychiatry. 2002;4(5):191–5.
32. Kroenke K, Spitzer R, Williams J. The PHQ-9: validity of a brief depression severity measure. J Gen Intern Med. 2001;16(9):606–13.
33. Zhong Q, Gelaye B, Fann JR, Sanchez SE, Williams MA. Cross-cultural validity of the Spanish version of PHQ-9 among pregnant Peruvian women: a Rasch item response theory analysis. J Affect Disord. 2014;158:148–53.
34. Rothman KJ, Greenland S, Lash TL: Modern Epidemiology. Philadelphia: Lippincott Williams & Wilkins; 2008.
35. Sacks D, Hadden D, Maresh M, Deerochanawong C, Dyer A, Metzger B, Lowe L, Coustan D, Hod M, Oats J, et al. Frequency of gestational diabetes mellitus at collaborating centers based on IADPSG consensus panel-recommended criteria: the Hyperglycemia and Adverse Pregnancy Outcome (HAPO) study. Diabetes Care. 2012;35(3):526–8.
36. Lavery JA, Friedman AM, Keyes KM, Wright JD, Ananth CV. Gestational diabetes in the United States: temporal changes in prevalence rates between 1979 and 2010. BJOG. 2017;24(5):804-13.
37. Koo BK, Lee JH, Kim J, Jang EJ, Lee CH. Prevalence of gestational diabetes mellitus in Korea: a National Health Insurance Database Study. PLoS One. 2016;11(4):e0153107.
38. Kumari A. Pregnancy outcome in women with morbid obesity. Int J Gynaecol Obstet. 2001;73(2):101–7.
39. Bianco A, Smilen S, Davis Y, Lopez S, Lapinski R, Lockwood C. Pregnancy outcome and weight gain recommendations for the morbidly obese woman. Obstet Gynecol. 1998;91(1):97–102.
40. Chu SY, Callaghan WM, Kim SY, Schmid CH, Lau J, England LJ, Dietz PM. Maternal obesity and risk of gestational diabetes mellitus. Diabetes Care. 2007;30(8):2070–6.
41. Kim SY, England L, Sappenfield W, Wilson HG, Bish CL, Salihu HM, Sharma AJ. Racial/ethnic differences in the percentage of gestational diabetes mellitus cases attributable to overweight and obesity, Florida, 2004-2007. Prev Chronic Dis. 2012;9:E88.

42. Group HSCR. Hyperglycaemia and Adverse Pregnancy Outcome (HAPO) study: associations with maternal body mass index. BJOG. 2010;117(5):575–84.
43. Hinkle SN, Buck Louis GM, Rawal S, Zhu Y, Albert PS, Zhang C. A longitudinal study of depression and gestational diabetes in pregnancy and the postpartum period. Diabetologia. 2016;59(12):2594–602.
44. Barakat S, Martinez D, Thomas M, Handley M. What do we know about gestational diabetes mellitus and risk for postpartum depression among ethnically diverse low-income women in the USA? Arch Womens Ment Health. 2014;17(6):587–92.
45. Ross GP, Falhammar H, Chen R, Barraclough H, Kleivenes O, Gallen I. Relationship between depression and diabetes in pregnancy: a systematic review. World J Diabetes. 2016;7(19):554–71.
46. O'Dwyer V, Farah N, Hogan J, O'Connor N, Kennelly MM, Turner MJ. Timing of screening for gestational diabetes mellitus in women with moderate and severe obesity. Acta Obstet Gynecol Scand. 2012;91(4):447–51.
47. Lutsiv O, McKinney B, Foster G, Taylor VH, Pullenayegum E, McDonald SD. Pregnancy complications associated with the co-prevalence of excess maternal weight and depression. Int J Obes. 2015;39(12):1710–6.

Relationship between threatened miscarriage and gestational diabetes mellitus

Hee Joong Lee[1], Errol Norwitz[2] and Banghyun Lee[3*]

Abstract

Background: Both threatened miscarriage and gestational diabetes mellitus (GDM) are common complications of pregnancy. However, only one pilot study has reported that these complications are not related. We aimed to investigate whether threatened miscarriage is one of the risk factors of GDM.

Methods: An unmatched case-control study of 1567 pregnant Korean women who underwent a two-step approach to diagnose GDM was retrospectively conducted. The eligible women were classified into normal ($n = 840$), borderline GDM ($n = 480$), and GDM ($n = 247$) groups. We analyzed the associations with threatened miscarriage in all groups with adjustment for confounding factors.

Results: The proportion of women who experienced threatened miscarriage was significantly lower in the GDM group than in the normal group (adjusted odds ratio (OR), 0.38; 95% confidence interval (CI), 0.18–0.78). It was significantly lower in the maternal hyperglycemia group (borderline GDM and GDM groups) than in the normal group (adjusted OR, 0.66; 95% CI, 0.47–0.91). The proportion of women who experienced threatened miscarriage was also significantly lower in the GDM group than in the normal (adjusted OR, 0.35; 95% CI, 0.17–0.70) and borderline GDM groups (adjusted OR, 0.46; 95% CI, 0.22–0.94). Moreover, the proportion of women who experienced threatened miscarriage significantly decreased according to the severity of glucose intolerance (adjusted OR, 0.94; 95% CI, 0.76–1.16).

Conclusion: This study demonstrates that threatened miscarriage is associated with decreased risk of GDM and the severity of glucose intolerance in Korean women. Additional studies are warranted to understand the pathophysiologic mechanisms that might exist between these frequent complications of pregnancy.

Keywords: Gestational diabetes mellitus, Threatened miscarriage, Borderline GDM, Maternal hyperglycemia

Background

Threatened miscarriage, which is defined as any vaginal bleeding that occurs during the first half of a pregnancy, occurs in an estimated 14–20% of all pregnant women (14.8% in Korean women) [1, 2]. Approximately 50% of women who experienced threatened miscarriage eventually suffer miscarriages [3, 4]. Bleeding that originates from the uteroplacental vessels between the chorionic membrane and the uterine wall is often considered to be the most common cause of vaginal bleeding in threatened miscarriage [3]. Depending on the severity of bleeding, miscarriage can occur [3]. Many studies have reported that threatened miscarriage is associated with an increased risk of adverse obstetric outcomes, such as antepartum hemorrhage, preterm delivery, cesarean delivery, preterm premature rupture of membrane (PPROM), pregnancy-induced hypertension, preeclampsia, placenta previa, and placenta abruption, and adverse perinatal outcomes, such as perinatal death, small-for-gestational-age (SGA) infants and low birth weight [1, 3, 5, 6].

Maternal hyperglycemia occurs when insulin secretion from pancreatic β cells is inadequate for the increased insulin requirements during pregnancy [7]. Gestational diabetes mellitus (GDM) is defined as any severity of maternal hyperglycemia with onset or first recognition during pregnancy [8, 9]. However, a fasting plasma

* Correspondence: banghyun.lee@gmail.com
[3]Department of Obstetrics and Gynecology, Hallym University Kangdong Sacred Heart Hospital, 150, Seongan-ro, Gangdong-gu, Seoul, Republic of Korea

glucose level > 7.0 mmol/L or a casual plasma glucose > 11.1 mmol/L meets the threshold for type 2 diabetes diagnosis [8]. The prevalence of GDM ranges between 1 and 14% depending on the risk level of the affected population (5.7–9.5% in Korean women) [9–12]. Borderline GDM is usually considered to be maternal hyperglycemia that does not meet the diagnostic criteria for GDM and type 2 diabetes [10]. Although no clear consensus has been reached, 1-h venous plasma glucose ≥7.8 or 7.2 mmol/L on a positive 50-g oral glucose challenge test (OGCT) is considered a minimum glucose level for borderline GDM diagnosis [13, 14]. Several studies have reported that borderline GDM occurs in approximately 7–9% of all pregnant women [10].

Progesterone is essential for establishment and maintenance of pregnancy [15, 16]. Low progesterone levels are associated with an increased risk of first trimester miscarriage [17]. Recently, some studies reported that progesterone therapy during early pregnancy in women with threatened miscarriage may reduce pregnancy loss and the risk of adverse obstetric and perinatal outcomes [17–20]. Insulin resistance in pregnancy normally increases during the second and third trimesters [21]. Several studies in rats, mice, and adipocytes have reported that progesterone induces insulin resistance by multiple mechanisms during pregnancy [22–24]. The use of 17-alpha hydroxyprogesterone caproate for preterm delivery prevention is associated with an increased risk of developing GDM [25, 26]. Therefore, we hypothesized that women with threatened miscarriage possess lower levels of progesterone throughout pregnancy than those without threatened miscarriage. As a result, women with threatened miscarriage may have less insulin resistance during the second and third trimesters of pregnancy than those without threatened miscarriage, followed by a lower risk for glucose intolerance.

Both threatened miscarriage and GDM are common complications of pregnancy. Whether threatened miscarriage is associated with GDM warrants evaluation. To our knowledge, only one small-scale pilot study performed in Europe has reported that no relationship exists between threatened miscarriage and GDM [27]. Therefore, in the present study, we aimed to investigate whether threatened miscarriage is a risk factor of GDM and to evaluate this relationship according to the severity of glucose intolerance.

Methods

This study was approved by the Institutional Review Board of The Catholic Medical Center at the Catholic University of Korea (No. XC14RIMI0013U) on February 1, 2014. Informed consent was waived. We reviewed the medical records of pregnant women who enrolled in the routine prenatal care program of Seoul or Uijeongbu St. Mary's Hospital at the Catholic University of Korea before 12 weeks of gestation and who gave birth in the same hospital from January 1, 2006 to October 31, 2013. Pregnant women who underwent a two-step approach to diagnose GDM were included [7]. The exclusion criteria were as follows: women who did not undergo a 100-g oral glucose tolerance test (OGTT) after a positive 50-g OGCT; women who had other causes of vaginal bleeding (e.g., post-coital bleeding, polyp, vaginitis) at the time of assessment; women with fetal anomalies, multifetal gestation, or overt diabetes mellitus; and non-Korean ethnicity. Because only 3 non-Korean women met the study criteria, they were excluded from this study.

The medical records of 1567 pregnant women who were eligible for the study were reviewed. A total of 247 pregnant women were diagnosed with GDM. Borderline GDM and normal groups included 480 and 840 pregnant women, respectively.

In Seoul and Uijeongbu St. Mary's Hospitals (the tertiary and secondary hospitals), the routine protocol to diagnose GDM was based on a two-step approach that consisted of a universal 50-g OGCT and a diagnostic 100-g OGTT [7]. A 50-g OGCT was performed at 24–28 weeks of gestation. Plasma glucose level > 7.8 mmol/L at 1-h post-glucose load without prior fasting was regarded as a positive GDM screening result, and a diagnostic 100-g OGTT was then recommended. In the diagnostic 100-g OGTT, the fasting plasma glucose levels were measured prior to glucose load ingestion, and three plasma glucose levels were measured at 1, 2, and 3 h following the glucose load ingestion. To diagnose GDM, we used the Carpenter and Coustan criteria, which included women with two or more plasma glucose measurements greater than the following thresholds: fasting glucose of ≥5.3 mmol/L, 1-h glucose of ≥10.0 mmol/L, 2-h glucose of ≥8.6 mmol/L, and 3-h glucose of ≥7.8 mmol/L [28]. Borderline GDM in women was defined as a positive OGCT and a negative diagnostic OGTT (in which plasma glucose measurements greater than the thresholds were absent or only one value was greater than the threshold). The pregnant women with GDM were managed with diet control, exercise, careful glucose monitoring, and medication (insulin therapy or oral hypoglycemic agents). In this study, 14.6% ($n = 36$) of the 247 women with GDM were managed with insulin (2 women were managed with oral hypoglycemic agents after insulin use for 2 months) and 85.4% ($n = 211$) were managed with diet control. The pregnant women with borderline GDM were managed with the same routine prenatal care as the healthy pregnant women, except for one woman who was administered with insulin.

Gestational age was calculated from the last menstrual period (LMP) and was confirmed by the crown-rump length (CRL), which was measured using ultrasound during the first trimester. If the CRL dating differed by more than 7 days from the LMP dating, gestational age was changed according to the CRL dating [27, 29]. Threatened miscarriage was defined as women whose medical records documented vaginal bleeding before 20 weeks of gestation [1]. Data regarding the amount of bleeding and the number of bleeding episodes were extracted from the medical records of the patients. Threatened miscarriage was classified as "light" if the bleeding was written as scanty or small amounts in the medical record; otherwise, it was classified as "heavy" [5]. Intrauterine hematoma was defined as a crescent-shaped echolucent area between the chorionic membranes and the placenta and/or the myometrium on ultrasound [1]. All eligible women were classified as either women who experienced threatened abortion ($n = 194$) or women who did not experience threatened miscarriage ($n = 1373$). One woman with GDM and two women with borderline GDM received weekly intramuscular injections of progesterone (250 mg, 1 to 3 times).

Pre-pregnancy body mass index (BMI) was calculated using the baseline weight (self-reported pre-pregnancy weight or weight measured at the first visit during early

Table 1 Clinical characteristics of the normal and GDM groups

	Total (n = 1087)	Normal (n = 840)	GDM (n = 247)	P^b	OR (95% CI)	P^c
Maternal age (years), mean ± SD	34.1 ± 3.9	33.9 ± 3.9	34.7 ± 4.0	0.003	1.06 (1.02–1.10)	0.003
< 35, n (%)	623 (57.3)	498 (59.3)	125 (50.6)	0.015	ref	0.016
≥35, n (%)	464 (42.7)	342 (40.7)	122 (49.4)		1.42 (1.07–1.89)	
Parity, n (%)				0.003		0.003
Primipara	613 (56.4)	494 (58.8)	119 (48.2)		ref	
Multipara	474 (43.6)	346 (41.2)	128 (51.8)		1.54 (1.16–2.04)	
Intrauterine hematoma, n (%)	80 (7.4)	72 (8.6)	8 (3.2)	0.005	0.36 (0.17–0.75)	0.007
Gestational age at birth (weeks), mean ± SD	38.6 ± 1.6	38.8 ± 1.4	38.0 ± 2.0	< 0.001	0.74 (0.68–0.82)	< 0.001
Preterm delivery (before 37 weeks), n (%)	78 (7.2)	45 (5.4)	33 (13.4)	< 0.001	2.72 (1.70–4.38)	< 0.001
Delivery methods, n (%)				< 0.001		
Normal delivery	718 (66.1)	588 (70.0)	130 (52.6)		ref	
Operative delivery (vacuum)	12 (1.1)	10 (1.2)	2 (0.8)		0.91 (0.20–4.18)	0.90
Primary cesarean section	170 (15.6)	121 (14.4)	49 (19.8)		1.83 (1.25–2.69)	0.002
Repeat cesarean section	187 (17.2)	121 (14.4)	66 (26.7)		2.47 (1.73–3.52)	< 0.001
PROM, n (%)	186 (17.1)	148 (17.6)	38 (15.4)	0.41	0.85 (0.58–1.25)	0.41
PPROM, n (%)	38 (3.5)	25 (3.0)	13 (5.3)	0.09	1.81 (0.91–3.60)	0.09
Preeclampsia, n (%)	19 (1.8)	8 (1.0)	11 (4.5)	0.001	4.85 (1.93–12.19)	0.001
Placenta previa, n (%)	27 (2.5)	17 (2.0)	10 (4.0)	0.07	2.04 (0.92–4.52)	0.08
Placenta abruption, n (%)	7 (0.6)	7 (0.8)	0 (0.0)	0.36	0.35 (0.00–1.81)	0.33
Still birth, n (%)	3 (0.3)	3 (0.4)	0 (0.0)	> 0.999	0.88 (0.00–5.84)	0.92
History of prior GDM, n (%)	53 (4.9)	1 (0.1)	52 (21.1)	< 0.001	58.4 (37.73- > 999.99)	< 0.001
50 g OGCT (mmol/L), mean ± SD (n = 972) [a]	124.4 ± 36.2	108.7 ± 17.1	172.1 ± 37.3	< 0.001	1.29 (1.23–1.36)	< 0.001
Pre-pregnancy BMI (kg/m^2), mean ± SD	21.2 ± 3.3	20.5 ± 2.4	23.5 ± 4.4	< 0.001	1.34 (1.27–1.40)	< 0.001
Birth weight (g), mean ± SD	3188.2 ± 480.9	3189.3 ± 456.0	3184.4 ± 558.3	0.97	1.00 (0.99–1.00)	0.89
SGA, n (%)	140 (12.9)	114 (13.6)	26 (10.5)	0.21	0.75 (0.48–1.18)	0.21
AGA, n (%)	903 (83.1)	698 (83.1)	205 (83.0)	0.97	0.99 (0.68–1.45)	0.97
LGA, n (%)	44 (4.1)	28 (3.3)	16 (6.5)	0.028	2.01 (1.07–3.78)	0.030
Macrosomia, n (%)	43 (4.1)	29 (3.5)	14 (5.7)	0.12	1.68 (0.87–3.23)	0.12
Progesterone therapy	1 (0.1)	0 (0.0)	1 (0.4)	0.23	3.40 (0.18-Infinity)	0.46
Insulin therapy	36 (3.3)	0 (0.0)	36 (14.6)	< 0.001	203.42 (45.29-Infinity)	< 0.001

SGA small for gestational age: <10th percentile, *AGA* appropriate for gestational age: 10th–90th percentile, *LGA* large for gestational age: >90th percentile, *Macrosomia* Estimated fetal weight ≥ 4 kg [25]

[a]Missing data are excluded from statistical analyses

[b]Chi-square test or Fisher's exact test for categorical variables and Wilcoxon rank sum test for continuous variables

[c]Univariate logistic regression

pregnancy when the pre-pregnancy weight was unknown) and measured height [14]. BMI was calculated as body mass in kg divided by height in m^2. SGA (<10th percentile), appropriate for gestational age (AGA) (10–90th percentile), large for gestational age (LGA) (>90th percentile), and macrosomia (estimated fetal weight ≥ 4000 g) were defined for birth weight [30].

In this study, the association between threatened miscarriage and glucose intolerance was compared between the normal and GDM groups, between the normal and maternal hyperglycemia (borderline GDM and GDM groups) groups, and among the normal, borderline GDM, and GDM groups.

All analyses were performed using SAS software, version 9.2 (SAS Institute, Cary, NC, USA). To confirm that continuous variables were normally distributed, we applied the Shapiro-Wilk test. For non-normal distributed data, the significance of the differences between groups was tested using the Wilcoxon rank sum test. The categorical responses between the groups were analyzed using the chi-square test or Fisher's exact test. The associations of the independent risk factors with each group

Table 2 Clinical characteristics of the normal and maternal hyperglycemia (Borderline GDM and GDM groups) groups

	Total (n = 1567)	Normal (n = 840)	Borderline GDM and GDM (n = 727)	P [b]	OR (95% CI)	P [c]
Maternal age (years), mean ± SD	33.8 ± 3.9	33.9 ± 3.9	33.7 ± 4.0	0.23	0.99 (0.96–1.01)	0.35
< 35, n (%)	931 (59.4)	498 (59.3)	433 (59.6)	0.91	ref	0.91
≥35, n (%)	636 (40.6)	342 (40.7)	294 (40.4)		0.99 (0.81–1.21)	
Parity, n (%)				0.11		0.11
Primipara	892 (56.9)	494 (58.8)	398 (54.7)		ref	
Multipara	675 (43.1)	346 (41.2)	329 (45.3)		1.18 (0.97–1.44)	
Intrauterine hematoma, n (%)	113 (7.2)	72 (8.6)	41 (5.6)	0.025	0.64 (0.43–0.95)	0.026
Gestational age at birth (weeks), mean ± SD	38.5 ± 1.7	38.8 ± 1.4	38.2 ± 2.0	< 0.001	0.81 (0.76–0.86)	< 0.001
Preterm delivery (before 37 weeks), n (%)	123 (7.9)	45 (5.4)	78 (10.7)	< 0.001	2.12 (1.45–3.11)	< 0.001
Delivery methods, n (%)				< 0.001		
Normal delivery	1015 (64.8)	588 (70.0)	427 (58.7)		ref	
Operative delivery (vacuum)	22 (1.4)	10 (1.2)	12 (1.7)		1.65 (0.71–3.86)	0.25
Primary cesarean section	246 (15.7)	121 (14.4)	125 (17.2)		1.42 (1.08–1.88)	0.013
Repeat cesarean section	284 (18.1)	121 (14.4)	163 (22.4)		1.86 (1.42–2.42)	< 0.001
PROM, n (%)	267 (17.0)	148 (17.6)	119 (16.4)	0.51	0.92 (0.70–1.19)	0.51
PPROM, n (%)	54 (3.5)	25 (3.0)	29 (4.0)	0.27	1.35 (0.79–2.33)	0.28
Preeclampsia, n (%)	35 (2.2)	8 (1.0)	27 (3.7)	< 0.001	4.01 (1.81–8.89)	0.001
Placenta previa, n (%)	35 (2.2)	17 (2.0)	18 (2.5)	0.56	1.23 (0.63–2.41)	0.55
Placenta abruption, n (%)	10 (0.6)	7 (0.8)	3 (0.4)	0.36	0.49 (0.13–1.91)	0.31
Still birth, n (%)	4 (0.3)	3 (0.4)	1 (0.1)	0.63	0.39 (0.04–3.71)	0.41
History of prior GDM, n (%)	58 (3.7)	1 (0.1)	57 (7.8)	< 0.001	71.20 (9.86–514.24)	< 0.001
50 g OGCT (mmol/L), mean ± SD (n = 1445) [a]	134.8 ± 34.3	108.7 ± 17.1	161.5 ± 25.9	< 0.001	1.42 (1.34–1.50)	< 0.001
Pre-pregnancy BMI (kg/m^2), mean ± SD	21.2 ± 3.3	20.5 ± 2.4	22.1 ± 4.0	< 0.001	1.18 (1.14–1.23)	< 0.001
Birth weight (g), mean ± SD	3186.7 ± 485.0	3189.3 ± 456.0	3183.6 ± 516.7	0.82	1.00 (0.99–1.00)	0.82
SGA, n (%)	187 (11.9)	114 (13.6)	73 (10.0)	0.032	0.71 (0.52–0.97)	0.032
AGA, n (%)	1319 (84.2)	698 (83.1)	621 (85.4)	0.21	1.19 (0.91–1.57)	0.21
LGA, n (%)	61 (3.9)	28 (3.3)	33 (4.5)	0.22	1.38 (0.83–2.31)	0.22
Macrosomia, n (%)	59 (3.8)	29 (3.5)	30 (4.1)	0.48	1.20 (0.72–2.03)	0.48
Progesterone therapy	3 (0.2)	0 (0.0)	3 (0.4)	0.10	4.46 (0.68-Infinity)	0.20
Insulin therapy	37 (2.4)	0 (0.0)	37 (5.1)	< 0.001	64.23 (14.36-Infinity)	< 0.001

SGA small for gestational age: <10th percentile, *AGA* appropriate for gestational age: 10th–90th percentile, *LGA* large for gestational age: >90th percentile, *Macrosomia* Estimated fetal weight ≥ 4 kg [25]

[a]Missing data are excluded from statistical analyses

[b]Chi-square test or Fisher's exact test for categorical variables and Wilcoxon rank sum test for continuous variables

[c]Univariate logistic regression

Table 3 Association between GDM and threatened miscarriage

	Total (*n* = 1087)	Normal (*n* = 840)	GDM (*n* = 247)	OR (95% CI)	*p*	Adjusted OR (95% CI)	*p*
Threatened miscarriage, n (%)					0.002		0.009
Negative	949 (87.3)	719 (85.6)	230 (93.1)	ref		ref	
Positive	138 (12.7)	121 (14.4)	17 (6.9)	0.44 (0.26–0.75)		0.38 (0.18–0.78)	
Amount of bleeding, n (%) (*n* = 137) [a]					0.11		0.69
Light	117 (85.4)	100 (83.3)	17 (100.0)	ref		ref	
Heavy	20 (14.6)	20 (16.7)	0 (0.0)	0.21 (0.00–1.05)		0.63 (0.00–3.46)	
Number of bleeding episodes, n (%) (*n* = 137) [a]					0.13		0.53
≤ 2	108 (78.8)	92 (76.7)	16 (94.1)	ref		ref	
≥ 3	29 (21.2)	28 (23.3)	1 (5.9)	0.21 (0.03–1.62)		0.50 (0.06–4.42)	

Statistical analyses were performed by univariable and multivariable logistic regression
The data were adjusted for maternal age (< 35 years, ≥35 years), parity, history of prior GDM, pre-pregnancy BMI, progesterone therapy, and insulin therapy
[a]Missing data are excluded from statistical analyses

were analyzed using logistic regression, with or without adjusting for confounding factors. Confounding factors included maternal age (< 35 years, ≥35 years), parity, history of prior GDM, gestational age at birth, and pre-pregnancy BMI, which are known risk factors for GDM [14, 31], and showed statistical significance in the current univariate analysis. According to a previous study, maternal age > 35 years was a risk factor for GDM [31]. Data were also adjusted for progesterone and insulin therapy based on their influence on the study result. Hosmer-Lemeshow goodness-of-fit test was performed ($P > 0.05$) to identify the most appropriate model. $P < 0.05$ was considered statistically significant.

Results

The clinical characteristics of the study population are presented in Tables 1 and 2. The GDM group showed a lower incidence of intrauterine hematoma and a lower gestational age at birth than the normal group. The absolute maternal age and the rates of women with a maternal age ≥ 35 years, multiparity, preterm delivery, cesarean section, preeclampsia, history of prior GDM, pre-pregnancy BMI, and LGA were higher in the GDM group than in the normal group. The absolute birth weight and the incidence rates of operative delivery, premature rupture of membrane (PROM), PPROM, placenta previa, placenta abruption, stillbirth, SGA, and AGA, and macrosomia did not differ between the groups (Table 1). Additionally, the maternal hyperglycemia (borderline GDM and GDM groups) group exhibited a lower incidence of intrauterine hematoma and SGA, and a lower gestational age at birth than the normal group. The preterm delivery, cesarean section, preeclampsia, history of prior GDM, and pre-pregnancy BMI were higher in the maternal hyperglycemia (borderline GDM and GDM

Table 4 Association between maternal hyperglycemia (Borderline GDM and GDM) and threatened miscarriage

	Total (*n* = 1567)	Normal (*n* = 840)	Borderline GDM and GDM (*n* = 727)	OR (95% CI)	*p*	Adjusted OR (95% CI)	*p*
Threatened miscarriage, n (%)					0.009		0.013
Negative	1373 (87.6)	719 (85.6)	654 (90.0)	ref		ref	
Positive	194 (12.4)	121 (14.4)	73 (10.0)	0.66 (0.49–0.90)		0.66 (0.47–0.91)	
Amount of bleeding, n (%) (*n* = 192) [a]					0.29		0.15
Light	164 (85.4)	100 (83.3)	64 (88.9)	ref		ref	
Heavy	28 (14.6)	20 (16.7)	8 (11.1)	0.63 (0.26–1.50)		0.66 (0.26–1.67)	
Number of bleeding episodes, n (%) (*n* = 192) [a]					0.022		0.14
≤ 2	157 (81.8)	92 (76.7)	65 (90.3)	ref		ref	
≥ 3	35 (18.2)	28 (23.3)	7 (9.7)	0.35 (0.15–0.86)		0.36 (0.14–0.93)	

Statistical analyses were performed by univariable and multivariable logistic regression
The data were adjusted for maternal age (< 35 years, ≥35 years), parity, history of prior GDM, pre-pregnancy BMI, progesterone therapy, and insulin therapy
[a]Missing data are excluded from statistical analyses

Table 5 Association between the severity of maternal hyperglycemia and threatened miscarriage: Multinomial logistic regression

	Normal (n = 840)	Borderline GDM (n = 480)	GDM (n = 247)	OR (95% CI)				Adjusted OR (95% CI)			
				Normal vs GDM	p	Borderline GDM vs GDM	p	Normal vs GDM	p	Borderline GDM vs GDM	p
Threatened miscarriage					0.002		0.044		0.003		0.034
Negative	719 (85.6)	424 (88.3)	230 (93.1)	ref		ref		ref		ref	
Positive	121 (14.4)	56 (11.7)	17 (6.9)	0.44 (0.26–0.75)		0.56 (0.32–0.99)		0.35 (0.17–0.70)		0.46 (0.22–0.94)	

Statistical analyses were performed by univariable and multivariable logistic regression
The data were adjusted for maternal age (< 35 years, ≥35 years), parity, history of prior GDM, pre-pregnancy BMI, progesterone therapy, and insulin therapy

groups) group than in the normal group. Other variables were not different between the groups (Table 2).

The proportion of women who experienced threatened miscarriage was significantly lower in the GDM group than in the normal group with or without adjusting for confounding factors (adjusted odds ratio (OR), 0.38; 95% confidence interval (CI), 0.18–0.78; $P = 0.009$) (Table 3). It was also significantly lower in the maternal hyperglycemia (borderline GDM and GDM groups) group than in the normal group (adjusted OR, 0.66; 95% CI, 0.47–0.91; $P = 0.013$) (Table 4). The amount of bleeding and the number of bleeding episodes in women who experienced threatened miscarriage were not different between the groups (Tables 3 and 4).

Threatened miscarriage showed significant associations among the normal, borderline GDM, and GDM groups. The proportion of women who experienced threatened miscarriage was significantly lower in the GDM group than in the normal group with or without adjusting for confounding factors (adjusted OR, 0.35; 95% CI, 0.17–0.70; $P = 0.003$). The proportion of women who experienced threatened miscarriage was also significantly lower in the GDM group than in the borderline GDM group with or without adjusting for confounding factors (adjusted OR, 0.46; 95% CI, 0.22–0.94; $P = 0.034$). Moreover, the proportion of women who experienced threatened miscarriage significantly decreased according to the severity of glucose intolerance with or without adjusting for confounding factors (adjusted OR, 0.94; 95% CI, 0.76–1.16; $P < 0.001$) (Tables 5 and 6).

Discussion

In this case-control study, we found that the women who experienced threatened miscarriage had a significantly decreased risk of GDM in current pregnancies. This finding was observed in the comparison between the normal and GDM groups, between the normal and maternal hyperglycemia (borderline GDM and GDM groups) groups, and among the normal, borderline GDM, and GDM groups. Moreover, threatened miscarriage showed an inverse correlation with the severity of glucose intolerance. Our data supported our initial hypothesis that low progesterone levels in women with threatened miscarriage might be associated with a low increase in insulin resistance during the second and third trimesters of pregnancy, followed by a low incidence of glucose intolerance. Our findings potentially aids in understanding these common complications of pregnancy. However, future prospective, large-scale studies are necessary to explore the relationship between threatened miscarriage and GDM.

A prospective pilot study based on a small population with a very low incidence of GDM [threatened miscarriage vs normal pregnancy, 3/69 (4.3%) vs 11/564 (2.0%), respectively] reported no relationship between threatened miscarriage and GDM [27]. By contrast, our study (normal pregnancy vs GDM with or without borderline GDM) retrospectively showed relatively lower incidences of GDM and maternal hyperglycemia (borderline GDM and GDM) in women who experienced threatened miscarriage [27]. However, in a large-scale retrospective study involving women who received intramuscular high-dosage progesterone therapy (the total accumulated dose was ≥500 mg) due to threatened miscarriage in the second and third months of pregnancy, the incidence of GDM was slightly higher in women with threatened miscarriage [37/532 (6.95%)] than in women with normal pregnancy [1141/21,054 (5.42%)], but it was not statistically significant [20]. In the same study, threatened miscarriage was

Table 6 Association between the severity of maternal hyperglycemia and threatened miscarriage: Ordinal logistic regression

	Normal (n = 840)	Borderline GDM (n = 480)	GDM (n = 247)	OR (95% CI)	p	Adjusted OR (95% CI)	p
Threatened miscarriage					0.003		< 0.001
Negative	719 (85.6)	424 (88.3)	230 (93.1)	ref		ref	
Positive	121 (14.4)	56 (11.7)	17 (6.9)	0.63 (0.47–0.86)		0.94 (0.76–1.16)	

Statistical analyses were performed by univariable and multivariable logistic regression
The data were adjusted for maternal age (< 35 years, ≥35 years), parity, history of prior GDM, pre-pregnancy BMI, progesterone therapy, and insulin therapy

not associated with an increased risk of adverse obstetric and perinatal outcomes, such as preterm delivery, hypertensive disorders in pregnancy, placenta previa, placenta abruption, live births, and low birth weight, compared with normal pregnancy [20]. These findings demonstrate that the risks of common adverse obstetric and perinatal outcomes of threatened miscarriage were affected by progesterone therapy. In particular, considering the effect of progesterone therapy, we speculate that threatened miscarriage in the previous study might be associated with a low risk of GDM, which corresponded with the results of our study that showed inverse correlation between threatened miscarriage and GDM (Tables 3, 5 and 6).

Intrauterine hematoma is detected in 18–39% of pregnant women who experience threatened miscarriage. It is associated with an increased risk of adverse obstetric outcomes, such as preterm delivery, pregnancy-induced hypertension, preeclampsia, placental abruption, and SGA, through mechanisms that are similar to those that result in threatened miscarriage [1, 3]. In the present study, the incidence of intrauterine hematoma (50.5%) in women with threatened miscarriage was higher than that described in previous reports [3]. Moreover, the incidence of intrauterine hematoma decreased in women with GDM and maternal hyperglycemia (borderline GDM and GDM) compared with the normal women, in accordance with the risk of threatened miscarriage (Tables 1 and 2).

The amount of vaginal bleeding during pregnancy is a subjective measurement. Consequently, distinguishing between light and heavy vaginal bleeding has not been effective [6]. In our study, although the data did not reach statistical significance, GDM and maternal hyperglycemia (borderline GDM and GDM) occurred less frequently in women with heavy bleeding than in women with light bleeding. They also occurred less frequently in women with higher bleeding levels (≥3) than in women with lower bleeding levels (≤2), which is in accordance with the risk of threatened miscarriage (Tables 3 and 4).

In our study, the GDM group displayed typical characteristics of women with GDM compared with the normal group, which is in accordance with prior reports (Table 1) [30–33]. However, compared with previous reports [34–36], we detected a similar birth weight, low pre-pregnancy BMI and rates of macrosomia/LGA, and a high rate of SGA in the study cohort. This result suggests inherent ethnic differences in which Koreans consider lean body shape as superior to obese, followed by excessive diet control and exercise (Table 1). Additionally, in contrast to prior studies that reported higher birth weight, higher macrosomia/LGA rates, and lower SGA rates in women with GDM [35–37], the birth weight and the incidence rate of SGA, LGA, or macrosomia were unchanged in women with GDM and maternal hyperglycemia (borderline GDM and GDM) compared with the normal women in our study (Tables 1 and 2). These findings could be explained by the low pre-pregnancy BMI and the low rates of macrosomia/LGA in our study groups in addition to the higher preterm delivery rate and the shorter gestational age at birth in women with GDM and maternal hyperglycemia (borderline GDM and GDM) compared with the normal women.

The significance of our study might be limited because definite mechanisms to elucidate the relationship between threatened miscarriage, and GDM and the severity of glucose intolerance were not clinically investigated. However, our study is important because it focused on their specific relationship, although it was performed using a retrospective design.

Conclusions

In this retrospective study, we demonstrated that GDM was less frequently observed in Korean women who experienced threatened miscarriage showing inverse relationship between threatened miscarriage and the severity of glucose intolerance. Further research is recommended to confirm these relationships and to evaluate the pathophysiologic mechanisms that interplay between these common obstetric complications. We believe that these interesting findings will help improved care for women with adverse obstetric outcomes.

Abbreviations

AGA: Appropriate for gestational age; BMI: Body mass index; CRL: Crown-rump length; GDM: Gestational diabetes mellitus; LGA: Large for gestational age; LMP: Last menstrual period; OGCT: Oral glucose challenge test; OGTT: Oral glucose tolerance test; PPROM: Preterm premature rupture of membrane; SGA: Small for gestational age

Acknowledgments

Statistical support was provided by the Catholic Research Coordinating Center of the Korea Health 21 Research & Development Project (No. A070001), Ministry of Health and Welfare, Republic of Korea.

Authors' contributions

HJL, EN, and BL participated in designing the research. HJL and BL participated in field data collection and conducted statistical analyses. BL wrote the manuscript, and HJL and EN read and commented on it. The final paper submitted for publication was read and approved by HJL, EN, and BL.

Competing interests

The authors declare that they have no competing interests.

Author details

[1]Department of Obstetrics & Gynecology, College of Medicine, The Catholic University of Korea, Seoul, Republic of Korea. [2]Department of Obstetrics & Gynecology, Tufts University School of Medicine, Boston, MA, USA. [3]Department of Obstetrics and Gynecology, Hallym University Kangdong Sacred Heart Hospital, 150, Seongan-ro, Gangdong-gu, Seoul, Republic of Korea.

References

1. Jauniaux E, Van Oppenraaij RH, Burton GJ. Obstetric outcome after early placental complications. Curr Opin Obstet Gynecol. 2010;22:452–7.
2. Park C, Kang MY, Kim D, Park J, Eom H, Kim EA. Prevalence of abortion and adverse pregnancy outcomes among working women in Korea: a cross-sectional study. PLoS One. 2017;12(8):e0182341.
3. van Oppenraaij RH, Jauniaux E, Christiansen OB, Horcajadas JA, Farquharson RG, Exalto N. Predicting adverse obstetric outcome after early pregnancy events and complications: a review. Hum Reprod Update. 2009;15:409–21.
4. Dadkhah F, Kashanian M, Eliasi G. A comparison between the pregnancy outcome in women both with or without threatened abortion. Early Hum Dev. 2010;86:193–6.
5. Weiss JL, Malone FD, Vidaver J, Ball RH, Nyberg DA, Comstock CH, et al. Threatened abortion: a risk factor for poor pregnancy outcome, a population based screening study. Am J Obstet Gynecol. 2004;190:745–50.
6. Saraswat L, Bhattacharya S, Maheshwari A, Bhattacharya S. Maternal and perinatal outcome in women with threatened miscarriage in the first trimester: a systematic review. BJOG. 2010;117:245–57.
7. Buchanan TA, Xiang AH, Page KA. Gestational diabetes mellitus: risks and management during and after pregnancy. Nat Rev Endocrinol. 2012;8:639–49.
8. American Diabetes Association. Gestational diabetes mellitus. Diabetes Care. 2003;26(suppl 1):s103–5.
9. No PB. 137: gestational diabetes mellitus. Obstet Gynecol. 2013;122(2 Pt 1):406–16.
10. Han S, Crowther CA, Middleton P. Interventions for pregnant women with hyperglycaemia not meeting gestational diabetes and type 2 diabetes diagnostic criteria. Cochrane Database Syst Rev. 2012;1:CD009037.
11. Mulla WR, Henry TQ, Homko CJ. Gestational diabetes screening after HAPO: has anything changed? Curr Diab Rep. 2010;10:224–8.
12. Koo BK, Lee JH, Kim J, Jang EJ, Lee CH. Prevalence of gestational diabetes mellitus in Korea: a National Health Insurance Database Study. PLoS One. 2016;11(4):e0153107.
13. Han S, Middleton PF, Bubner TK, Crowther CA. Women's views on their diagnosis and management for borderline gestational diabetes mellitus. J Diabetes Res. 2015;2015:209215.
14. Park TC, Lee BH, Norwitz ER, Lee HJ. Maternal hyperglycemia and the 100-g oral glucose tolerance test. Taiwan J Obstet Gynecol. 2015;54(2):137–42.
15. Nakajima ST, Nason FG, Badger GJ, Gibson M. Progesterone production in early pregnancy. Fertil Steril. 1991;55:516–21.
16. Mesiano S, Wang Y, Norwitz ER. Progesterone receptors in the human pregnancy uterus: do they hold the key to birth timing? Reprod Sci. 2011; 18:6–19.
17. Qureshi NS. Treatment options for threatened miscarriage. Maturitas. 2009; 65(Suppl 1):S35–41.
18. Carp H. A systematic review of dydrogesterone for the treatment of recurrent miscarriage. Gynecol Endocrinol. 2015;31:422–30.
19. Wahabi HA, Fayed AA, Esmaeil SA, Al Zeidan RA. Progestogen for treating threatened miscarriage. Cochrane Database Syst Rev. 2011;(12):CD005943. https://doi.org/10.1002/14651858.CD005943.pub4. Review.
20. Duan L, Yan D, Zeng W, Yang X, Wei Q. Effect of progesterone treatment due to threatened abortion in early pregnancy for obstetric and perinatal outcomes. Early Hum Dev. 2010;86:41–3.
21. Carr DB, Gabbe S. Gestational diabetes: detection, management, and implications. Clin Diabetes. 1998;16:4–11.
22. Ryan EA, Enns L. Role of gestational hormones in the induction of insulin resistance. J Clin Endocrinol Metab. 1988;67:341–7.
23. Wada T, Hori S, Sugiyama M, Fujisawa E, Nakano T, Tsuneki H, et al. Progesterone inhibits glucose uptake by affecting diverse steps of insulin signaling in 3T3-L1 adipocytes. Am J Physiol Endocrinol Metab. 2010;298:E881–8.
24. Picard F, Wanatabe M, Schoonjans K, Lydon J, O'Malley BW, Auwerx J. Progesterone receptor knockout mice have an improved glucose homeostasis secondary to beta -cell proliferation. Proc Natl Acad Sci U S A. 2002;99:15644–8.
25. Egerman R, Ramsey R, Istwan N, Rhea D, Stanziano G. Maternal characteristics influencing the development of gestational diabetes in obese women receiving 17-alpha-hydroxyprogesterone caproate. J Obes. 2014;2014:563243.
26. Rebarber A, Istwan NB, Russo-Stieglitz K, Cleary-Goldman J, Rhea DJ, Stanziano GJ, et al. Increased incidence of gestational diabetes in women receiving prophylactic 17alpha-hydroxyprogesterone caproate for prevention of recurrent preterm delivery. Diabetes Care. 2007;30:2277–80.
27. Calleja-Agius J, Calleja N, Brincat M, Spiteri D. Obstetric outcome in cases of threatened spontaneous abortion. Int J Gynaecol Obstet. 2010;110:75–6.
28. Carpenter MW, Coustan DR. Criteria for screening tests for gestational diabetes. Am J Obstet Gynecol. 1982;144:768–73.
29. Scorza WE, Vintzileos A. First and second trimester sonography: an American perspective. Int J Fertil Menopausal Stud. 1996;41(3):288–92.
30. Metzger BE, Lowe LP, Dyer AR, Trimble ER, Chaovarindr U, Coustan DR, et al. Hyperglycemia and adverse pregnancy outcomes. N Engl J Med. 2008;358:1991–2002.
31. Galtier F. Definition, epidemiology, risk factors. Diabetes Metab. 2010;36:628–51.
32. Beucher G, Viaris de Lesegno B, Dreyfus M. Maternal outcome of gestational diabetes mellitus. Diabetes Metab. 2010;36(6 Pt 2):522–37.
33. Riskin-Mashiah S, Damti A, Younes G, Auslander R. Pregestational body mass index, weight gain during pregnancy and maternal hyperglycemia. Gynecol Endocrinol. 2011;27:464–7.
34. Most O, Langer O. Gestational diabetes: maternal weight gain in relation to fetal growth, treatment modality, BMI and glycemic control. J Matern Fetal Neonatal Med. 2012;25:2458–63.
35. Hillier TA, Pedula KL, Vesco KK, Schmidt MM, Mullen JA, LeBlanc ES, et al. Excess gestational weight gain: modifying fetal macrosomia risk associated with maternal glucose. Obstet Gynecol. 2008;112:1007–14.
36. Ellerbe CN, Gebregziabher M, Korte JE, Mauldin J, Hunt KJ. Quantifying the impact of gestational diabetes mellitus, maternal weight and race on birthweight via quantile regression. PLoS One. 2013;8:e65017.
37. Gonzalez Gonzalez NL, Goya M, Bellart J, Lopez J, Sancho MA, Mozas J, et al. Obstetric and perinatal outcome in women with twin pregnancy and gestational diabetes. J Matern Fetal Neonatal Med. 2012;25:1084–9.

10

Screening of differentially expressed proteins from syncytiotrophoblast for severe early-onset preeclampsia in women with gestational diabetes mellitus using tandem mass tag quantitative proteomics

Xiaotong Sun[1,2], Tao Qu[3], Xiyan He[2], Xueping Yang[2], Nan Guo[2], Yan Mao[2], Xianghong Xu[3], Xiaodong Sun[4], Xuehong Zhang[1,5,6*] and Weihua Wang[7*]

Abstract

Background: Previous studies have revealed that women with gestational diabetes mellitus (GDM) have an increased risk of developing preeclampsia (PE). The possible reason is the abnormal lipid metabolism caused by GDM that leads to dysfunction of vascular endothelial cells and atherosclerosis, resulting in the onset of PE. However, studies focusing on the pathogenesis of PE in syncytiotrophoblast of GDM patients are lacking. This study aimed to compare differentially expressed proteins from syncytiotrophoblast between women with GDM and women with GDM with subsequently developed PE.

Methods: Syncytiotrophoblast samples were obtained from pregnant women immediately after delivery. To explore the protein expression changes of syncytiotrophoblast that might explain the pathogenesis of PE in women with GDM, quantitative proteomics was performed using tandem mass tag (TMT) isobaric tags and liquid chromatography-tandem mass spectrometry. Bioinformatics analysis was performed to enrich the biological processes that these differentially expressed proteins were involved in.

Results: A total of 28,234 unique peptides and 4140 proteins were identified in all samples. Among them, 23 differentially expressed proteins were identified between patients with GDM and patients with GDM with subsequently developed PE. Therein, 11 proteins were upregulated and 12 proteins were downregulated. Two relative proteins (FLT1 and PABPC4) were independently verified using immunoblotting analysis. Bioinformatic results indicated that the onset of PE in patients with GDM is a multifactorial disorder, involving factors such as apoptosis, transcriptional misregulation, oxidative stress, lipid metabolism, cell infiltration and migration, and angiogenesis.

Conclusion: These results indicated that the inadequacy of endometrium infiltration, angiogenic disorder, and oxidative stress in syncytiotrophoblast are more likely to occur in patients with GDM and may be the potential mechanisms leading to such patients secondarily developing severe early-onset PE.

Keywords: Preeclampsia, Gestational diabetes mellitus, Syncytiotrophoblast, TMT technology, Biomarkers

* Correspondence: zhangxueh@lzu.edu.cn; wangweihua11@yahoo.com
[1]The First Clinical Medical College, Lanzhou University, Lanzhou, China
[7]Houston Fertility Laboratory, Houston, TX, USA
Full list of author information is available at the end of the article

Background

Preeclampsia (PE), which is one of the major causes of maternal and perinatal mortality or serious morbidity, is a common pregnancy-specific placental disease, affecting at least 5% of pregnant women [1–3]. PE is characterised by new-onset maternal hypertension and proteinuria after 20 weeks' gestation [3, 4]. According to the onset time, PE can be divided into two subtypes: early-onset subtype, occurring before 34 weeks of gestation, and late-onset subtype, occurring from 34 weeks [5]. Although the known pathogenesis of PE is so diverse and complex that no hypothesis has so far covered all the causes, recent studies suggest that the early-onset and late-onset subtypes arise from different etiopathogenic causes. Early-onset PE is associated with abnormal placental function, mainly manifested in the insufficient invasion of the maternal myometrium by the trophoblast cells, which results in uterine spiral artery remodelling disorder and placental superficial implantation. Late-onset PE is associated with maternal predisposition to arterial diseases, developed due to interfering endothelial function by obesity, diabetes, lipid metabolism dysfunction, and inflammation [1, 6–8].

Gestational diabetes mellitus (GDM) also is a pregnancy-specific disease, characterised by the new onset of any degree of glucose intolerance during pregnancy [9]. Although GDM and PE share several similar risk factors such as increased pre-pregnancy body mass index (BMI) and maternal age as well as multiple gestation pregnancies, GDM was found to be an independent risk factor for PE [10, 11]. Women with GDM have an increased risk of developing PE [12–14]. One reason is that abnormal lipid metabolism caused by GDM leads to dysfunction of vascular endothelial cells and atherosclerosis [15]. This reason is consistent with the pathogenesis of late-onset PE.

Recently, high-throughput proteomic technology has been widely applied to screen differentially expressed proteins in different tissues of the placenta, plasma, syncytiotrophoblast extracellular vesicles, and umbilical artery from patients with PE [3, 16–19]. These studies partly revealed the potential pathogenesis of PE and identified candidate biomarkers to predict the occurrence of PE during pregnancy. Li et al. found that the level of plasma fatty acid-binding protein 4 (FABP4) in patients with PE in the GDM group was significantly higher than that in the GDM group, suggesting that plasma FABP4 level could predict the occurrence of PE in women with GDM [20]. However, no studies using high-throughput proteomic analysis to screen differentially expressed proteins between patients with GDM and patients with GDM with subsequently developed PE have been conducted. Therefore, this study aimed to establish a comparative proteomics of the syncytiotrophoblast in patients with GDM and patients with GDM with subsequently developed PE using the tandem mass tag (TMT) quantitative technology, in the hope of identifying candidate biomarkers for predicting PE from patients with GDM and providing targets for future therapy in women with PE with GDM.

Methods

Sample collection

This study was approved by the Ethical Committee of the Gansu Provincial Hospital. All study participants agreed to the sample collection and provided written informed consent. The inclusion criteria for all participants were the following: informed consent to participate in this study, age between 18 and 35 years, singleton pregnancy, absence of diabetes mellitus, hypertension, kidney disease, cardiovascular disease before pregnancy, and not taking any medication. A total of 24 patients with GDM were diagnosed according to a 75-g oral glucose tolerance test (OGTT) at 24–28 weeks of gestation (fasting ≥ 5.1 mmol/L, 2 h ≥ 8.5 mmol/L). All pregnant women with GDM were treated with diet without insulin intervention. Among them, 9 patients developed severe PE according to systolic blood pressure (SBP) ≥160 mmHg and/or diastolic blood pressure (DBP) ≥110 mmHg and proteinuria > 3 g/24 h and selected as cases.

Placental samples of the 9 patients with GDM and 9 patients with PE with GDM were obtained after the participants' delivery at the Gansu Provincial Hospital. The syncytiotrophoblasts were separated from the placental samples within 30 min, frozen immediately in liquid nitrogen, and stored at – 80 °C.

Protein extraction

Three samples from the 9 patients with GDM or 9 patients with PE with GDM were randomly selected as one biological parallel. An equal amount of syncytiotrophoblast sample from each patient was pooled and ground into powder in liquid nitrogen. All of the mixed samples were homogenised using homogeniser in SDT1 buffer (4% SDS, 1 mmol DTT, 100 mmol Tris–HCl, pH 7.6). Protein extraction was performed by sonication (Power 80 W, work 10 s, interval 10 s, cycle 10 times) on ice and then was boiled for 15 min. The crude extract was centrifuged at 14,000 g for 40 min to collect the supernatant. The supernatant was filtered with 0.22-μm filters and quantified with the BCA Protein Assay Kit (Bio-Rad, USA). The filtrates were stored at – 80 °C for future use.

Protein digestion and TMT labelling

Protein digestion was performed using filter-aided sample preparation (FASP) procedure as described before [19]. Briefly, 200 μg of total proteins from each pool was diluted in 30 μl SDT2 buffer (4% SDS, 100 mmol DTT, 150 mmol Tris–HCl, pH 8.0), boiled for 5 min, and cooled to 25 °C. The proteins were washed using washing buffer (8 M urea,

150 mmol Tris–HCl, pH 8.0) by repeated ultrafiltration (Microcon units, 10 kD) at 14,000 g for 15 min to remove the low-molecular-weight components. Each filter was added in 100 μl iodoacetamide (100 mM iodoacetamide in washing buffer) for blocking reduced cysteine residues, incubated in darkness for 30 min, and then centrifuged to discard the filtrate. The filter was washed three times using 100 μl washing buffer and 100 μl of 100 mM TEAB buffer. Then, 4-μg trypsin (Promega, USA), revolved in 40-μl TEAB buffer, was added to digest the protein suspension overnight at 37 °C. Finally, the resulting peptides were collected via centrifugation, and the concentrations were calculated according to OD280.

About 100 μg of each resulting peptide mixture was labelled using TMT reagent according to the manufacturer's instructions (Thermo Fisher Scientific, USA). Specifically, three syncytiotrophoblast samples from patients with GDM were labelled with 128 N, 128C, and 129 N isobaric TMT tags, while the other three syncytiotrophoblast samples from patients with PE with GDM were labelled with 129C, 130 N, and 130C isobaric TMT tags, respectively. After TMT labelling, the digested sample was fractionated into 10 fractions, and the excess label and salts were removed, according to Pierce High pH Reversed-Phase Fractionation Kit Manual (Thermo Fisher Scientific).

Liquid chromatography–mass spectrometry/mass spectrometry analysis

Each fraction, dissolved into solution A (0.1% formic acid), was loaded into a reverse phase trap column (Thermo Scientific Acclaim PepMap100, 100 μm × 2 cm, nanoViper C18) connected to the C18-reversed phase analytical column (Thermo Scientific Easy Column, 10 cm long, 75-μm inner diameter, 3-μm resin) and separated with a linear gradient of solution B (84% acetonitrile and 0.1% formic acid) at a flow rate of 300 nL/min. The linear gradient was processed as follows: 0–55% solution B for 80 min, 55–100% solution B for 5 min, and 100% solution B for 5 min.

Ten fractions from each sample were analysed using liquid chromatography–mass spectrometry/mass spectrometry (LC-MS/MS) by Q Exactive Mass Spectrometer coupled to Easy nLC (Thermo Scientific) in positive ion mode for 90 min. MS data was acquired using a data-dependent top10 method, dynamically choosing the most abundant precursor ions from the survey scan (300–1800 m/z) for higher-energy collisional dissociation (HCD) fragmentation. The instrument parameters were set as follows: automatic gain control target was 3e6; dynamic exclusion duration, 40 s; resolution for survey scans, 70,000 at m/z 200; resolution for HCD spectra, 35,000 at m/z 200; and isolation width, 2 m/z. Normalised collision energy was 30 eV, and the underfill ratio was 0.1%.

Data analysis

The acquired MS spectra were analysed using MASCOT search engine (version 2.2; Matrix Science, London, UK) embedded into Proteome Discoverer 1.4 (Thermo Electron, San Jose, CA, USA). The parameters were set as follows: peptide mass tolerance was ±20 ppm, fragment mass tolerance was 0.1 Da, and max missed cleavages were set to 2. TMT-10plex was set as fixed modifications, and oxidation was set as variable modifications. False discovery rate of peptides was set to be < 0.01. All peptide ratios were normalised by the median protein ratio, and the median protein ratio was defined as 1 after the normalisation.

Protein identification and bioinformatic analysis

For identification of differentially expressed proteins, the fold change should be > 1.2 or < 0.83 with a P value (student's t-test) < 0.05. The gene ontology (GO) annotation of differentially expressed proteins was blasted against SwissProt database (human) using the NCBI BLAST+ client software. Functional annotation was searched against the online Kyoto Encyclopedia of Genes and Genomes (KEGG) database (http://geneontology.org/). GO enrichment and KEGG pathway enrichment were performed based on the Fisher' exact test. Hierarchical clustering was analysed using Cluster 3.0 (http://bonsai.hgc.jp/~mdehoon/software/cluster/software.htm) and the Java Treeview software. The protein–protein interaction (PPI) networks were analysed using IntAct Molecular Interaction Database (http://www.ebi.ac.uk/intact/) and visualised using Cytoscape software.

Immunoblotting

For immunoblotting analysis, syncytiotrophoblast tissue was homogenised in RIPA buffer containing protease inhibitors and quantified with the BCA Protein Assay Kit. The protein bands were detected and imaged using a capillary-based western blot automated system ProteinSimple WES with anti-vascular endothelial growth factor receptor 1 (FLT1, 1:1000, Proteintech, 13,687–1-AP), anti-polyadenylate-binding protein 4 (PABPC4, 1:1000, Proteintech, 14,960–1-AP), and anti-glyceraldehyde-3-phosphate dehydrogenase (GAPDH, 1:1000, Proteintech, 10,494–1-AP).

Results

Characteristics of the patients

Table 1 shows the clinical characteristics of patients with GDM and patients with GDM with subsequently developed PE. The maternal age, parity, pregnancy BMI at 12 week, gestation age at delivery, gestation age at 75-g OGTT, and glucose concentrations of 0 and 2 h OGTT in patients with GDM did not differ significantly from those in patients with GDM with subsequently developed PE. Systolic and diastolic blood pressures, as well as insulin concentration, were significantly higher in patients with GDM with subsequently developed PE than that in patients with GDM (P < 0.05). The

Table 1 Clinical characteristics of patients with GDM and patients with GDM with subsequently developed PE (GDM/PE)

	GDM	GDM/PE	*P* value
Sample size (*n*)	9	9	
Maternal age (years)	32.67 ± 5.12	30.22 ± 3.90	0.107
Parity	0.44 ± 0.53	0.33 ± 0.47	0.681
Pregnancy BMI at 12 week (kg/m^2)	25.76 ± 2.56	25.93 ± 2.14	0.824
Gestation age at delivery (wk)	38.49 ± 0.98	33.97 ± 1.05	< 0.001*
Gestation age at 75-g OGTT (wk)	24.70 ± 040	24.81 ± 0.49	1.100
OGTT 0 h glucose (mmol/L)	5.46 ± 0.64	5.31 ± 0.27	0.533
OGTT 2 h glucose (mmol/L)	7.36 ± 1.12	8.43 ± 1.39	0.027*
Insulin (mU/L)	11.73 ± 1.79	15.17 ± 3.09	0.046*
Maximum SBP (mmHg)	131.33 ± 5.70	186.44 ± 11.59	< 0.001*
Maximum DBP (mmHg)	85.22 ± 4.58	121.89 ± 9.46	< 0.001*
Proteinuria (g/24 h)	0.01 ± 0.01	5.56 ± 1.65	< 0.001*

*$P < 0.05$

protein contents in a 24-h urine collection in all of the patients with GDM with subsequently developed PE were 5.56 ± 1.65 g, while those in all of the patients with GDM were 0.01 ± 0.01 g. It is worth noting that, without medication, all of the diagnoses of PE in patients with GDM in our study were severe and before 34 weeks (data not shown), suggesting that GDM promotes the development of severe early-onset PE.

Protein identification

A total of 28,234 unique peptides and 4140 proteins were identified in all samples. According to protein identification criteria, 23 differentially expressed proteins were found in comparison between the patients with PE with GDM and patients with GDM (Table 2). Among them, 11 proteins were upregulated, and 12 proteins were downregulated. The K-means clustering of these differentially expressed proteins is shown in a heat map (Fig. 1).

Immunoblotting verification

To verify the expression levels of differentially expressed proteins discovered by TMT analysis, immunoblotting was performed to investigate the expression patterns of FLT1 and PABPC4, two proteins in the same samples. GAPDH was chosen as an internal control. The results showed that FLT1 was expressed at higher levels, while PABPC4 was expressed at lower levels in PE with GDM groups than in GDM groups (Fig. 2), suggesting that the immunoblotting results were in line with TMT proteomics results.

Bioinformatic analysis

Figure 3 shows the top 20 rankings of biological process, molecular function, and cellular component based on GO annotation. The main biological process of these differentially expressed proteins was regulation of extrinsic apoptotic signalling pathway, regulation of transcription from RNA polymerase, cellular modified amino acid metabolic process, selenium compound metabolic process, establishment or maintenance of polarity of follicular epithelium, and animal organ senescence. The main molecular function of these proteins was associated with methylselenol reductase activity, 15-hydroxyprostaglandin dehydrogenase activity, diamine oxidase activity, histamine oxidase activity, and icosanoid receptor activity. The main cellular component was ribonuclease H2 complex, CHOP–activating transcription factor 3 complex, actomyosin, actin portion, and cornified envelope. By KEGG pathway analysis, 4 differentially expressed proteins were enriched into histidine metabolism and transcriptional misregulation in cancer pathways (Fig. 4). By PPI analysis, 7 differentially expressed proteins (WDR1, FLT1, MUC1, ANXA4, ERO1A, ATF3, and PABPC4) interacted with each other and enriched into a larger protein interaction network. The other 10 differentially expressed proteins (KIF1BP, NDUFV3, and GSTA3; ASPSCR1 and MRGBP; AHCYL2 and TCHH; TXNRD1; RNASEH2C; and PAPP-A2) enriched into different protein interaction network, respectively (Fig. 5). These results suggested that occurrence of PE in women with GDM is the result of multiple pathway dysfunction.

Discussion

Although studies have revealed that GDM is one of the risk factors for developing PE, the pathogenesis remains unclear. To clarify the molecular mechanisms and search the potential biomarkers for PE screening from women with GDM, we identified and quantified differentially expressed proteins from women with GDM with subsequently developed PE compared with GDM women. The results showed that a total of 23 proteins expressed differentially between the two groups. These proteins involved in different biological functions and signalling

Table 2 The differentially expressed proteins identified in syncytiotrophoblast from patients with GDM with subsequently developed PE and patients with GDM

Protein name	Accession No	Gene name	Fold change	*P* value
WD repeat-containing protein 1	O75083	WDR1	1.600	0.026
Vascular endothelial growth factor receptor 1	P17948	FLT1	1.377	0.031
15-hydroxyprostaglandin dehydrogenase	P15428	HPGD	1.366	0.015
Ribonuclease H2, subunit C	E9PKP0	RNASEH2C	1.339	0.001
Amine oxidase	D3DX03	ABP1	1.311	0.003
cDNA FLJ51917	B4DNZ4	N/A	1.261	0.040
Mucin 1	B6ECB2	MUC1	1.256	0.049
Annexin A4	P09525	ANXA4	1.251	0.049
cDNA FLJ38330	Q8N959	N/A	1.235	0.045
Pappalysin-2	Q9BXP8	PAPPA2	1.221	0.015
ERO1-like protein 1 alpha	Q96HE7	ERO1A	1.205	0.011
KIF 1-binding protein	Q96EK5	KIF1BP	0.826	0.047
Activating transcription factor 3	Q7Z567	ATF3	0.823	0.041
Thioredoxin reductase 1	E9PIR7	TXNRD1	0.822	0.027
cDNA FLJ16285	B3KV96	N/A	0.815	0.035
NADH dehydrogenase flavoprotein 3	P56181	NDUFV3	0.815	0.010
Glutathione S-transferase A3	Q5JW85	GSTA3	0.802	0.045
Tether containing UBX domain for GLUT4	J3QL04	ASPSCR1	0.795	0.037
Trichohyalin	Q07283	TCHH	0.789	0.044
Solute carrier family 13	Q59HF0	N/A	0.781	0.009
MRG/MORF4L-binding protein	Q9NV56	MRGBP	0.776	0.042
Adenosylhomocysteinase 2	Q96HN2	AHCYL2	0.746	0.028
Polyadenylate-binding protein 4	B1ANR0	PABPC4	0.744	0.025

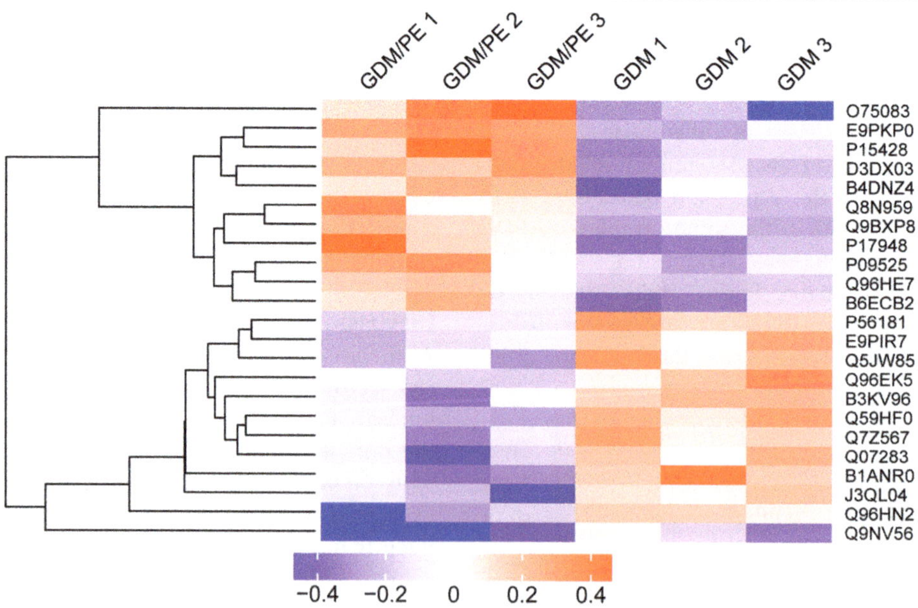

Fig. 1 K-means clustering of differentially expressed proteins identified in human syncytiotrophoblast

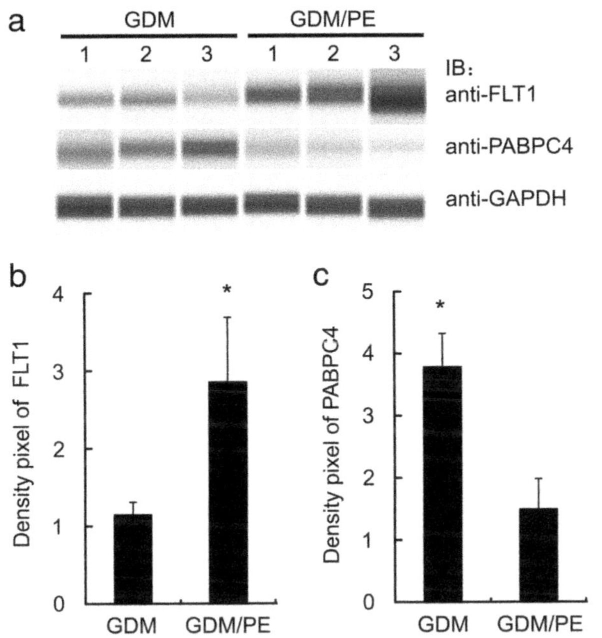

Fig. 2 Immunoblotting analysis with anti-FLT1, anti-PABPC4 and anti-GAPDH antibodies was performed on patients with GDM and patients with GDM with subsequently developed PE (**a**). Comparison of protein expression levels of FLT1 (**b**) and PABPC4 (**c**) in patients with GDM with subsequently developed PE and patients with GDM groups. The Y-axis represents the relative quantification of target proteins normalised to GAPDH. The minimum mean of band density pixels was taken as 1

pathway implied that multiple mechanisms contribute to the development of PE from women with GDM.

Of the 23 differentially expressed proteins, 7 have been reported to be implicated in the onset of PE. In our study, 5 of these proteins have upregulated expression, such as FLT1, MUC1, ANXA4, PAPP-A2, and HPGD. Two proteins were downregulated, such as ATF3 and TXNRD1.

As a transcriptional repressor, ATF3 is induced rapidly when cells are exposed to a wide range of stress stimuli. The increased ATF3 prevents cells from tumour necrosis factor alpha (TNF-α)-induced apoptosis by inhibiting tumour suppressor gene p53 transcription and cleavage of procaspase 3. Thus, ATF3 may maintain the survival of endothelial cells during vascular inflammation and atherosclerosis [21]. In preeclamptic placentas, both mRNA and protein expression levels of ATF3 were decreased. This reduction was likely to occur after prolonged hypoxia. The decrease of ATF3 expression increased cytokine interleukin 6, TNF-α, and nuclear factor kappaB (NF-κB) expression as well as Flt-1 secretion [22]. FLT1 is produced in the placenta and can be detected in the placenta, amniotic fluid, and serum [23–25]. The function of FLT1 is to antagonise vascular endothelial growth factor (VEGF) effects on the formation of placental vasculature and maternal endothelial cell function [24]. The increase of FLT1 protein level is an important risk factor leading to impaired placental angiogenesis [26]. In fact, the expression level of FLT1 in serum of the large number of women with PE were significantly elevated [27–31], while after 48 h of delivery, the level of FLT1 in serum decreased dramatically [32, 33]. Patients with GDM tend to develop dysfunction of vascular endothelial cells and atherosclerosis, leading to PE [15]. Therefore, ATF3–FLT1 axis may be the primary pathogenesis of women with GDM to secondarily developed PE.

MUC1, with a large mucin-like extracellular domain, locates on the surface of cells. Overexpression of MUC1 reduces cell–cell interactions and inhibits integrin-mediated cell adhesion to the extracellular matrix [34]. Immunohistochemical and immunoblotting analysis showed that the expression levels of MUC1 in the syncytiotrophoblast and extravillous trophoblast cells (EVT) of severe preeclamptic placentas were increased. MUC1 overexpression suppressed cell–matrix adhesion and EVT invasion [35], probably leading to insufficient infiltration of syncytiotrophoblast cells into the endometrium.

ANXA4 is a Ca^{2+}-dependent phospholipid binding protein, specifically expressing on the basal surface of syncytiotrophoblast. The increased activity of phospholipase A2 would lead to more arachidonic acid decomposing into thromboxane A2, which results in coagulation subsequently. Therefore, after delivery, ANXA4 enters the maternal bloodstream and prevent the activation of blood coagulation [36]. In gallbladder cancer tissues, the ANXA4 gene was highly expressed. Moreover, the elevated ANXA4 expression correlated well with invasion depth in patients with gallbladder cancer. One reason is that upregulated expression of ANXA4 promotes tumour cell growth, migration, and invasion by activating NF-κB pathway [37]. NF-κB plays important roles in the cell proliferation, inflammation, angiogenesis, apoptosis, invasion, and cellular adhesion, which also are important features in pathogenesis of PE. Using 2D electrophoresis combined with MALDI-TOF-MS, ANXA4 was identified as one of the 11 upregulated expressed proteins from preeclamptic placenta compared to that of normal pregnancy. This result is the first finding that there is a relationship between upregulated ANXA4 and the occurrence of PE [38]. In our study, ANXA4 also has upregulated expression in patients with GDM with subsequently developed PE compared to patients with GDM. The involved common mechanism should be further studied in detail.

Insulin-like growth factors (IGFs) and their binding proteins (IGFBPs) play important roles during establishment of pregnancy and placental development by mediating cell communication between trophoblasts and deciduae, as well as promoting trophoblast invasion [39]. PAPP-A2, also named pregnancy-associated plasma protein-A2, is capable of cleaving IGFBP5 specifically to regulate its biological function [40]. Both mRNA and protein expression levels of PAPP-A2 were upregulated in severe early-onset preeclamptic placentas and

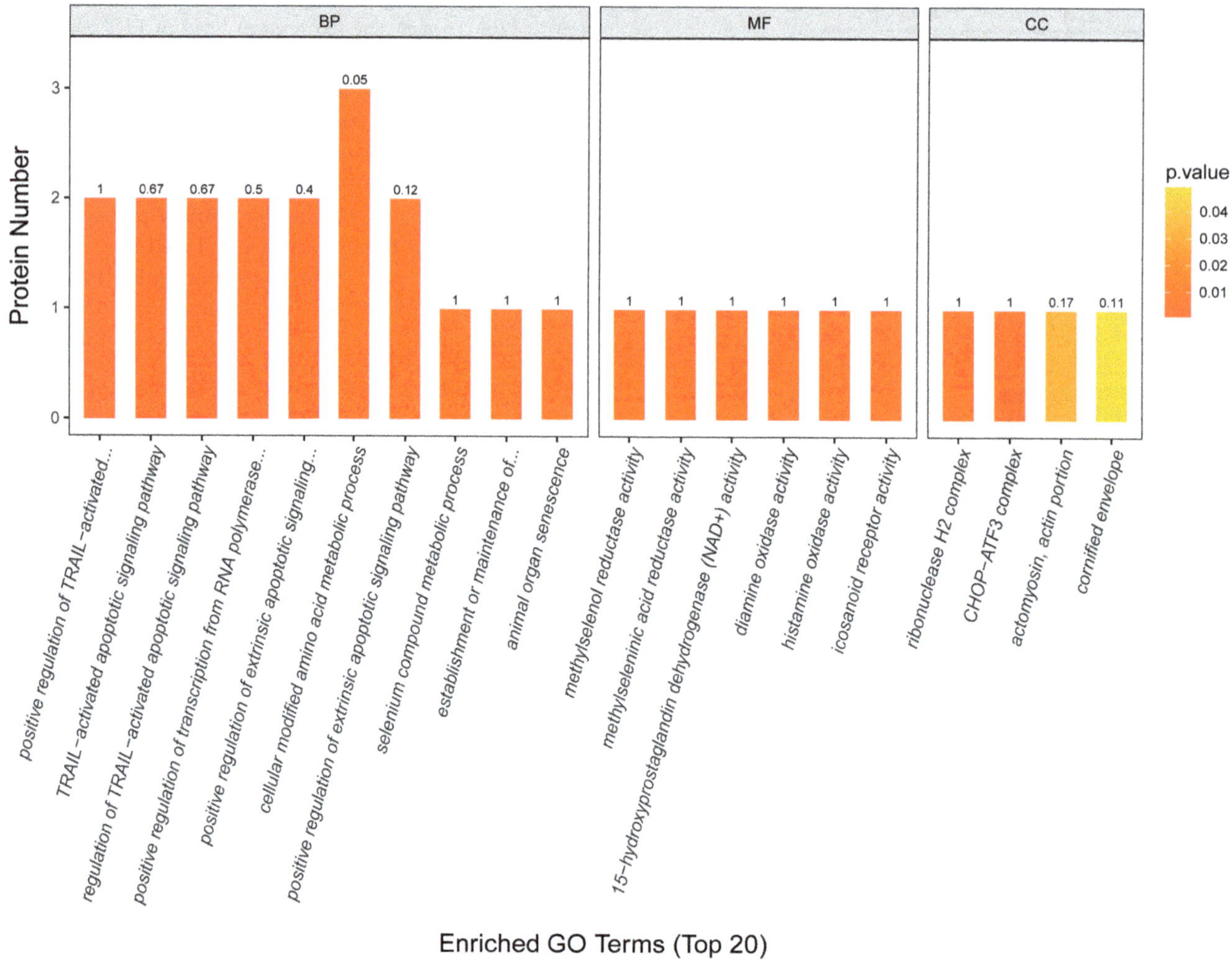

Fig. 3 Bioinformatics analysis of the differentially expressed proteins. The top 20 rankings of biological process, molecular function, and cellular component that significantly changed based on GO analysis. The number on each bar represents the proportion of the differentially expressed proteins annotated to a GO category to the overall proteins annotated to the same GO category

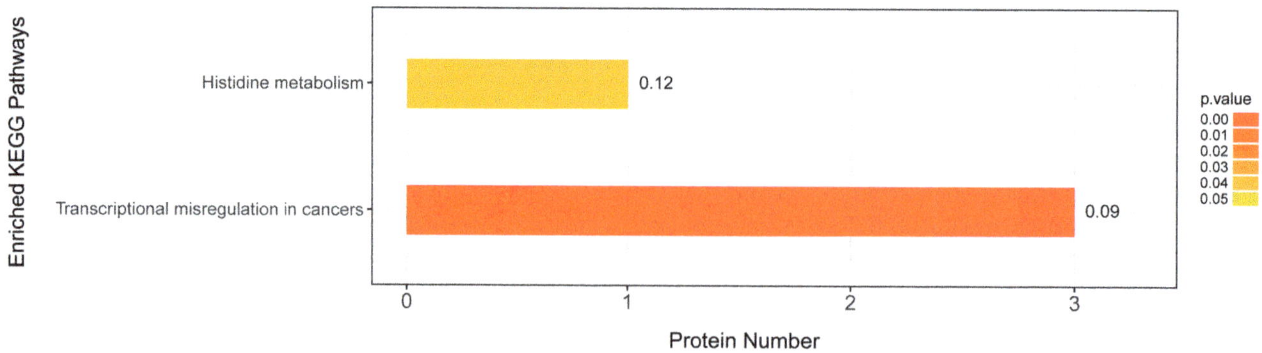

Fig. 4 KEGG pathway enrichment of differentially expressed proteins. The number on each bar represents the proportion of differentially expressed proteins annotated to a KEGG pathway to the overall proteins annotated to the same KEGG pathway

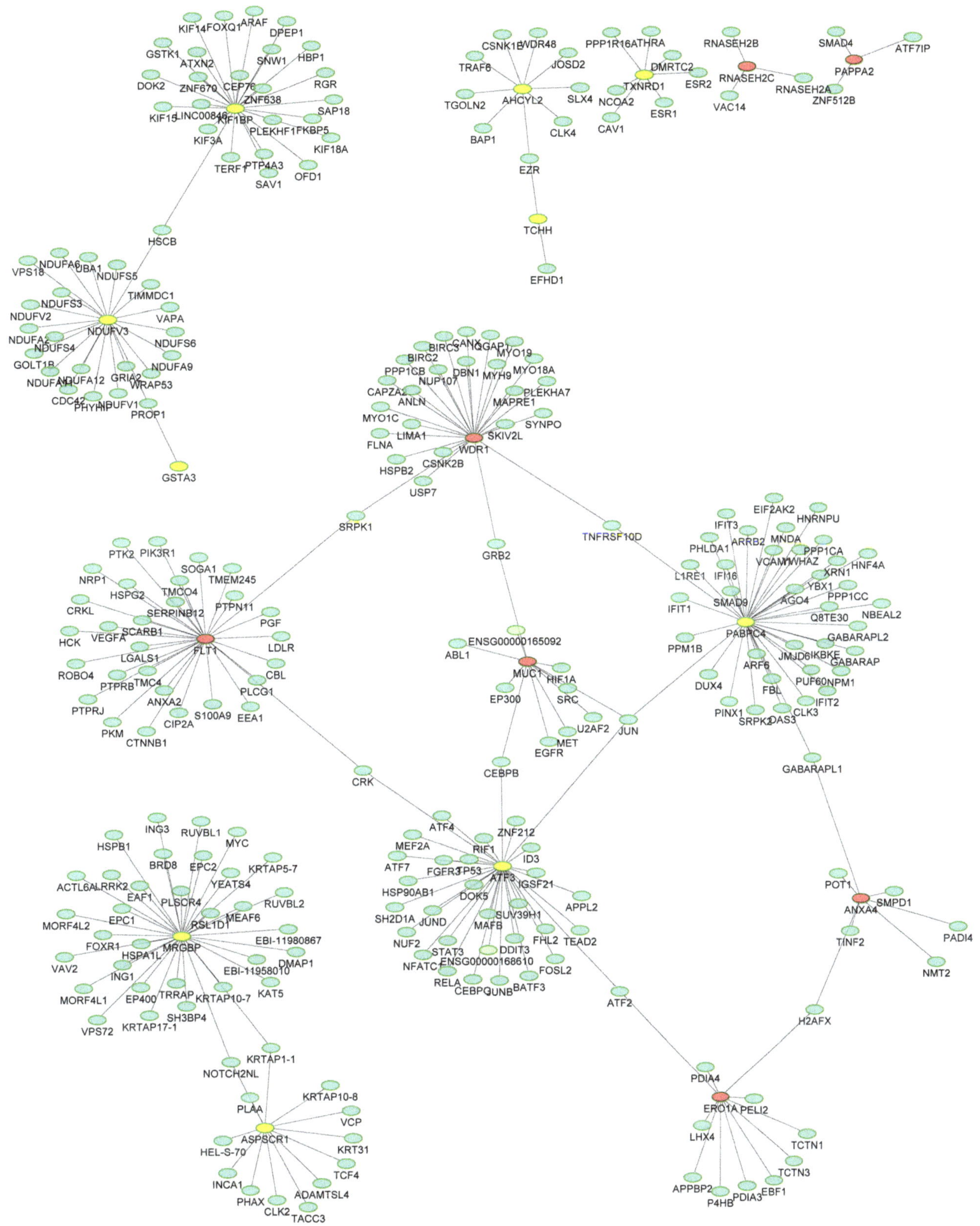

Fig. 5 The protein interaction network of differentially expressed proteins. Red spot indicates upregulated protein, yellow spot indicates downregulated protein

localised to the syncytiotrophoblast [41]. The upregulated PAPP-A2 may degrade IGFBP5 and then inhibit trophoblast invasion. However, a study has also shown that hypoxia and TNF-α, but not oxidative stress, contributed to the upregulation of PAPPA2, suggesting that PAPPA2 is upregulated as a consequence, rather than a cause of PE [42]. Due to the increased concentration of PAPP-A2 in serum in agreement with that in placenta, PAPP-A2 has a potential as a biomarker for the onset of PE [43].

Oxidative stress damages placental tissue resulting in intrauterine growth retardation and foetal distress, involving in the pathogenesis of PE. Thioredoxin reductase was located in the cytoplasm and mitochondria of cytotrophoblasts and deciduae in the placenta. It may protect the placenta against oxidative stress by reducing reactive oxygen species [44]. The decreased protein expression level of TXNRD1 may be attributed to patients with GDM with PE.

As a cancer suppressor, the expression level of HPGD is decreased in several tumour cells. The decreased HPGD blocks the production of the prostaglandin E2 (PGE2) metabolite, which can promote cancer progression by modulating tumour cells of proliferation, migration, invasion, angiogenesis, and apoptosis [45]. In a previous study, the mRNA level of HPGD in the placenta of patients with PE was decreased [46], while in our study, the protein level of HPGD was increased, implying that gene expression of HPGD might be regulated by negative feedback. Therefore, the increased HPGD protein in our study may also interfere syncytiotrophoblast cells of proliferation, migration, invasion, angiogenesis, and apoptosis. This finding is worthy of further investigation.

In addition, ERO1A, upregulated in our study, was strongly induced by hypoxia, involving in oxidative endoplasmic reticulum protein folding and inhibition of VEGF-driven angiogenesis [47]. Although the function of inhibiting VEGF-driven angiogenesis is similar to that of FLT1, the relationship between ERO1A and onset of PE remains unknown. More studies are required to investigate whether ERO1A is involved in the pathogenesis of PE and can be used as a potential biomarker.

Subsequently, we selected two proteins, FLT1, involved in the key processes as mentioned above, and PABPC4, verified by immunoblotting analysis. The expression pattern of these proteins was consistent with the proteomics results. Finally, bioinformatic analysis revealed that the differentially expressed proteins mainly enriched to apoptosis function and transcriptional misregulation in cancer pathways. These results implied that the regulation mechanism of syncytiotrophoblast on the invasion and migration of endometrium may be similar to that of tumour cells. Patients with GDM are more likely to have misregulation of transcription, angiogenic disorder, and oxidative stress, which lead to insufficient infiltration of syncytiotrophoblast cells and dysfunction of apoptosis, subsequently leading to the onset of severe early-onset PE. Further research and verification are needed to explore the possible.

Limitation of our study was that the sample size was small, for it is a little difficult to recruit more patients with strict inclusion criteria. A large number of experimental samples from different hospitals will be required to verify and obtain further arguments in future study. Moreover, proteomics studies of placental tissue are not the only way to confirm our findings, protein-related studies of fetal appendages such as blood, urine, and amniotic fluid are also feasible. Therefore, we hope that there will be more research on preeclampsia in the future.

Conclusion

In this study, we performed TMT proteomic analysis on syncytiotrophoblast to compare the differentially expressed proteins. Twenty-three protein expressions were identified as significant differences between patients with GDM and patients with GDM with subsequently developed PE. Some of these differentially expressed proteins have been confirmed to be involved in the development of PE. Bioinformatic results indicated that the onset of PE form GDM patients also is a multifactorial disorder, involving in apoptosis, transcriptional misregulation, oxidative stress, cell infiltration and migration, angiogenesis, etc. Our results show that the inadequacy of endometrium infiltration, dysfunction of apoptosis, angiogenic disorder, and oxidative stress in syncytiotrophoblast cells more likely occur in GDM patients. These processes may be the potential mechanisms leading to GDM patients to secondarily developed severe early-onset PE. Thus, these proteins can also be considered as candidate biomarkers for predicting the onset of PE from women with GDM or as an intervention target for preventing GDM from developing into PE.

Abbreviations

BMI: Body mass index; DBP: Diastolic blood pressure; EVT: Extravillous trophoblast cells; FABP4: Fatty acid-binding protein 4; FASP: Filter-aided sample preparation; FLT1: Vascular endothelial growth factor receptor 1; GAPDH: Glyceraldehyde-3-phosphate dehydrogenase; GDM: Gestational diabetes mellitus; GO: Gene ontology; HCD: Higher-energy collisional dissociation; HPGD: 15-hydroxyprostaglandin dehydrogenase; IGFBPs: Insulin-like growth factor binding proteins; IGFs: Insulin-like growth factors; KEGG: Kyoto encyclopedia of genes and genomes; LC-MS/MS: Liquid chromatography–mass spectrometry/ mass spectrometry; NF-κB: Nuclear factor kappaB; OGTT: Oral glucose tolerance test; PABPC4: Polyadenylate-binding protein 4; PE: Preeclampsia; PGE2: Prostaglandin E2; PPI: Protein–protein interaction; SBP: Systolic blood pressure; TMT: Tandem mass tag; TNF-α: Tumour necrosis factor alpha; VEGF: Vascular endothelial growth factor

Acknowledgements

We thank all mothers for consenting to participate in this study and provide their information, and Editage for providing professional writing services.

Funding

This research was supported by Gansu Provincial Commission of Health and Family Planning (No. GSWSKY2016–48), Gansu Provincial Hospital (No. 17GSSY2–3 and 16GSSY4–4), and Lanzhou science and technology program (No. 2017-4-68).

Authors' contributions
XS1 conceived the study design, interviewed mother for each case, and wrote the manuscript. TQ performed the experiments and analysed the data. XH and XY collected samples for each case and reviewed relevant background research. NG and YM reviewed medical records and assisted in analysis of the data. XX assisted in interpretation of medical record data. XS2 advised in designing the study. XZ and WW advised in designing the study and revised the manuscript. All authors read and approved the final manuscript.

Consent for publication
All mothers provided written informed consent to publish their individual information.

Competing interests
The authors declare that they have no competing interests.

Author details
[1]The First Clinical Medical College, Lanzhou University, Lanzhou, China. [2]Department of Obstetrics, Gansu Provincial Hospital, Lanzhou, China. [3]Department of Biotherapy Center, Gansu Provincial Hospital, Lanzhou, China. [4]Department of Endocrinology, Affiliated Hospital of Weifang Medical University, Weifang, China. [5]The Reproductive Medicine Special Hospital of the First Hospital of Lanzhou University, Lanzhou, China. [6]Key Laboratory for Reproductive Medicine and Embryo of Gansu, Lanzhou, China. [7]Houston Fertility Laboratory, Houston, TX, USA.

References

1. Steegers EA, von Dadelszen P, Duvekot JJ, Pijnenborg R. Pre-eclampsia. Lancet. 2010;376(9741):631–44.
2. Saleem S, McClure EM, Goudar SS, Patel A, Esamai F, Garces A, Chomba E, Althabe F, Moore J, Kodkany B, et al. A prospective study of maternal, fetal and neonatal deaths in low- and middle-income countries. Bull World Health Organ. 2014;92(8):605–12.
3. Auer J, Camoin L, Guillonneau F, Rigourd V, Chelbi ST, Leduc M, Laparre J, Mignot TM, Vaiman D. Serum profile in preeclampsia and intra-uterine growth restriction revealed by iTRAQ technology. J Proteome. 2010;73(5):1004–17.
4. Montoro MN, Kjos SL, Chandler M, Peters RK, Xiang AH, Buchanan TA. Insulin resistance and preeclampsia in gestational diabetes mellitus. Diabetes Care. 2005;28(8):1995–2000.
5. von Dadelszen P, Magee LA, Roberts JM. Subclassification of preeclampsia. Hypertens Pregnancy. 2003;22(2):143–8.
6. Nadeau-Vallee M, Obari D, Palacios J, Brien ME, Duval C, Chemtob S, Girard S. Sterile inflammation and pregnancy complications: a review. Reproduction. 2016;152(6):R277–92.
7. Nelson DB, Ziadie MS, McIntire DD, Rogers BB, Leveno KJ: Placental pathology suggesting that preeclampsia is more than one disease. Am J Obstet Gynecol 2014, 210(1):66 e61–67.
8. Villa PM, Marttinen P, Gillberg J, Lokki AI, Majander K, Orden MR, Taipale P, Pesonen A, Raikkonen K, Hamalainen E, et al. Cluster analysis to estimate the risk of preeclampsia in the high-risk prediction and prevention of preeclampsia and intrauterine growth restriction (PREDO) study. PLoS One. 2017;12(3):e0174399.
9. Singh A, Subramani E, Datta Ray C, Rapole S, Chaudhury K. Proteomic-driven biomarker discovery in gestational diabetes mellitus: a review. J Proteome. 2015;127(Pt A):44–9.
10. Schneider S, Freerksen N, Rohrig S, Hoeft B, Maul H. Gestational diabetes and preeclampsia--similar risk factor profiles? Early Hum Dev. 2012;88(3):179–84.
11. Mrema D, Lie RT, Ostbye T, Mahande MJ, Daltveit AK. The association between pre pregnancy body mass index and risk of preeclampsia: a registry based study from Tanzania. BMC Pregnancy Childbirth. 2018;18(1):56.
12. Nerenberg KA, Johnson JA, Kaul P. Risk of preeclampsia in pregnant women with gestational diabetes in Alberta. Pregnancy Hypertens. 2012;2(3):323–4.
13. Ostlund I, Haglund B, Hanson U. Gestational diabetes and preeclampsia. Eur J Obstet Gynecol Reprod Biol. 2004;113(1):12–6.
14. Phaloprakarn C, Tangjitgamol S. Risk assessment for preeclampsia in women with gestational diabetes mellitus. J Perinat Med. 2009;37(6):617–21.
15. Llurba E, Casals E, Dominguez C, Delgado J, Mercade I, Crispi F, Martin-Gallan P, Cabero L, Gratacos E. Atherogenic lipoprotein subfraction profile in preeclamptic women with and without high triglycerides: different pathophysiologic subsets in preeclampsia. Metabolism. 2005;54(11):1504–9.
16. Qi WH, Zheng MY, Li C, Xu L, Xu JE. Screening of differential proteins of placenta tissues in patients with pre-eclampsia by iTRAQ proteomics techniques. Minerva Med. 2017;108(5):389–95.
17. Kolla V, Jeno P, Moes S, Lapaire O, Hoesli I, Hahn S. Quantitative proteomic (iTRAQ) analysis of 1st trimester maternal plasma samples in pregnancies at risk for preeclampsia. J Biomed Biotechnol. 2012;2012:305964.
18. Li H, Han L, Yang Z, Huang W, Zhang X, Gu Y, Li Y, Liu X, Zhou L, Hu J, et al. Differential proteomic analysis of Syncytiotrophoblast extracellular vesicles from early-onset severe preeclampsia, using 8-Plex iTRAQ labeling coupled with 2D Nano LC-MS/MS. Cell Physiol Biochem. 2015;36(3):1116–30.
19. Pan HT, Guo MX, Xiong YM, Ren J, Zhang JY, Gao Q, Ke ZH, Xu GF, Tan YJ, Sheng JZ, et al. Differential proteomic analysis of umbilical artery tissue from preeclampsia patients, using iTRAQ isobaric tags and 2D nano LC-MS/MS. J Proteome. 2015;112:262–73.
20. Li B, Yang H, Zhang W, Shi Y, Qin S, Wei Y, He Y, Yang W, Jiang S, Jin H. Fatty acid-binding protein 4 predicts gestational hypertension and preeclampsia in women with gestational diabetes mellitus. PLoS One. 2018;13(2):e0192347.
21. Kawauchi J, Zhang C, Nobori K, Hashimoto Y, Adachi MT, Noda A, Sunamori M, Kitajima S. Transcriptional repressor activating transcription factor 3 protects human umbilical vein endothelial cells from tumor necrosis factor-alpha-induced apoptosis through down-regulation of p53 transcription. J Biol Chem. 2002;277(41):39025–34.
22. Kaitu'u-Lino TJ, Brownfoot FC, Hastie R, Chand A, Cannon P, Deo M, Tuohey L, Whitehead C, Hannan NJ, Tong S. Activating transcription factor 3 is reduced in Preeclamptic placentas and negatively regulates sFlt-1 (soluble fms-like tyrosine kinase 1), soluble Endoglin, and Proinflammatory cytokines in placenta. Hypertension. 2017;70(5):1014–24.
23. He B, Yang X, Li Y, Huang D, Xu X, Yang W, Dai Y, Zhang H, Chen Z, Cheng W. TLR9 (toll-like receptor 9) agonist suppresses angiogenesis by differentially regulating VEGFA (vascular endothelial growth factor a) and sFLT1 (soluble vascular endothelial growth factor receptor 1) in preeclampsia. Hypertension. 2018;71(4):671–80.
24. Koga K, Osuga Y, Yoshino O, Hirota Y, Ruimeng X, Hirata T, Takeda S, Yano T, Tsutsumi O, Taketani Y. Elevated serum soluble vascular endothelial growth factor receptor 1 (sVEGFR-1) levels in women with preeclampsia. J Clin Endocrinol Metab. 2003;88(5):2348–51.
25. Vuorela P, Helske S, Hornig C, Alitalo K, Weich H, Halmesmaki E. Amniotic fluid--soluble vascular endothelial growth factor receptor-1 in preeclampsia. Obstet Gynecol. 2000;95(3):353–7.
26. Ahmad S, Ahmed A. Elevated placental soluble vascular endothelial growth factor receptor-1 inhibits angiogenesis in preeclampsia. Circ Res. 2004;95(9):884–91.
27. Levine RJQC, Maynard SE, Yu KF, Epstein FH, Karumanchi SA. Serum sFlt1 concentration during preeclampsia and mid trimester blood pressure in healthy nulliparous women. Am J Obstet Gynecol. 2006;194:1034–41.
28. Palmer KRK-LT, Hastie R, Hannan NJ, Ye L, Binder N, Cannon P, Tuohey L, Johns TG, Shub A, et al. Placental-specific sFLT-1 e15a protein is increased in preeclampsia, antagonizes vascular endothelial growth factor signaling, and has antiangiogenic activity. Hypertension. 2015;66:1251–9.
29. Levine RJMS, Qian C, Lim K-H, England LJ, Yu KF, Schisterman EF, Thadhani R, Sachs BP, Epstein FH, et al. Circulating Angiogenic factors and the risk of preeclampsia. N Engl J Med. 2004;350:672–83.
30. Shibata ERA, Powers RW, Larkin RW, Gilmour C, Bodnar LM, Crombleholme WR, Ness RB, Roberts JM, Hubel CA. Soluble fms-like tyrosine kinase 1 is increased in preeclampsia but not in normotensive pregnancies with small-for-gestational-age neonates: relationship to circulating placental growth factor. Endocrinol Metab J Clin. 2005;90:4895–903.

31. Souders CAMS, Yan J, Wang Y, Boatright NK, Sedan J, Balyozian D, Cheslock PS, Molrine DC, Simas TA. Circulating levels of sFlt1 splice variants as predictive markers for the development of preeclampsia. Int J Mol Sci. 2015; 16:12436–53.
32. McKeeman GCAJ, Caldwell CM, Hunter AJ, McClure N. Soluble vascular endothelial growth factor receptor-1 (sFlt-1) is increased throughout gestation in patients who have preeclampsia develop. Am J Obstet Gynecol. 2004;191:1240–6.
33. Chaiworapongsa TRR, Espinoza J, Bujold E, Mee Kim Y, Goncalves LF, Gomez R, Edwin S. Evidence supporting a role for blockade of the vascular endothelial growth factor system in the pathophysiology of preeclampsia. Young Investigator Award. Am J Obstet Gynecol. 2004;190:1541–7.
34. Wesseling J, van der Valk SW, Vos HL, Sonnenberg A, Hilkens J. Episialin (MUC1) overexpression inhibits integrin-mediated cell adhesion to extracellular matrix components. J Cell Biol. 1995;129(1):255–65.
35. Shyu MK, Chen CW, Lin NY, Liao WC, Chen CH, Lin CJ, Huang HC, Lee JJ, Huang MJ, Tseng GF, et al. MUC1 expression is elevated in severe preeclamptic placentas and suppresses trophoblast cell invasion via beta1-integrin signaling. J Clin Endocrinol Metab. 2011;96(12):3759–67.
36. Masuda J, Takayama E, Satoh A, Ida M, Shinohara T, Kojima-Aikawa K, Ohsuzu F, Nakanishi K, Kuroda K, Murakami M, et al. Levels of annexin IV and V in the plasma of pregnant and postpartum women. Thromb Haemost. 2004;91(6):1129–36.
37. Yao HS, Sun C, Li XX, Wang Y, Jin KZ, Zhang XP, Hu ZQ. Annexin A4-nuclear factor-kappaB feedback circuit regulates cell malignant behavior and tumor growth in gallbladder cancer. Sci Rep. 2016;6:31056.
38. Yang JI, Kong TW, Kim HS, Kim HY. The proteomic analysis of human placenta with pre-eclampsia and Normal pregnancy. J Korean Med Sci. 2015;30(6):770–8.
39. Gratton RJ, Asano H, Han VK. The regional expression of insulin-like growth factor II (IGF-II) and insulin-like growth factor binding protein-1 (IGFBP-1) in the placentae of women with pre-eclampsia. Placenta. 2002;23(4):303–10.
40. Overgaard MT, Boldt HB, Laursen LS, Sottrup-Jensen L, Conover CA, Oxvig C. Pregnancy-associated plasma protein-A2 (PAPP-A2), a novel insulin-like growth factor-binding protein-5 proteinase. J Biol Chem. 2001;276(24):21849–53.
41. Macintire K, Tuohey L, Ye L, Palmer K, Gantier M, Tong S, Kaitu'u-Lino TJ. PAPPA2 is increased in severe early onset pre-eclampsia and upregulated with hypoxia. Reprod Fertil Dev. 2014;26(2):351–7.
42. Wagner PK, Otomo A, Christians JK. Regulation of pregnancy-associated plasma protein A2 (PAPPA2) in a human placental trophoblast cell line (BeWo). Reprod Biol Endocrinol. 2011;9:48.
43. Kloverpris S, Gaidamauskas E, Rasmussen LC, Overgaard MT, Kronborg C, Knudsen UB, Christiansen M, Kumar A, Oxvig C. A robust immunoassay for pregnancy-associated plasma protein-A2 based on analysis of circulating antigen: establishment of normal ranges in pregnancy. Mol Hum Reprod. 2013;19(11):756–63.
44. Ejima K, Nanri H, Toki N, Kashimura M, Ikeda M. Localization of thioredoxin reductase and thioredoxin in normal human placenta and their protective effect against oxidative stress. Placenta. 1999;20(1):95–101.
45. Backlund MG, Mann JR, Holla VR, Buchanan FG, Tai HH, Musiek ES, Milne GL, Katkuri S, DuBois RN. 15-Hydroxyprostaglandin dehydrogenase is down-regulated in colorectal cancer. J Biol Chem. 2005;280(5):3217–23.
46. Schoof E, Girstl M, Frobenius W, Kirschbaum M, Dorr HG, Rascher W, Dotsch J. Decreased gene expression of 11beta-hydroxysteroid dehydrogenase type 2 and 15-hydroxyprostaglandin dehydrogenase in human placenta of patients with preeclampsia. J Clin Endocrinol Metab. 2001;86(3):1313–7.
47. May D, Itin A, Gal O, Kalinski H, Feinstein E, Keshet E. Ero1-L alpha plays a key role in a HIF-1-mediated pathway to improve disulfide bond formation and VEGF secretion under hypoxia: implication for cancer. Oncogene. 2005;24(6):1011–20.

11

Associations of physical activity and sedentary behavior during pregnancy with gestational diabetes mellitus among Asian women in Singapore

Natarajan Padmapriya[1*], Jonathan Y. Bernard[2], Shen Liang[3], See Ling Loy[4], Shirong Cai[1], Iris Shen Zhe[1], Kenneth Kwek[4,5], Keith M. Godfrey[6,7], Peter D. Gluckman[2,8], Seang Mei Saw[9], Yap-Seng Chong[1,2], Jerry Kok Yen Chan[4,5], Falk Müller-Riemenschneider[9,10] and on behalf of the GUSTO Study Group

Abstract

Background: Few studies have investigated physical activity (PA) and sedentary behavior (SB) in relation to fasting (FG) and 2-h postprandial plasma glucose (2hPG) levels and gestational diabetes mellitus (GDM); we investigated these associations among Asian pregnant women.

Methods: As part of the Growing Up in Singapore Towards healthy Outcomes cohort study, PA and SB (sitting and television times) were assessed by interviewer-administered questionnaire. During 75 g oral glucose tolerance tests at 26–28 weeks' gestation we measured FG, 2hPG levels and GDM (FG ≥ 7.0 mmol/L and/or 2hPG ≥ 7.8 mmol/L). Associations were analysed by multiple linear and logistic regression.

Results: Among the 1083 women studied, 18.6% had GDM. SB was not associated with FG, 2hPG and GDM. Higher categories of PA were associated with lower 2hPG and a lower likelihood of GDM (p-trend < 0.05), but not with FG levels. Compared to insufficiently active women, highly active women had lower 2hPG levels [β (95% CI): -0.32 (−0.59, −0.05), $p = 0.020$) and were less likely to have GDM [OR: 0.56 (0.32–0.98), $p = 0.040$]. Stratified analysis revealed no associations among under/normal-weight women, but significant associations among overweight/obese women; in those with BMI ≥23 kg/m^2, sufficiently active and highly active women were less likely to have GDM [OR: 0.52, (0.29–0.93), $p = 0.028$, and OR: 0.34, (0.15–0.77), $p = 0.010$, respectively].

Conclusion: Higher PA was associated with lower 2hPG levels and a lower prevalence of GDM, particularly in overweight/obese women. Further studies are warranted to confirm these findings, and to examine the effectiveness of PA promotion strategies for the prevention of gestational hyperglycemia.

Keywords: Physical activity, Sedentary behavior, Gestational diabetes mellitus, Maternal glucose levels, Pregnancy

Background

Gestational diabetes mellitus (GDM) is defined by the onset or first detection of any degree of glucose intolerance during pregnancy [1]. It has been reported that almost 17.8% of all pregnancies are affected by GDM [2]; this rate ranges from 1 to 25.5% depending on the population studied and the diagnostic tests performed [2, 3]. GDM is associated with a higher risk of complications for both mother and offspring, including caesarean section, preeclampsia, perinatal morbidity, including macrosomia, neonatal hypoglycemia and jaundice [4], and developing type 2 diabetes later in life for mothers and offspring [5]. This emphasises the importance of research on modifiable factors to prevent GDM.

Physical activity (PA) is one of the modifiable lifestyle factors known to have direct and indirect impacts on insulin sensitivity and glucose homeostasis [6–8]. At least 150 min of moderate intensity PA per week is recommended for healthy pregnant women [9, 10], in

* Correspondence: obgnp@nus.edu.sg
[1]Department of Obstetrics & Gynaecology, Yong Loo Lin School of Medicine, National University of Singapore, Singapore, Singapore

line with the World Health Organization (WHO) recommendation for health benefit in general adult populations [11, 12]. Evidence suggests that regular PA during pregnancy may be inversely associated with the risk of GDM [6, 13–20]. The literature also highlights the role of pre-pregnancy body mass index (BMI) as a strong predictor of GDM [21, 22]. However, to our knowledge few studies have examined the association between PA and GDM according to pre-pregnancy BMI and their results were inconsistent [23–25].

Engaging in prolonged sedentary behavior (SB) may have an effect on metabolic health regardless of PA [26]. SB is defined as any waking behavior in a sitting or reclining posture with less than or equal to 1.5 metabolic equivalent tasks (METs) of energy expenditure [27]. A recent meta-analysis reported that prolonged sedentary time is independently associated with deleterious health outcomes, including type 2 diabetes [28]. However, the influence of sedentary behavior (SB) during pregnancy on GDM is poorly understood and the results of existing studies are inconsistent [24, 29, 30].

The majority of previous studies on PA and SB have been conducted in Western populations [17, 23–25, 29, 30], and only a few studies have been conducted among Asian women [31, 32]. However, Asian populations appear to be at a higher risk of developing GDM [21, 33–35], highlighting the public health relevance of examining the association of PA and SB with GDM in Asian women. Moreover, previous studies have investigated the association of PA and SB with gestational glycaemia mainly based on an established glycemic level cut-off points for GDM diagnosis [36]. However, the international multicenter Hyperglycemia and Adverse Pregnancy Outcomes (HAPO) study reported that maternal fasting and stimulated glucose levels even below previous GDM cut-off points were linearly associated with increased adverse pregnancy and neonatal outcomes [37]. This suggests the need to additionally investigate continuous maternal glucose levels regardless of GDM cut-off points.

Based on the above evidence and gaps in the existing literature, we examined the associations of PA and SB during pregnancy with maternal glycemic levels and GDM among Asian women. Additionally, we investigated the magnitude of these associations according to pre-pregnancy BMI subgroups.

Methods

Study design and population

The Growing Up in Singapore Towards healthy Outcomes (GUSTO) mother-offspring cohort study recruited pregnant women attending their first-trimester antenatal dating ultrasound scan clinics at two major public maternity units in Singapore, KK Women's and Children's Hospital (KKH) and National University Hospital (NUH) from June 2009 to September 2010. Pregnant women aged 18 years and above, major ethnic groups (Chinese, Malay and Indian), Singapore citizen or permanent residents who had the intention of delivering in KKH/NUH and staying in Singapore for at least next 5 years, and who had agreed to donate their birth tissues were invited to participate in the study. Women who had type I diabetes mellitus, or who were receiving chemotherapy or psychotropic drugs were excluded. The GUSTO study was designed to investigate the early determinants of child health and development. More details on the study are available elsewhere [38, 39]. The study protocol was approved by the ethics committees of the hospitals involved: SingHealth Centralized Institutional Review Board and the National Healthcare Group Domain Specific Review Board in Singapore. All participants gave written informed consent.

Data collection

As part of interviewer-administered questionnaires at recruitment, women were asked about their age, ethnicity, educational level, pre-pregnancy weight, family history of diabetes, and maternal history of GDM in previous pregnancies. When seen at 26–28 weeks gestation, women were asked questions about cigarette smoking during pregnancy and whether they were exposed to cigarette smoking at home or in their workplace during pregnancy; answers were combined to determine active/passive cigarette smoking during pregnancy.

Participants' dietary energy intake was ascertained based on a 24-h dietary recall; this was administered by trained interviewers at a face-to-face interview at 26–28 weeks of gestation. Various portion sizes of standardized household measuring utensils and food pictures were used to assist women in quantifying their food and beverage intake. Nutrient analysis software (Dietplan, version 7, Forestfield Software) with a food composition database of locally available foods was used to calculate total daily energy intake. Additionally, for food items not found in the database, nutrient information was obtained from food labels or the USDA national nutrient database [19].

Parity data was collected from hospital medical records. Height (to the nearest 0.1 cm) and weight (to 0.01 kg) were measured by trained research staff using a stadiometer (SECA model 213, Hamburg, Germany) and a weighing scale (SECA model 803), respectively. Self-reported pre-pregnancy weight, and height measured at the 26–28 weeks gestational visit were used to calculate pre-pregnancy BMI (kg/m^2). BMI was categorized as underweight, normal weight, overweight and obese (<18.5, 18.5–23, 23–27.5 and ≥27.5, respectively) according to Asian cut-offs [40–42]. Gestational weight gain until 26–28 weeks was calculated by subtracting self-reported pre-pregnancy weight from the weight measured at 26–28 weeks' gestation [43].

Assessment of maternal blood glucose concentrations

Participants underwent a 75-g oral glucose tolerance testing (OGTT) at 26–28 weeks' gestation; overnight fasting (8–10 h) and 2-h postprandial blood specimens were collected. Colorimetry [Advia 2400 Chemistry system (Siemens Medical Solutions Diagnostics) and Beckman LX20 Pro analyzer (Beckman Coulter)] were used to measure both fasting glucose (FG) and 2-h postprandial glucose (2hPG) concentrations. Glucose concentrations were used to classify GDM according to the 1999 WHO standard criteria: ≥7.0 mmol/L for FG and/or ≥7.8 mmol/L for 2hPG [36, 44].

Assessment of physical activity and sedentary behavior

PA questions were part of a structured questionnaire administered by trained interviewers at 26–28 weeks' gestation; the questionnaire included questions on physical activities during the past 6 months of pregnancy. The detailed measurement of PA and SB in the cohort has been reported elsewhere [45]. Briefly, total physical activities were categorized as light-moderate (leaves the person tired but not exhausted, e.g. walking, gardening and golf), moderate (leaves the person exhausted but not breathless, e.g. brisk walking, easy swimming and dancing) and vigorous intensity (makes the heart beat rapidly and leaves the person breathless, e.g. jogging, vigorous swimming, cycling and aerobics). The participants reported the frequency and duration of the three different intensity levels of all physical activities. Frequency was categorized in the questionnaire as never, once every 2–3 months, once a month, once a fortnight, 1–2 times per week, 3–6 times per week, once a day, and more than once a day. Based on these categories an average frequency per week was converted into 0, 0.1, 0.25, 0.5, 1.5, 4.5, 7, and 10.5 times per week, respectively. Women reported an average duration of each period of activity, and the answers were standardized to the nearest 0.5 h. Total hours spent in each intensity level of PA per week was derived by multiplying frequency per week and duration per episode.

An absolute metabolic equivalent task (MET) value was assigned for light-moderate, moderate and vigorous intensity activities (3.3, 4.0 and 8.0, respectively), adapted from the protocol for the International Physical Activity Questionnaire (IPAQ) short form, with 1.0 MET corresponding to resting energy expenditure [46]. Energy expended on each level of PA intensity in MET-hours per week was calculated by multiplying total hours spent on specific intensity per week with its corresponding MET value. Energy expended per week in all three PA intensity levels were summed to estimate total energy expenditure (TEE) on PA per week (light-moderate + moderate + vigorous MET-hours/week), which was then converted into MET-minutes per week. TEE on PA was categorized into insufficiently active (<600 MET-minutes/week), sufficiently active (600 to <3000 MET-minutes/week), and highly active (≥3000 MET-minutes/week). This approach is based on the WHO PA recommendation of a minimum of 600 MET-minutes per week for health benefits in adults [11, 12], and on the IPAQ definition of at least 3000 MET-minutes per week for highly active adults [46]. For example, women who engaged in 30 min of moderate intensity PA at least for 5 days per week were classified as sufficiently active, and women who additionally engaged in 120 min of light-moderate intensity PA daily were classified as highly active.

Sedentary behavior was determined by asking participants to report total sitting time per day during the past 6 months of pregnancy during an interview at 26–28 weeks of gestation; the answers were standardized to the nearest 0.5 h. A separate question determined time spent watching television per day; answers were categorized as none, less than an hour, 1–2 h, 2–3 h, 3–4 h, 4–5 h, and more than 5 h. Based on these categories, an average television viewing duration was converted into 0, 0.5, 1.5, 2.5, 3.5, 4.5 and 5.5 h per day, respectively. In the absence of cut-offs for SB, daily total sitting time during pregnancy was categorized into tertiles to define low, medium and high total sitting time (<7, 7–10, ≥10 h/day, respectively). Higher television viewing time per day during pregnancy was determined based on an upper tertile, which was ≥3 h per day in this sample. This category corresponds with the existing literature, in which 20 or more hours of television viewing time per week during pre-pregnancy has been associated with GDM [47].

Statistical analysis

Frequencies and percentages were calculated for categorical variables, and means and standard deviations for continuous variables. Differences between women with and without GDM were compared using an independent t-test for continuous variables and chi-square tests for categorical variables. Multivariable linear regression was used to investigate the associations of PA, total sitting time and television time with FG and 2hPG concentrations. Multivariable logistic regression was used to assess the associations of PA, total sitting time and television time with GDM. Based on the literature, models were adjusted for following confounders: maternal age, ethnicity, education, pre-pregnancy BMI (continuous), parity at recruitment, history of GDM in previous pregnancy, family history of diabetes, dietary energy intake, exposure to active/passive smoking during pregnancy and pregnancy weight gain at 26–28 gestational visit [24, 48–50]. Additionally, PA and total sitting time, and PA and television viewing time were mutually adjusted in separate models, to explore the independent associations of PA, total sitting time, and television viewing time with all outcome measures. The magnitude of these associations according to pre-pregnancy BMI subgroups was tested by stratifying regressions according to BMI subgroups, though the interaction between PA/SB and BMI subgroups on FG/2hPG/GDM was not statistically significant ($p > 0.05$). BMI subgroups were combined into two groups, under/normal weight and overweight/obese to enhance statistical power. Based on the observed standard deviations, a targeted statistical power of ≥80% and a type I error of 5%, our study is powered to detect differences of 0.05 and 0.14 mmol/L for fasting and 2-h glucose, respectively. For a subgroup of 100 participants, the differences that could be detected were 0.14 and 0.43 mmol/L, respectively. All association tests were two-tailed, and confidence intervals were calculated at the 95% level. All statistical analyses were performed using Statistical Package for the Social Sciences v19 (IBM, Chicago, IL, USA).

Results

There were 1236 women eligible for the study; among them, 1083 (87.6%) participants completed the OGTT and answered PA and SB questions and were thus included in the present analysis (Fig. 1). Excluded women were similar to included subjects in relation to their age, education, parity, BMI, history of GDM, family history of diabetes and dietary energy intake (p > 0.05), but they were more likely to be of Malay or Indian ethnicity ($p = 0.033$). In our sample 18.6% ($n = 201$) of the women had been diagnosed with GDM; these women were more likely to be older, of Indian ethnicity, highly educated, to have a higher BMI and a history of GDM and to not report active/passive smoking during pregnancy ($p < 0.05$) (Table 1).

Associations of PA and SB during pregnancy with maternal blood glucose levels

PA and television time during pregnancy were not significantly associated with FG levels in the overall sample and in BMI subgroups (Table 2). Total sitting time was inversely associated with FG levels in the unadjusted model (overall $p = 0.029$; p for trend =0.035), however, after adjustment this was attenuated with no linear trend (overall $p = 0.074$; p for trend = 0.183). Associations with 2hPG are shown in Table 3. Higher PA during pregnancy was associated with lower 2hPG (p for trend = 0.016). Compared with insufficiently active women, highly active women had lower 2hPG levels [β (95% CI): -0.32 (−0.59, −0.05), $p = 0.020$]. However, a sufficient level of PA was not significantly associated with 2hPG levels [β: −0.16 (−0.37, 0.04), $p = 0.116$]. Stratified analysis revealed associations only among overweight/obese women, but not among underweight/normal weight women (β: −0.51 (−1.00, −0.01), $p = 0.044$, and −0.17 (−0.49, 0.15), $p = 0.291$, respectively).

Compared to women with low sitting time, women with high sitting time had significantly higher 2hPG levels; this association was no longer apparent after adjusting for potential confounders in the overall sample [unadjusted β 95% CI: 0.24 (0.001, 0.48), $p = 0.049$, adjusted β: 0.17 (−0.06, 0.40), $p = 0.137$; p for trend = 0.189]. Among under/normal weight women, those categorized as having medium and high sitting time had higher 2hPG as compared to women with low sitting time [adjusted β 95% CI: 0.31, (0.02, 0.60), $p = 0.037$, and 0.25 (−0.01, 0.52), $p = 0.062$, respectively]; however, there was no linear association (p for trend = 0.099). Sitting time was not associated with 2hPG among overweight/obese women. Television time during pregnancy was not associated with the 2hPG level.

Associations of PA and SB with GDM

Table 4 shows that PA during pregnancy was inversely associated with the likelihood of having GDM (p for trend = 0.041): compared with insufficiently active women, highly active women were less likely to have GDM [adjusted OR (95% CI): 0.56 (0.32–0.98), $p = 0.040$]. However, a sufficient level of PA was not associated with GDM in the overall sample (OR: 0.82 (0.56–1.20), $p = 303$). Among overweight/obese women, sufficiently active and highly active women during pregnancy were less likely to have GDM as compared to insufficiently active women [adjusted OR: 0.52 (0.29–0.93), $p = 0.028$, and 0.34 (0.15–0.77), $p = 0.010$, respectively; p for trend = 0.004]. Among under/normal weight women on the other hand, PA during pregnancy was not associated with GDM [OR: 1.18 (0.71–1.98), $p = 0.526$, and 0.89 (0.42–1.90), $p = 0.766$, for sufficiently and highly active women, respectively]. Compared to women in the low sitting time group, women in the medium and high sitting groups had increased odds of having GDM, but this was not statistically significant [OR: 1.45 (0.90, 2.34), $p = 131$ and 1.42 (0.90, 2.22), p = 131, respectively]. There was no evidence for associations of television viewing time with GDM.

The findings were substantively similar in terms of magnitude and statistical significance after PA and total sitting time, and PA and television viewing time were mutually adjusted in separate models to examine independent associations of PA, total sitting time and television time with FG and 2hPG levels and GDM (data not shown).

Discussion

In our study, levels of PA were inversely associated with 2hPG levels and the likelihood of having GDM, but not with FG levels. Compared to insufficiently active women, highly active women had lower 2hPG levels and were less likely to develop GDM. These associations were stronger among overweight/obese women; compared to

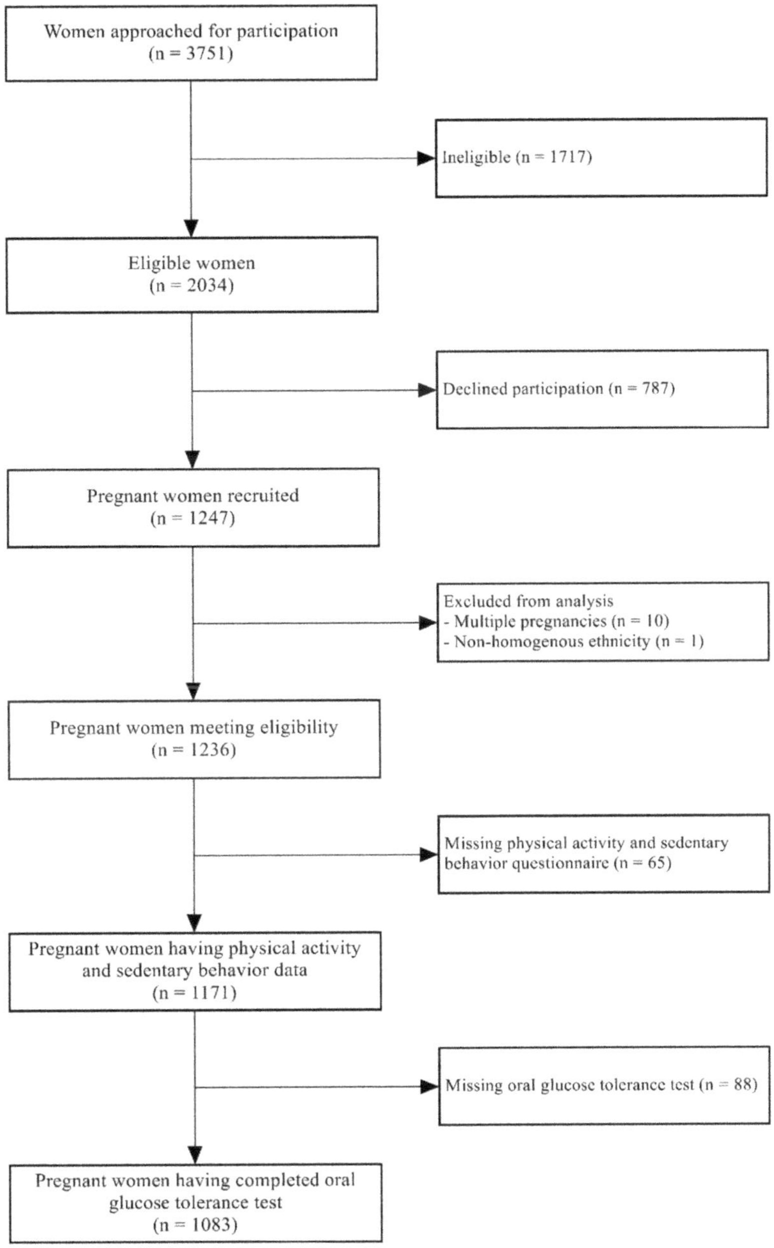

Fig. 1 Study flow diagram

insufficiently active women, sufficiently and highly active women were less likely to have GDM. Total sitting time was not associated with FG and 2hPG level, or with GDM. Some possible differences between the BMI subgroups were noted, but they were not consistent and require further investigation. Television viewing time was also not associated with glucose levels and GDM.

Our study in a multi-ethnic Asian population generally supports results of a previous meta-analysis reporting inverse associations between PA during pregnancy and risk of developing GDM [6]. Demspsy et al., observed similar results, indicating that women who engaged in any recreational PA during pregnancy experienced a 48% reduction in GDM risk compared with inactive women [49]. There are a limited number of observational studies that examined the association of PA and maternal glucose concentration in the absence of GDM [24, 32]. Chasen-Taber et al. reported a 50% lower risk of abnormal glucose tolerance among women with high levels of moderate-intensity activity as compared with women in the lowest quartile during pregnancy [32]. Higher levels of PA were associated with a lower 2hPG level in our study, which indicates the importance of PA on glucose tolerance in pregnant women; as a

Table 1 Characteristics of pregnant women according to GDM in the GUSTO cohort study (*n* = 1083)

	GDM absent *n* = 882 (81.4%)	GDM present *n* = 201 (18.6%)	*p*-value
Mean age in years (SD)	30.3 (5.1)	32.5 (4.7)	<0.001
Ethnicity (n, %)			0.001
Chinese	494 (56.0)	126 (62.7)	
Malay	245 (27.8)	31 (15.4)	
Indian	143 (16.2)	44 (21.9)	
Education (n, %)			0.008
No-formal/Primary/Secondary	279 (31.6)	46 (22.9)	
GCE 'A' levels/polytechnic/Diploma/ Technical education	312 (35.4)	72 (35.8)	
University	278 (31.5)	83 (41.3)	
Missing data	13 (1.5)	0 (0.0)	
BMI in kg/m^2 (n, %)			<0.001
< 18.5	105 (11.9)	16 (7.9)	
18.5–23	431 (48.9)	81 (40.3)	
23.0–27.5	179 (20.3)	54 (26.9)	
≥ 27.5	97 (11.0)	43 (21.4)	
Missing data	70 (7.9)	7 (3.5)	
Parity at recruitment (n, %)			0.128
0	407 (46.1)	85 (42.3)	
≥ 1	463 (52.5)	116 (57.7)	
Missing data	12 (1.4)	0 (0.0)	
History of GDM (n, %)			
No	834 (94.6)	181 (90.0)	<0.001
Yes	18 (2.0)	18 (9.0)	
Missing data	30 (3.4)	2 (1.0)	
Family history of diabetes (n, %)			
No	603 (68.4)	133 (66.2)	0.072
Yes	253 (28.7)	67 (33.3)	
Missing data	26 (2.9)	1 (0.5)	
Dietary energy intake in kcal (Mean, SD)	1881.3 (604.5)	1815.2 (520.7)	0.118
Missing data (n,%)	6 (0.7)	2 (1.0)	
Active/ passive smoking during pregnancy (n, %)			0.001
No	503 (57.0)	138 (68.6)	
Yes	350 (39.7)	52 (25.9)	
Missing data	29 (3.3)	11 (5.5)	
Pregnancy weight gain at week 26–28 (Mean, SD)	8.7 (4.5)	8.0 (4.4)	0.061
Missing (n,%)	79 (9.0)	7 (3.5)	
Physical activity during pregnancy (n, %)			0.125
Insufficiently active	289 (32.8)	78 (38.8)	
Sufficiently active	415 (47.1)	95 (47.3)	
Highly active	167 (18.9)	25 (12.4)	
Missing data	11 (1.2)	3 (1.5)	
Total sitting time during pregnancy (n, %)			0.193
Low (<7 h/day)	252 (28.6)	43 (21.4)	
Medium (7–10 h/day)	239 (27.1)	62 (30.8)	
High (≥10 h/day)	389 (44.1)	95 (47.3)	
Missing data	2 (0.2)	1 (0.5)	
Total television viewing time (n, %)			0.066
Low (<3 h/day)	593 (67.2)	142 (70.6)	
High (≥3 h/day)	289 (32.8)	58 (28.9)	
Missing data	0 (0.0)	1 (0.5)	

GDM gestational diabetes mellitus, *SD*, standard deviation, *GCE 'A' levels* General Certificate of Education-Advance levels, *BMI* body mass index
p-values were determined by Chi-square or independent t-test

consequence it may also have an effect in preventing adverse pregnancy outcome. For instance, two United Kingdom (UK) cohort studies have reported that higher maternal glucose levels within the non-diabetes range were consistently related to adverse pregnancy outcome [51].

The stratified analysis further highlights that these associations were mainly observed in overweight/obese women. Pre-pregnancy BMI may be an effect modifier for the association of level of PA with glucose concentration and GDM. However, this effect was evaluated in only four previous studies [24, 25, 49, 52]. In contrast to our results, the majority of previous studies indicated either no difference in the association between PA and GDM according to maternal BMI [49] or that the association was only found among women with a pre-pregnancy BMI of <25 kg/m^2 [24]. Deierlein AL et al. reported that women with a pre-pregnancy BMI of <25 kg/m^2 who engaged in any recreational moderate and vigorous physical activities during pregnancy had a 48% reduced risk of hyperglycemia compared to women who reported no moderate and vigorous activity [52]. The inconsistency between studies might be related to methodological issues, such as study design, population and assessment methods, but also highlights the need for further investigation of these observations. A potential biological mechanism behind the observed associations may be that skeletal muscle contraction as a result of PA may trigger glucose uptake and promote insulin sensitivity [24, 53]. PA-induced reductions in fat mass and increases in muscle mass may also lead to improved glucose tolerance and increased insulin sensitivity. Adipose tissue may also play a significant role in glucose clearance in physically active individuals, especially in obese individuals where this tissue can be considerable

Table 2 Associations of physical activity and sedentary behavior with fasting glucose levels (mmol/l) during pregnancy in the GUSTO study

Variables	Overall sample					Underweight/Normal weight			Overweight/obese			P for interaction
	n	Unadjusted		Adjusted[a]		Adjusted[b]			Adjusted[b]			
		β (95% CI)	*P*-value	β (95% CI)	*P*-value	n	β (95% CI)	*P*-value	n	β (95% CI)	*P*-value	
Physical activity			0.759		0.806			0.525			0.863	0.933
Insufficiently active	325	Reference		Reference		202	Reference		123	Reference		
Sufficiently active	436	0.01 (−0.06, 0.08)	0.822	0.01 (−0.06, 0.08)	0.754	284	0.03 (−0.03, 0.10)	0.321	152	−0.001 (−0.15, 0.15)	0.988	
Highly active	160	0.04 (−0.06, 0.13)	0.463	0.03 (−0.06, 0.12)	0.512	99	0.04 (−0.05, 0.13)	0.350	61	0.05 (−0.15, 0.25)	0.631	
p for trend			0.492		0.520			0.286			0.681	
Total sitting time			**0.029**		0.074			0.106			0.202	0.457
Low (<7 h/day)	251	Reference		Reference		153	Reference		98	Reference		
Medium (7–10 h/day)	265	0.02 (−0.06, 0.11)	0.627	0.04 (−0.04, 0.13)	0.304	160	0.06 (−0.01, 0.14)	0.111	105	0.002 (−0.17, 0.18)	0.980	
High (≥10 h/day)	417	−0.07 (−0.15, 0.003)	0.060	−0.04 (−0.12, 0.04)	0.285	277	−0.01 (−0.08, 0.06)	0.843	140	−0.13 (−0.30, 0.04)	0.144	
p for trend			**0.035**		0.183			0.598			0.119	
Television time			0.446		0.367			0.134			0.791	0.399
Low (<3 h/day)	640	Reference		Reference		411	Reference		229	Reference		
High (≥3 h/day)	294	0.03 (−0.04, 0.09)		0.03 (−0.04, 0.10)		180	0.05 (−0.02, 0.11)		114	−0.02 (−0.17, 0.13)		

β beta-coefficient, *CI* confidence interval, *BMI* body mass index

A[a]Adjusted for maternal age, ethnicity, education, pre-pregnancy BMI, parity at recruitment, history of GDM in previous pregnancy, family history of diabetes, dietary energy intake, active/passive smoking during pregnancy and pregnancy weight gain at 26–28 gestational visit

B[b]Adjusted for maternal age, ethnicity, education, parity at recruitment, history of GDM in previous pregnancy, family history of diabetes, dietary energy intake, active/passive smoking during pregnancy and pregnancy weight gain at 26–28 gestational visit

p-values were determined by multivariable linear regression

enough to contribute to improved glucose metabolism following physical training [49].

In our study, there was no evidence for an association of sedentary behavior with glucose levels and GDM. Nonetheless, we observed consistent increased odds of having GDM in women sitting for ≥7 h/day, but this was not led to statistical significant, which may be due to a lack of statistical power. A previous study that used television viewing time as one of the measures of sedentary behavior also reported no association with abnormal glucose tolerance and GDM risk [24], while another study found that longer sitting time was associated a with

Table 3 Associations of physical activity and sedentary behavior with 2-h-postprandial glucose levels (mmol/l) during pregnancy in the GUSTO study

Variables	Overall sample					Underweight/Normal weight			Overweight/obese			P for interaction
	n	Unadjusted		Adjusted[a]		Adjusted[b]			Adjusted[b]			
		β (95% CI)	*P*-value	β (95% CI)	*P*-value	n	β (95% CI)	*P*-value	n	β (95% CI)	*P*-value	
Physical activity			**0.032**		0.056			0.570			0.109	0.607
Insufficiently active	325	Reference		Reference		202	Reference		123	Reference		
Sufficiently active	436	−0.13 (−0.35, 0.08)	0.222	−0.16 (−0.37, 0.04)	0.116	284	−0.07 (−0.31, 0.17)	0.576	152	−0.28 (−0.66, 0.10)	0.152	
Highly active	160	**−0.38 (−0.67, −0.10)**	**0.009**	**−0.32 (−0.59, −0.05)**	**0.020**	99	−0.17 (−0.49, 0.15)	0.291	61	**−0.51 (−1.00, −0.01)**	**0.044**	
p for trend			**0.010**		**0.016**			0.295			**0.036**	
Total sitting time			0.091		0.172			0.082			0.885	0.547
Low (<7 h/day)	251	Reference		Reference		153	Reference		98	Reference		
Medium (7–10 h/day)	265	0.25 (−0.01, 0.52)	0.056	0.23 (−0.02, 0.47)	0.073	160	**0.31 (0.02, 0.60)**	**0.037**	105	0.10 (−0.34, 0.55)	0.652	
High (≥10 h/day)	417	**0.24 (0.001, 0.48)**	**0.049**	0.17 (−0.06, 0.40)	0.137	277	0.25 (−0.01, 0.52)	0.062	140	0.02 (−0.41, 0.45)	0.931	
p for trend			0.069		0.189			0.099			0.971	
Television time			0.284		0.649			0.925			0.571	
Low (<3 h/day)	640	Reference		Reference		411	Reference		229	Reference		0.363
High (≥3 h/day)	294	−0.11 (−0.32, 0.10)		0.05 (−0.15, 0.25)		180	−0.01 (−0.25, 0.23)		114	0.11 (−0.26, 0.47)		

β beta-coefficient, *CI* confidence interval, *BMI* body mass index

A[a]Adjusted for maternal age, ethnicity, education, pre-pregnancy BMI, parity at recruitment, history of GDM in previous pregnancy, family history of diabetes, dietary energy intake, active/passive smoking during pregnancy and pregnancy weight gain at 26–28 gestational visit

b[b]Adjusted for maternal age, ethnicity, education, parity at recruitment, history of GDM in previous pregnancy, family history of diabetes, dietary energy intake, active/passive smoking during pregnancy and pregnancy weight gain at 26–28 gestational visit

p-values were determined by multivariable linear regression

Table 4 Associations of physical activity and sedentary behavior during pregnancy with GDM in the GUSTO study

Variables	Overall sample					Underweight/Normal weight			Overweight/obese			P for interaction
	Cases n (%)	Unadjusted		Adjusted[a]		Adjusted[b]			Adjusted[b]			
		OR (95% CI)	*P*-value	OR (95% CI)	*P*-value	Cases n (%)	OR (95% CI)[a]	*P*-value	Cases n (%)	OR (95% CI)[a]	*P*-value	
Physical activity			0.107		0.118			0.673			**0.015**	0.098
Insufficiently active	71 (21.8)	1.0		1.0		30 (14.9)	1.0		41 (33.3)	1.0		
Sufficiently active	86 (19.7)	0.88 (0.62, 1.25)	0.475	0.82 (0.56, 1.20)	0.303	50 (17.6)	1.18 (0.71, 1.98)	0.526	36 (23.7)	**0.52 (0.29, 0.93)**	**0.028**	
Highly active	22 (13.8)	**0.57 (0.34, 0.96)**	**0.035**	**0.56 (0.32, 0.98)**	**0.040**	12 (12.1)	0.89 (0.42, 1.90)	0.766	10 (16.4)	**0.34 (0.15, 0.77)**	**0.010**	
p for trend			**0.045**		**0.041**			0.975			**0.004**	
Total sitting time			0.197		0.246			0.532			0.304	0.660
Low (<7 h/day)	39 (15.5)	1.0		1.0		19 (12.4)	1.0		20 (20.4)	1.0		
Medium (7–10 h/day)	55 (20.8)	1.42 (0.91, 2.24)	0.126	1.45 (0.90, 2.34)	0.131	24 (15.0)	1.29 (0.65, 2.56)	0.476	31 (29.5)	1.71 (0.86, 3.40)	0.123	
High (≥10 h/day)	87 (20.9)	1.43 (0.95, 2.17)	0.089	1.42 (0.90, 2.22)	0.131	49 (17.7)	1.42 (0.77, 2.63)	0.261	38 (27.1)	1.38 (0.71, 2.69)	0.341	
p for trend			0.114		0.172			0.271			0.438	
Television time			0.287		0.885			0.248			0.304	0.052
Low (<3 h/day)	130 (20.3)	1.0		1.0		73 (17.8)	1.0		57 (24.9)	1.0		
High (≥3 h/day)	51 (17.3)	0.82 (0.58, 1.18)		1.03 (0.70, 1.51)		19 (10.6)	0.71 (0.40, 1.26)		32 (28.1)	1.33 (0.77, 2.29)		

GDM gestational diabetes mellitus, *BMI* body mass index, *OR* odds ratio, *CI* confidence interval
A[a]Adjusted for maternal age, ethnicity, education, pre-pregnancy BMI, parity at recruitment, history of GDM in previous pregnancy, family history of diabetes, dietary energy intake, active/passive smoking during pregnancy and pregnancy weight gain at 26–28 gestational visit
B[b]Adjusted for maternal age, ethnicity, education, parity at recruitment, history of GDM in previous pregnancy, family history of diabetes, dietary energy intake, active/passive smoking during pregnancy and pregnancy weight gain at 26–28 gestational visit
p-values were determined by multivariable logistic regression

higher risk of developing gestational diabetes [30]. These inconsistencies warrant further research.

GUSTO is the first multi-ethnic birth cohort study in Asia investigating the associations of PA, total sitting time and television time during pregnancy with blood glucose levels and GDM. PA and SB data were collected as part of a structured questionnaire, administered by trained interviewers to mitigate the likelihood of systematic reporting errors. Standardized objective methods were used to quantify maternal blood glucose levels, and to determine GDM. Nevertheless, limitations of our study should be considered when interpreting our findings. Firstly, PA and SB data were limited to subjects' self-reports with potential recall bias due to their complexity, and the questionnaire has not been validated locally against objective methods. Hence, some women might have misclassified their PA intensity categories. Secondly, assigned MET values and categorization of total MET values are suggested for an adult, and not specifically for pregnant women. However, we believe that the magnitude of imprecision is acceptable as the PA assessment was restricted to the first two trimesters of pregnancy. Thirdly, the prevalence of GDM was determined by 1999 WHO diagnostic criteria because only FG and 2hPG data were available, and more recent definitions could not be applied [36]. However, this study also examined the associations of PA and SB with maternal glucose concentrations, which are not influenced by these cut-off criteria for diagnosis. Fourthly, pre-pregnancy BMI was derived from self-reported weight which might have led to misclassification of some women in BMI categories. However, the literature suggests that pre-pregnancy BMI category by self-reported and measured weight are identical for most women [54] Finally, the generalizability of our results is limited because our cohort was not representative of the general Singaporean population [39].

Conclusions

PA was inversely associated with 2hPG levels and GDM, but not associated with FG levels. Highly active women during pregnancy had significantly lower levels of 2hPG and were less likely to be diagnosed with GDM, especially among those who were overweight/obese. Overweight/obese women with the minimum recommended or higher levels of PA were less likely to have GDM. In contrast, there was little evidence of an association between SB (total sitting time or TV viewing time) and glucose levels in our study. These findings suggest the importance of recommending or maintaining sufficiently high levels of physical activity during pregnancy to reduce the risk of adverse pregnancy outcomes for mothers and their offspring due to hyperglycemia. More prospective longitudinal studies and further trials are warranted, combining subjective and objective assessment of PA and SB with activity specific information, and more precise assessment of GDM, to confirm these findings. This knowledge will help to develop more effective health promotion strategies to prevent hyperglycemia among Asian women.

Abbreviations

2hPG: 2-h postprandial glucose; BMI: Body mass index; CI: Confidence interval; FG: Fasting glucose; GDM: Gestational diabetes mellitus; GUSTO: Growing Up in Singapore Towards healthy Outcomes; IPAQ: International Physical Activity Questionnaire; KKH: KK Women's and Children's Hospital; MET: metabolic equivalent tasks; NUH: National University Hospital; OGTT: Oral Glucose Tolerance Testing; OR: Odds ratio; PA: Physical activity; SB: Sedentary behavior; UK: United Kingdom; WHO: World Health Organization

Acknowledgments

We would like to thank GUSTO study group, operational managers, research fellows, study coordinators and data management team. We greatly appreciate the voluntary participation of all participants and cooperation of maternity units in KK Women's and Children's Hospital and National University Hospital and their staff. The GUSTO study group includes Allan Sheppard, Amutha Chinnadurai, Anne Eng Neo Goh, Anne Rifkin-Graboi, Anqi Qiu, Arijit Biswas, Bee Wah Lee, Birit F.P. Broekman, Boon Long Quah, Borys Shuter, Chai Kiat Chng, Cheryl Ngo, Choon Looi Bong, Christiani Jeyakumar Henry, Cornelia Yin Ing Chee, Yam Thiam Daniel Goh, Doris Fok, Fabian Yap, George Seow Heong Yeo, Helen Chen, Hugo P S van Bever, Iliana Magiati, Inez Bik Yun Wong, Ivy Yee-Man Lau, Jeevesh Kapur, Jenny L. Richmond, Joanna D. Holbrook, Joshua J. Gooley, Kok Hian Tan, Krishnamoorthy Niduvaje, Leher Singh, Lin Lin Su, Lourdes Mary Daniel, Lynette Pei-Chi Shek, Marielle V. Fortier, Mark Hanson, Mary Foong-Fong Chong, Mary Rauff, Mei Chien Chua, Michael Meaney, Mya Thway Tint, Neerja Karnani, Ngee Lek, Oon Hoe Teoh, P. C. Wong, Pratibha Agarwal, Rob M. van Dam, Salome A. Rebello, Shang Chee Chong, Shu-E Soh, Sok Bee Lim, Chin-Ying Stephen Hsu, Victor Samuel Rajadurai, Walter Stunkel, Wee Meng Han, Wei Wei Pang, Yin Bun Cheung, Yiong Huak Chan and Yung Seng Lee.

Funding

This research is supported by the Singapore National Research Foundation under its Translational and Clinical Research (TCR) Flagship Programme and administered by the Singapore Ministry of Health's National Medical Research Council (NMRC), Singapore- NMRC/TCR/004-NUS/2008; NMRC/TCR/012-NUHS/2014. Additional funding is provided by the Singapore Institute for Clinical Sciences, Agency for Science Technology and Research (A*STAR), Singapore. KMG is supported by the National Institute for Health Research through the NIHR Southampton Biomedical Research Centre and by the European Union's Seventh Framework Programme (FP7/2007–2013), projects EarlyNutrition and ODIN under grant agreement numbers 289,346 and 613,977. JKYC received salary support from the Ministry of Health's National Medical Research Council, Singapore (NMRC/CSA/043/2012).

Authors' contributions

Conceived and designed the experiments: KK, PDG, KMG, SMS and YSC. Performed the experiments: ISZ and NP. Analyzed the data: NP, JYB, FMR, SL, SLL, SC and JKYC. Wrote the paper: NP, JYB and FMR. All authors read and approved the final manuscript.

Consent for publication

All participants gave written consent to publish the data collected.

Competing interests

PDG, KMG and YSC report receiving reimbursement for speaking at conferences sponsored by companies selling nutritional products. PDG, KMG and YSC report being part of an academic consortium that has received research funding from Abbott Nutrition, Nestle and Danone. No other disclosures were reported. This does not alter the authors' adherence to BMC policies on sharing data and materials.

Author details

[1]Department of Obstetrics & Gynaecology, Yong Loo Lin School of Medicine, National University of Singapore, Singapore, Singapore. [2]Singapore Institute for Clinical Sciences, Agency for Science and Technology Research (A*STAR), Singapore, Singapore. [3]Biostatistics Unit, Yong Loo Lin School of Medicine, National University of Singapore, Singapore, Singapore. [4]KK Women's and Children's Hospital, Singapore, Singapore. [5]Duke-National University of Singapore, Singapore, Singapore. [6]Medical Research Council Lifecourse Epidemiology Unit, Southampton, UK. [7]NIHR Southampton Biomedical Research Centre, University of Southampton, Southampton, UK. [8]Liggins Institute, University of Auckland, Auckland, New Zealand. [9]Saw Swee Hock School of Public Health, National University of Singapore, Singapore, Singapore. [10]Institute for Social Medicine, Epidemiology and Health Economics, Charite University Medical Centre, Berlin, Germany.

References

1. The Expert Committee on the Diagnosis Classification of Diabetes Mellitus. Report of the expert committee on the diagnosis and classification of diabetes mellitus. Diabetes Care. 2003;26(Supplement 1):S5–S20.
2. Sacks DA, Hadden DR, Maresh M, Deerochanawong C, Dyer AR, Metzger BE, Lowe LP, Coustan DR, Hod M, Oats JJ, et al. Frequency of gestational diabetes mellitus at collaborating centers based on IADPSG consensus panel-recommended criteria: the hyperglycemia and adverse pregnancy outcome (HAPO) study. Diabetes Care. 2012;35(3):526–8.
3. American Diabetes A. Diagnosis and classification of diabetes mellitus. Diabetes Care. 2014, 37 Suppl 1(1):S81-S90.
4. Samoa R, Fujimoto W, Wotring A. Gestational diabetes in high-risk populations.(DIABETES ADVOCACY). Clinical Diabetes. 2013;31(2):90.
5. Damm P. Future risk of diabetes in mother and child after gestational diabetes mellitus. Int J Gynaecol Obstet. 2009;104(Suppl 1):S25–6.
6. Tobias DK, Zhang C, van Dam RM, Bowers K, FB H. Physical activity before and during pregnancy and risk of gestational diabetes mellitus: a meta-analysis. Diabetes Care. 2011;34(1):223–9.
7. Retnakaran R, Qi Y, Sermer M, Connelly PW, Zinman B, Hanley AJ. Pre-gravid physical activity and reduced risk of glucose intolerance in pregnancy: the role of insulin sensitivity. Clin Endocrinol. 2009;70(4):615–22.
8. Gradmark A, Pomeroy J, Renstrom F, Steiginga S, Persson M, Wright A, Bluck L, Domellof M, Kahn SE, Mogren I, et al. Physical activity, sedentary behaviors, and estimated insulin sensitivity and secretion in pregnant and non-pregnant women. BMC Pregnancy Childbirth. 2011;11(1):44.
9. U.S. Department of Health and Human Services. 2008 Physical Activity Guidelines for Americans. In.: https://health.gov/paguidelines/guidelines/summary.aspx; 2008.
10. Committee Opinion No. 650 summary: physical activity and exercise during pregnancy and the postpartum period. Obstet Gynecol 2015, 126(6):1326-1327.
11. World Health Organization. Global recommendations on physical activity for health. In.: http://whqlibdoc.who.int/publications/2010/9789241599979_eng.pdf?ua=1; 2010.
12. World Health Organization. Global Physical Activity Questionnaire (GPAQ) Analysis Guide. In.: http://www.who.int/chp/steps/resources/GPAQ_Analysis_Guide.pdf.
13. Dempsey FC, Butler FL, Williams FA. No need for a pregnant pause: physical activity may reduce the occurrence of gestational diabetes mellitus and preeclampsia. Exerc Sport Sci Rev. 2005;33(3):141–9.
14. Dawes J. The role of exercise in the prevention and treatment of gestational diabetes mellitus. Strength Cond J. 2006;28(3):66–8.
15. Mottola MF. The role of exercise in the prevention and treatment of gestational diabetes mellitus. Curr Sports Med Rep. 2007;6(6):381–6.
16. Colberg SR, Castorino K, Jovanovic L. Prescribing physical activity to prevent and manage gestational diabetes. World J Diabetes. 2013;4(6):256–62.
17. Dempsey JC, Sorensen TK, Williams MA, Lee IM, Miller RS, Dashow EE, Luthy DA. Prospective study of gestational diabetes mellitus risk in relation to maternal recreational physical activity before and during pregnancy. Am J Epidemiol. 2004;159(7):663–70.

18. Padayachee C, Coombes JS. Exercise guidelines for gestational diabetes mellitus. World J Diabetes. 2015;6(8):1033–44.
19. Loy SL, Ng MJ, Cheung YB, Godfrey KM, Calder PC, Lek N, Yap F, Muller-Riemenschneider F, Natarajan P, Chong YS, et al. Plasma omega-3 fatty acids in pregnancy are inversely associated with postpartum weight retention in a multiethnic Asian cohort. Am J Clin Nutr. 2017;22(10):151258.
20. Chasan-Taber L, Schmidt MD, Pekow P, Sternfeld B, Manson JE, Solomon CG, Braun B, Markenson G. Physical activity and gestational diabetes mellitus among Hispanic women. J Women's Health (2002). 2008;17(6):999–1008.
21. van der Ploeg HP, van Poppel MN, Chey T, Bauman AE, Brown WJ. The role of pre-pregnancy physical activity and sedentary behaviour in the development of gestational diabetes mellitus. J Sci Med Sport. 2011;14(2):149–52.
22. Ogonowski J, Miazgowski T, Kuczynska M, Krzyzanowska-Swiniarska B, Celewicz Z. Pregravid body mass index as a predictor of gestational diabetes mellitus. Diabet Med. 2009;26(4):334–8.
23. Deierlein AL, Siega-Riz AM, Evenson KR. Physical activity during pregnancy and risk of hyperglycemia. J Women's Health (Larchmt). 2012;21(7):769–75.
24. Oken E, Ning Y, Rifas-Shiman SL, Radesky JS, Rich-Edwards JW, Gillman MW. Associations of physical activity and inactivity before and during pregnancy with glucose tolerance. Obstet Gynecol. 2006;108(5):1200–7.
25. Dye TD, Knox KL, Artal R, Aubry RH, Wojtowycz MA. Physical activity, obesity, and diabetes in pregnancy. Am J Epidemiol. 1997;146(11):961–5.
26. Owen N, Healy GN, Matthews CE, Dunstan DW. Too much sitting: the population health science of sedentary behavior. Exerc Sport Sci Rev. 2010; 38(3):105–13.
27. Sedentary Behaviour Research N. Letter to the editor: standardized use of the terms "sedentary" and "sedentary behaviours". Appl Physiol Nutr Metab. 2012;37(3):540–2.
28. Biswas A, PI O, Faulkner GE, Bajaj RR, Silver MA, Mitchell MS, Alter DA. Sedentary time and its association with risk for disease incidence, mortality, and hospitalization in adults: a systematic review and meta-analysis. Ann Intern Med. 2015;162(2):123–32.
29. Gollenberg AL, Pekow P, Bertone-Johnson ER, Freedson PS, Markenson G, Chasan-Taber L. Sedentary behaviors and abnormal glucose tolerance among pregnant Latina women. Med Sci Sports Exerc. 2010;42(6):1079–85.
30. Sukumar N, Farmer J, Venkataraman H, Saravanan P. Longer duration of sitting down in pregnancy is associated with gestational diabetes, greater weight gain and depressive symptoms. Endocr Abstr. 2015;38
31. Anjana RM, Sudha V, Lakshmipriya N, Anitha C, Unnikrishnan R, Bhavadharini B, Mahalakshmi MM, Maheswari K, Kayal A, Ram U, et al. Physical activity patterns and gestational diabetes outcomes – the wings project. Diabetes Res Clin Pract. 2016;116:253–62.
32. Chasan-Taber L, Silveira M, Lynch KE, Pekow P, Braun B, Manson JE, Solomon CG, Markenson G. Physical activity before and during pregnancy and risk of abnormal glucose tolerance among Hispanic women. Diabete Metab. 2014;40(1):67–75.
33. Jenum AK, Morkrid K, Sletner L, Vangen S, Torper JL, Nakstad B, Voldner N, Rognerud-Jensen OH, Berntsen S, Mosdol A, et al. Impact of ethnicity on gestational diabetes identified with the WHO and the modified International Association of Diabetes and Pregnancy Study Groups criteria: a population-based cohort study. Eur J Endocrinol. 2012;166(2):317–24.
34. Cheung NW, Wasmer G, Al-Ali J. Risk factors for gestational diabetes among Asian women. Diabetes Care. 2001;24(5):955–6.
35. Chu SY, Abe K, Hall LR, Kim SY, Njoroge T, Qin C. Gestational diabetes mellitus: all Asians are not alike. Prev Med. 2009;49(2–3):265–8.
36. World Health Organization. Diagnostic Criteria and Classification of Hyperglycaemia First Detected in Pregnancy. In.: http://apps.who.int/iris/bitstream/10665/85975/1/WHO_NMH_MND_13.2_eng.pdf; 2013.
37. Group HSCR, Metzger BE, Lowe LP, Dyer AR, Trimble ER, Chaovarindr U, Coustan DR, Hadden DR, McCance DR, Hod M, et al. Hyperglycemia and adverse pregnancy outcomes. N Engl J Med. 2008;358(19):1991–2002.
38. Soh SE, Chong YS, Kwek K, Saw SM, Meaney MJ, Gluckman PD, Holbrook JD, Godfrey KM, Group GS. Insights from the growing up in Singapore towards healthy outcomes (GUSTO) cohort study. Ann Nutr Metab. 2014;64(3–4):218–25.
39. Soh SE, Tint MT, Gluckman PD, Godfrey KM, Rifkin-Graboi A, Chan YH, Stunkel W, Holbrook JD, Kwek K, Chong YS, et al. Cohort profile: growing up in Singapore towards healthy outcomes (GUSTO) birth cohort study. Int J Epidemiol. 2014;43(5):1401–9.
40. World Health Organization. BMI classification. In.: WHO:Global Database on Body Mass Index, http://www.euro.who.int/en/health-topics/disease-prevention/nutrition/a-healthy-lifestyle/body-mass-index-bmi.
41. WHO Expert Consultation. Appropriate body-mass index in Asian populations and its implications for policy and intervention strategies. Lancet. 2004;363(9403):157–63.
42. Identification, assessment, and management of overweight and obesity: summary of updated NICE guidance. In: BMJ. vol. 349:g6608: http://www.bmj.com/content/349/bmj.g6608/rr/805398; 2014.
43. Chen LW, Lim AL, Colega M, Tint MT, Aris IM, Tan CS, Chong YS, Gluckman PD, Godfrey KM, Kwek K, et al. Maternal folate status, but not that of vitamins B-12 or B-6, is associated with gestational age and preterm birth risk in a multiethnic Asian population. J Nutr. 2015;145(1):113–20.
44. Chong Y-S, Cai S, Lin H, Soh SE, Lee Y-S, Leow MK-S, Chan Y-H, Chen L, Holbrook JD, Tan K-H, et al. Ethnic differences translate to inadequacy of high-risk screening for gestational diabetes mellitus in an Asian population: a cohort study. BMC Pregnancy Childbirth. 2014;14(1):1–7.
45. Padmapriya N, Shen L, Soh SE, Shen Z, Kwek K, Godfrey KM, Gluckman PD, Chong YS, Saw SM, Muller-Riemenschneider F. Physical activity and sedentary behavior patterns before and during pregnancy in a multi-ethnic sample of Asian women in Singapore. Matern Child Health J. 2015;19(11):2523–35.
46. IPAQ Research Committee: Guidelines for data processing and analysis of the international physical activity questionnaire (IPAQ). 2005.
47. Zhang C, Solomon CG, Manson JE, FB H. A prospective study of pregravid physical activity and sedentary behaviors in relation to the risk for gestational diabetes mellitus. Arch Intern Med. 2006;166(5):543–8.
48. Redden SL, LaMonte MJ, Freudenheim JL, Rudra CB. The association between gestational diabetes mellitus and recreational physical activity. Matern Child Health J. 2011;15(4):514–9.
49. Dempsey JC, Butler CL, Sorensen TK, Lee IM, Thompson ML, Miller RS, Frederick IO, Williams MA. A case-control study of maternal recreational physical activity and risk of gestational diabetes mellitus. Diabetes Res Clin Pract. 2004;66(2):203–15.
50. Dunstan DW, Salmon J, Owen N, Armstrong T, Zimmet PZ, Welborn TA, Cameron AJ, Dwyer T, Jolley D, Shaw JE, et al. Physical activity and television viewing in relation to risk of undiagnosed abnormal glucose metabolism in adults. Diabetes Care. 2004;27(11):2603–9.
51. Ong KK, Diderholm B, Salzano G, Wingate D, Hughes IA, MacDougall J, Acerini CL, Dunger DB. Pregnancy insulin, glucose, and BMI contribute to birth outcomes in nondiabetic mothers. Diabetes Care. 2008;31(11):2193–7.
52. Deierlein AL, Siega-Riz AM, Evenson KR. Physical activity during pregnancy and risk of hyperglycemia. J Women's Health. 2012;21(7):769–75.
53. Michelle F. Mottola S-MR: Exercise Guidelines for Women with Gestational Diabetes In.: InTech, Available from: http://www.intechopen.com/books/gestational-diabetes/exercise-guidelines-for-women-with-gestationaldiabetes; 2011.
54. Bannon AL, Waring ME, Leung K, Masiero JV, Stone JM, Scannell EC, Moore Simas TA. Comparison of self-reported and measured pre-pregnancy weight: implications for gestational weight gain counseling. Matern Child Health J. 2017;2(10):017–2266.

12

Factors influencing timely initiation and completion of gestational diabetes mellitus screening and diagnosis - a qualitative study from Tamil Nadu, India

Karoline Kragelund Nielsen[1,2*], Thilde Rheinländer[1], Anil Kapur[3], Peter Damm[4], Veerasamy Seshiah[5] and Ib C. Bygbjerg[1]

Abstract

Background: In 2007, universal screening for gestational diabetes mellitus (GDM) was introduced in Tamil Nadu, India. To identify factors hindering or facilitating timely initiation and completion of the GDM screening and diagnosis process, our study investigated how pregnant women in rural and urban Tamil Nadu access and navigate different GDM related health services.

Methods: The study was carried out in two settings: an urban private diabetes centre and a rural government primary health centre. Observations of the process of screening and diagnosis at the health centres as well as semi-structured interviews with 30 pregnant women and nine health care providers were conducted. Data was analysed using qualitative content analysis.

Results: There were significant differences in the process of GDM screening and diagnosis in the urban and rural settings. Several factors hindering or facilitating timely initiation and completion of the process were identified. Timely attendance required awareness, motivation and opportunity to attend. Women had to attend the health centre at the right time and sometimes at the right gestational age to initiate the test, wait to complete the test and obtain the test report in time to initiate further action. All these steps and requirements were influenced by factors within and outside the health system such as getting right information from health care providers, clinic timings, characteristics of the test, availability of transport, social network and support, and social norms and cultural practices.

Conclusions: Minimising and aligning complex stepwise processes of prenatal care and GDM screening delivery and attention to the factors influencing it are important for further improving and expanding GDM screening and related services, not only in Tamil Nadu but in other similar low and middle income settings. This study stresses the importance of guidelines and diagnostic criteria which are simple and feasible on the ground.

Keywords: Gestational diabetes, Screening, India, Health care services, Antenatal care, Guidelines, Qualitative research

* Correspondence: kani@sund.ku.dk
[1]Department of Public Health, University of Copenhagen, Oester Farimagsgade 5, 1014 Copenhagen, Denmark
[2]Steno Diabetes Center Copenhagen, Niels Steensens Vej 6, 2820 Gentofte, Denmark
Full list of author information is available at the end of the article

Background

Gestational diabetes mellitus (GDM) increases the risk of various adverse pregnancy outcomes, as well as the risk of future diabetes in both the mother and offspring [1–4]. According to estimates from the International Diabetes Federation, approximately 21.4 million live births are annually affected by hyperglycaemia in pregnancy of which 84% are affected by GDM [5]. Despite the increased focus on GDM screening and diagnosis in recent years, also in low and middle income countries [6–8], very little is known about the barriers and challenges faced by women in this process, and how to implement or improve GDM screening and care on a large scale in such settings [9].

Based on work on diabetes and chronic disease management, *Mol* [10] showed that what may seem a simple process – the patient being informed about the use of a medical technology (e.g. blood sugar measurement), which he/she then uses to monitor his/her disease – is far from straightforward. *Mol* argues that the problem is not in the decision-making process (the patient was given the information and choice to do the blood sugar measurement or not), but in actually 'doing' the blood sugar measurement [10]. In order for the 'doing' to take place, the circumstances have to be right, and the technology has to be appropriate for the patient [11]. These issues are rarely taken into consideration when evaluating the use of diagnostic devices or test procedures and receive little attention despite the significant impact they have [11]. Thus, applying *Mol's* notions of 'doing' to analyse the GDM screening process can provide us with a deeper understanding of women's GDM screening experiences and behaviours.

India and in particular the South Indian state of Tamil Nadu (TN) is a highly relevant setting for such analysis: 65 million people in India are estimated to have diabetes [5] and the country continues to struggle with high maternal mortality and morbidity, accounting for 19% of worldwide maternal deaths [12]. A high prevalence rate of GDM (14%) has been identified in TN, and has subsequently been noted in other areas of India as well [13–15]. This led the Government of TN to introduce GDM screening as part of routine antenatal care (ANC) services at government health centres in 2007, applying the criteria recommended by the Diabetes in Pregnancy Study Group India (DIPSI) [16], i.e. a single-step test using a 75 g oral glucose tolerance test (OGTT) with diagnosis being made if the two hour value is 140 mg/dl or more. Screening for GDM is typically done in the 24–28th weeks of gestation, but sometimes also at the first ANC visit and it may also be repeated later in pregnancy. Additionally, awareness campaigns and capacity building initiatives targeted at both the government and the private health care system were carried out.

The health care system in TN as in rest of India is complex; involving a mixture of public and private health care providers (HCPs), practising different systems of medicine (modern, Ayurveda, Unani and Siddha). In TN, only 53% of the population uses the public health sector; with higher rates in rural settings, and among the poor [17]. The organisation of ANC services is also complex, with different levels of services, facilities and specialisations in rural and urban areas, and in the public and private sector. There are no clear-cut referral systems, and women's use of ANC services depend on their practical access, willingness and ability to pay for services. Many women attend both public and private health care services [18]. Other factors that determine utility of maternal health services in India include women finding the service relevant to themselves and their fetus/child, quality of care [19], their socio-economic status [20–22], distance to health facility, literacy, parity, obstetric history [23], husband's knowledge and attitude towards services [24], family traditions, financial constraints, behaviour of HCPs [25], and women's autonomy [26]. Thus, accessing and utilising services is much more complex than merely a question of awareness.

Implementing timely and effective detection and management of GDM in TN requires a good understanding of how women navigate their way through the complex health system. Therefore, our study investigated factors that might influence timely initiation and completion of the GDM screening and diagnosis process in a sample of urban and rural women in TN.

Methods

Study area

The study was carried out in two areas of TN: Chennai city and Thiruvallur district representing two different settings for GDM screening: a private urban and a government rural centre [27].

Chennai is the state capital, is currently experiencing substantial economic growth and is home to a growing middle class. In Chennai city, the study was conducted at a private diabetes hospital catering mainly to the urban middle class.

In Thiruvallur district, the study was conducted at a government primary health centre and its surroundings, located in a semi-rural area approximately 40 km north of Chennai city. However, most pregnant women attending ANC here reside in rural areas. While some inhabitants in the area work in Chennai, many are farmers, daily wagers or workers at the local factories. The villages are connected to the main roads via small paved or dirt roads.

Data collection, analysis and ethical considerations

Data for this study was collected between January 2013 and September 2014 as part of a larger study on GDM [27].

The study was qualitative with triangulation of several data sources and methods: observations at health facilities, and interviews with pregnant women and HCPs. This approach aimed at providing a holistic picture of the investigated phenomenon, while increasing validity and reducing the risk of bias [28].

Around 120 h of observation were conducted (by the lead author KKN) at the two health centres, with a focus on the screening process and patterns of actions as well as verbal and non-verbal interactions. Detailed note-taking was done. Observations provided contextual knowledge about the health system and organisation of services and highlighted issues from a third party perspective that informants (users and provider of services) take for granted and therefore do not mention in interviews [29].

Semi-structured interviews were conducted with 30 pregnant women attending ANC at the rural government primary health centre (18 women) and the private urban diabetes centre (12 women). An overview of the women is presented in Table 1. A purposive sampling strategy was used, and all the pregnant women had or were supposed to have undergone GDM screening procedures at the health centres during their current pregnancy. They were recruited at the health facility, through the local village health nurses or through referral from other pregnant women. Recruitment was continued until theoretical saturation was reached. The interviews took place at a private area of the health centre or at the women's homes and focused on their experiences with and perceptions of GDM screening services (Additional file 1).

Additionally, interviews with nine HCPs were carried out (four laboratory technicians, two village health nurses, one physician, and two private practicing gynaecologists/obstetricians). These HCPs were selected based on having a crucial role in the screening process. The interviews focused on their experiences in providing GDM screening services and challenges and opportunities in doing so (Additional file 2). A few village health nurses approached for interview declined, stating lack of time as the reason.

Informants fluent in English were interviewed by KKN, but the majority of interviews were conducted with support of a trained research assistant fluent in both English and Tamil. The overall purpose of the study was described to the participants, and verbal informed consent obtained prior to the interview, including approval for audio recording the interview. Verbal consent was chosen over written consent as obtaining written consent was seen as counterproductive to the informal and comfortable atmosphere we were trying to create to facilitate rapport and building trust between the researchers and informants [30]. The verbal informed consent was given in the presence of KKN and the research assistant. Ethical approval for the study, including the use of verbal informed consent, was given by the Institutional Ethics Committee at Dr. Seshiah Diabetes Research Institute and Dr. Balaji Diabetes Care Centre in Chennai.

The interviews, most lasting between 30 and 60 min, were transcribed verbatim and translated into English. The interview guides for the research intended to explore a number of overall topics, e.g. experience with the process, social support and informants' knowledge and expectations of the GDM test. An iterative-inductive analysis process [31] was followed, starting during fieldwork, which allowed follow-up and collection of additional data on emerging issues. Qualitative content analysis of interview and observation data was done by KKN, who read through and organised data into meaning units, categories and themes [32]. The coding was done using the software programme NVivo 10 (QSR International Pty Ltd. 1999–2012). First step of the analysis was to describe the differences in GDM screening and diagnosis procedures and compare these with government order instructions. Next step of the analysis identified two overall steps with two and three sub-steps, respectively. At each sub-step there were certain requirements or 'doing' as well as factors influencing women's navigation of the process (Fig. 1).

Results

Procedures for GDM screening and diagnosis

Data from observations and interviews with HCPs was synthesised on the actual procedures of GDM screening in the urban and rural health systems and compared to government order instructions on screening for hyperglycaemia in pregnancy (see Table 2). This analysis revealed several differences in GDM screening approaches: 1) different testing 'procedures' 2) different timing of GDM testing and 3) different diagnostic criteria and procedures.

At the rural government centre, GDM screening was carried out by a government employed laboratory technician as well as by a private-non-profit employed laboratory technician, working for a larger study on GDM (see Balaji et al. 2014). As shown in Table 1, the GDM screening process differed somewhat between the two categories of laboratory technicians at the rural centre. For testing by the government laboratory technician, the women had to attend in the fourth, sixth and eight months of pregnancy, whereas no specific

Table 1 Characteristics of the pregnant women interviewed

	Area	Age	Education	Gestational age at first test
Woman 1	Urban	35	Graduate	2.5 months
Woman 2	Urban	23	12th Grade	4.5 months
Woman 3	Urban	31	Postgraduate	1.5 months
Woman 4	Urban	29	Postgraduate	1.5 months
Woman 5	Urban	23	Graduate	2 months
Woman 6	Urban	26	Postgraduate	2 months
Woman 7	Urban	25	Postgraduate	1 month
Woman 8	Urban	20	12th Grade	9 months
Woman 9	Urban	38	8th Grade	2 months
Woman 10	Urban	28	Postgraduate	3 months
Woman 11	Urban	25	Postgraduate	1 month
Woman 12	Urban	26	Graduate	3 months
Woman 13	Rural	28	12th Grade	8 months
Woman 14	Rural	25	8th Grade	7 months, but did not complete
Woman 15	Rural	23	9th Grade	5 months
Woman 16	Rural	22	10th Grade	7 months
Woman 17	Rural	21	10th Grade	3.5 months
Woman 18	Rural	22	Graduate	3 months, but did not complete 6 months when it was completed
Woman 19	Rural	22	9th Grade	4 months
Woman 20	Rural	20	7th Grade	4 months
Woman 21	Rural	22	10th Grade	5 months, but did not complete
Woman 22	Rural	24	Postgraduate	6 months
Woman 23	Rural	23	12th Grade	7 months
Woman 24	Rural	25	10th Grade	4 months, but did not complete 6 months when it was completed
Woman 25	Rural	26	12th Grade	7 months
Woman 26	Rural	25	10th Grade	4 months, but did not complete 5 months when it was completed
Woman 27	Rural	25	8th Grade	6 months
Woman 28	Rural	23	10th Grade	5 months
Woman 29	Rural	22	10th Grade	4 months
Woman 30	Rural	21	10th Grade	3 months

gestational age was required for testing by the private-non-profit rural laboratory technician or at the urban site. A 75 g OGTT was used at all sites. A fasting venous sample was collected both at the urban centre and by the private-non-profit employed laboratory technician at the rural centre. At these two sites plasma glucose was also estimated at one and two hours after intake of the glucose solution. At the urban centre both of these were measured in venous samples, whereas the private-non-profit employed laboratory technician at the rural centre measured the one hour plasma glucose with a calibrated glucometer (capillary sample), and the two hour measurement was on venous blood sample. The government employed laboratory technician only took one sample: a two hour venous sample after ingestion of 75 g glucose load. At the urban centre the women were asked to wait for the results of their test and were given the results the same day, whereas women attending the rural centre got the results after a couple of days to weeks later. These differences are important and have consequences for large scale implementation as described later.

Analysis of the observational and interview data showed that at all sites two main steps had to be completed in order to ensure timely screening and diagnosis: 1) attending the health centre, and 2) initiating, completing and getting the test report. The

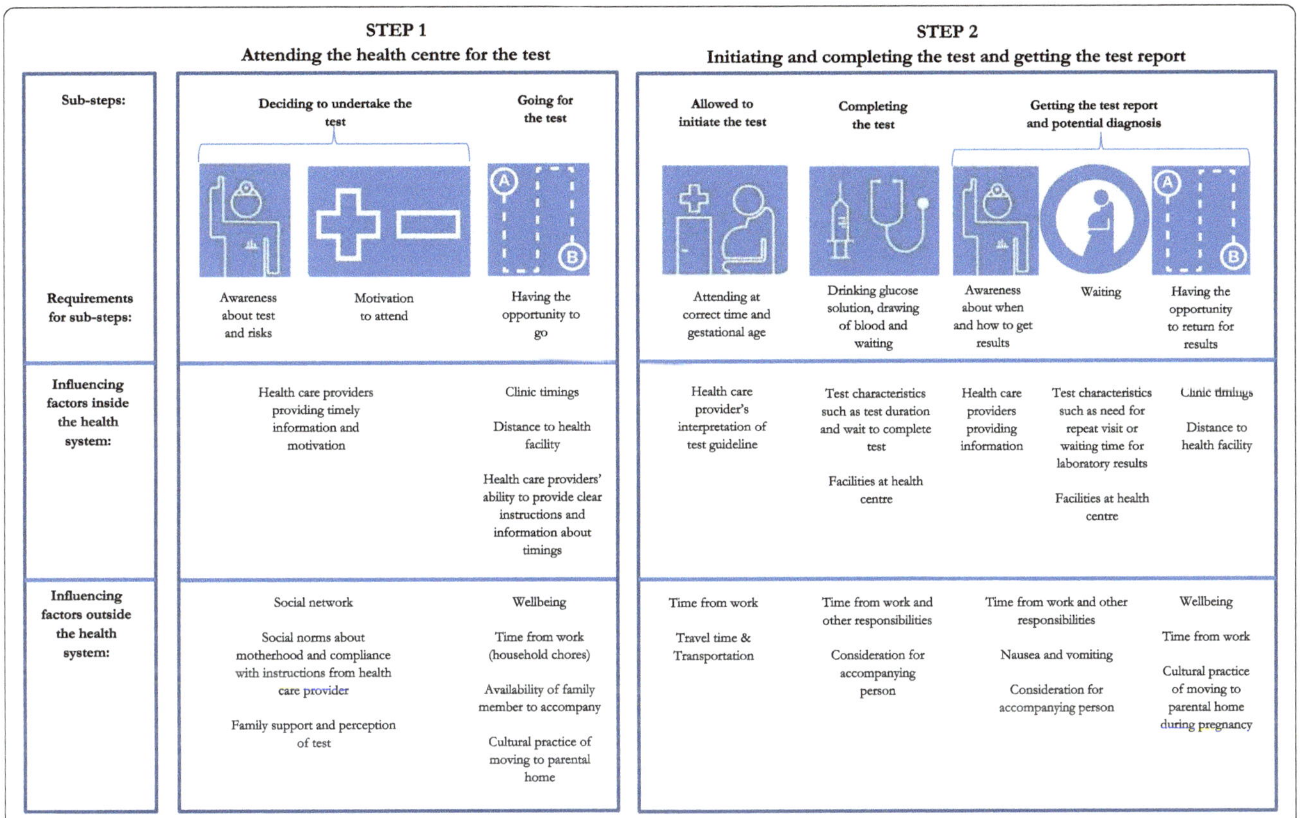

Fig. 1 Steps, sub-steps, and requirements in the GDM screening and diagnosis process, and influencing factors within and outside the health system

government employed laboratory technician at the rural centre required an extra step where a second test was administered; which meant a repetition of the two main steps (Table 2). Each step had sub-steps and certain requirements or 'doing' for completion, and various factors outside and within the health system influenced whether such 'doing' took place (see Fig. 1 and Table 3).

Overall, interview data showed that women's experiences of the screening process often differed based on rural or urban contexts. This was partly influenced by the differences in the screening procedures, but also by differences in infrastructure and access, and socio-economic backgrounds of the women as described in the following sections.

Step 1: Attending the health centre for the test

The first step in the process had two sub-steps: 1.a deciding to undertake the test and 1.b actually going for the test.

1.a). Deciding to undertake the test: Awareness and motivation

The analysis of the interviews with pregnant women and the HCPs identified that being *aware* of the test, including whether and why one had to undertake it, was the first requirement for deciding to go for the test. In practice, this meant that the pregnant women had to receive (correct) information about the test. This was usually done by the HCPs, i.e. the gynaecologist/obstetrician, if the women attended the urban diabetes centre, and the local village health nurse or the laboratory technician, if the women attended the rural government primary health centre. According to HCPs, this information is always provided, usually at the first ANC visit. However, six of the interviewed women from the rural area said they had not been informed about taking the test from their HCP – or if they had, it was only late in their pregnancy. Most of them had heard about the test from family or neighbours, or from other pregnant women attending ANC at the health centre or at the local *balwadi* (community pre-school and health post). A 26 year old woman from the rural area gave the following account of how she found out about the GDM screening test:

> *"Last week when I went for the regular check-up, I saw the other women sitting in a group for some test. So I asked them what test they were taking. They said "sugar test", and then I said "every month they take it, right? With the regular blood test?" The women said "yes". She [the village health nurse] hasn't told me anything. She comes here to give*

Table 2 Procedures for GDM screening and diagnosis synthesised based on observations, interviews, and available written information, versus instructions from government order on screening

		Private urban centre	Government rural centre - performed by private-non-profit laboratory technician	Government rural centre -performed by government l aboratory technician	Government order on screening for hyperglycaemia in pregnancy
Step 1: Attending the health centre for the test	*Informed and referred for the test*	Via the gynaecologist/ obstetrician	Via the village health nurse	Via the village health nurse	Not mentioned
Step 2: Initiating, completing and getting the report of the test	*Attending days*	Fasting on Mondays-Saturdays	Fasting on Tuesdays	No-fasting on Thursdays	1) Irrespective of whether she has taken her breakfast or not
	Attending time	Morning	Morning	Morning	2) Not mentioned
	Gestational age at attendance	No specific gestational age required, but testing is recommended in each trimester	No specific gestational age required, but testing is recommended in each trimester	4th, 6th and 8th month of pregnancy	3) Gestational week 24–28
	Flow of the testing procedure	1) Register 2) Consultation with doctor 3) Pay bill 4) Give fasting venous sample 5) Drink prepared glucose solution 6) Wait 1 h 7) Give 1 h venous sample 8) Wait 1 h 9) Give 2 h venous sample 10) Have breakfast and wait for results	1) Register 2) Give fasting venous sample 3) Mix and drink glucose solution 4) Wait 1 h 5) Give 1 h capillary sample 6) Wait 1 h 7) Give 2 h venous sample 8) Go home or wait for regular ANC check-ups	1) Register 2) Drink prepared glucose solution 3) Wait 2 h 4) Give 2 h venous sample 5) Go home	4) Registration not mentioned 5) Drink 75 g glucose solution 6) Wait 2 h 7) Give 2 h venous blood sample
	Getting the test report	On the day of the test. Around 1.5–2 h after 2 h sample	Usually 1 week later	If plasma glucose value is 140 mg/dl or more laboratory technician informs village health nurse who informs woman to come back fasting for a second test	Not mentioned
Diagnosis	*Steps of confirming test/s step to be completed*	A second test not requested as diagnosis is based on first test	A second test not requested as diagnosis is based on first test	1) Register 2) Fasting venous blood sample 3) Have breakfast consisting of 4 idlys (lentil and rice cakes). 4) Wait 1.5 h 5) Give 1.5 h venous sample 6) Go home	A second test not requested as diagnosis is based on first test
	Diagnostic cut-off levels used	2 h plasma glucose value ≥140 mg/dl (7.8 mmol/l)	2 h plasma glucose value ≥140 mg/dl (7.8 mmol/l)	Fasting plasma glucose value ≥110 mg/dl (6.1 mmol/l) 1.5 h plasma glucose value ≥140 mg/ dl (7.8 mmol/l)) Both values have to be above the cut-off	2 h plasma glucose value ≥140 mg/dl (7.8 mmol/l)

us the vaccination and that's all. We never see her in that hospital. She never helps us... We ourselves go and find out things." (Woman no. 25, rural area).

This woman had been tested for GDM for the first time three days before the interview at seven months into her pregnancy. Two other women from the rural area similarly had the first test done in 7th and 8th month, having not been informed about the test earlier. In the rural area, not receiving timely information about the test would thus delay or rule out testing entirely, clearly illustrating how dependent screening is on proper

Table 3 Barriers and facilitators for completing the two steps of the GDM screening process

Steps	Barriers	Facilitators
Step 1 Attending the health centre	• Not being informed (timely) about test by HCP • Weak or lack of social network	• Being informed (timely) about test by HCP • Strong social network • Strong motivation • Awareness of risk • Social norms about pregnancy and motherhood • Belief in importance of compliance with instructions from health care providers
	• Unsupportive family • Work • Feeling unwell • Being away from home	• Family in support of test • Conducive clinic timings
	• Lack of family member to accompany or help with household work	• Family member to accompany or help with household work
Step 2 Initiating, completing and getting the report of the screening and diagnostic test in a timely manner	• Not being aware of test time schedule • Lack of or delayed transportation and heavy traffic • No help with household work • Inflexible interpretation of timing of test in terms of gestational age	• Awareness of test time schedule • Available and timely transportation and conducive traffic • Help with household work
	• Glucose solution eliciting vomiting • Procedure stating that test has to be cancelled and done another day when women vomit	• Adding lemon drops to glucose solution
	• Long waiting time • Uncomfortable physical ambience of health centre and attitude of staff • Health care provider not informing the women about how and when the results will be available • Health care provider not informing the women about the results within a reasonable time period • Barriers mentioned under step 1 when women have to return to the health centre again	• Comfortable physical ambience of health centre and attitude of staff • Health services being free of charge • HCP informing the women about how and when the results will be available • HCP providing the results to the women over the phone or in-person in the village

and timely information by HCPs. On the other hand, it also reveals the importance of social network of women, and how they can function as facilitators; in this case for conveying information about the screening test, and, thus, compensate for the shortcomings of the health system. In the urban area, women also relied on their social network such as family and friends – but mainly when choosing obstetrician or maternity clinic, rather than as sources of screening information.

The second requirement for initiating testing was *motivation* to attend for testing. Once aware of the possibility for getting tested, most interviewed women displayed great motivation for the test. The motivation and decision to undertake the test was strongly influenced by the HCPs advice. Around 1/3 of all the women said they did the test mainly because their HCP had sent them for it and because they considered it to be compulsory.

> *"The doctor made this report, and that I have followed. Because it was just a blood test. When the doctor was saying "take it" and wrote it in the report and everything, that way I knew [about the GDM screening test]. The doctor has written this, so I follow their rules."* (Woman no. 3, urban area).

> *"I asked her [the village health nurse] what to do. She said that "tomorrow everyone will be doing the test. You too go and do it"."* (Woman no. 13, rural area).

Motivation was also strongly linked to the fear of the consequences of GDM and a strong desire to do whatever possible for the fetus' health. By doing the test, women saw an opportunity to prevent a danger at an early stage. Not taking the test was considered hazardous, risking harmful effects to the baby.

> *"We should do the sugar test. Only if we do it, we would have a healthy baby... If not, the baby would be born very big... We would have to do a caesarean, and if we have sugar, the place where the stitches are being put, would not heal fast. So we have to do a sugar test to check if we have sugar. Because if we have sugar even the baby would get it. If we do the test it's for the good of the child."* (Woman no. 15, rural area).

The prominence of motherhood was also mentioned in many interviews as a motivator for testing. Women stressed their new role as responsible mothers, and how GDM could potentially hamper the delivery of a healthy baby, and thereby risk the discontinuation of the family. Not handling this risk, could also lead to social stigma through gossip, particularly in the rural area, as aptly described by one woman: *"Becoming a mother is a big thing. So then if there is a problem [such as GDM] it would be sad only. It is like going through pain and then having another generation, and then if we don't deliver the baby well, the neighbours and all would talk badly about us."* (Woman no. 29, rural area).

Finally, deciding to attend the test was strongly influenced by the family. Almost all women from the rural area and around half of the urban women lived in joint families, typically with their in-laws, as is common in India. Many women in both areas said that their families would encourage and endorse them to undertake not only the GDM screening test, but all other tests and scans required during pregnancy.

> *"My parents, my husband, my mother-in-law, father-in-law, they all said "take all the tests, because this is the time to get the whatever, so you should be very careful this time. So whatever the doctor say, you should take that test. Whatever they say, you should follow that"."* (Woman no. 5, urban area).

Many women explained that they had to seek the approval of their husband and/or mother-in-law before going to the test, who had given it willingly – particularly as the testing was instructed by the HCP as part of routine ANC.

> *"For them it was just like "okay this is the protocol now. These tests are done for everybody, so it is good. You can rule it out now or take care from now". So they have been quite understanding about it as well."* (Woman no. 4, urban area).

Only two of the interviewed women (women no. 18 and 25, both from the rural area and newly married) gave accounts of how family members had been less enthusiastic about the test. The family was either concerned about the risk of evil spirits when pregnant women travel or about the drawing of blood. Low haemoglobin level is known in Tamil language as having 'less blood', and anaemia among women is very prevalent in this population. Thus, 'drawing of blood' seemed contradictory to these family members according to the pregnant women. Yet, both women also had family members supporting them in attending the test, and eventually the women disregarded the concerns and attended the GDM screening test. These findings highlight that having a supportive, well-informed family is clearly an important facilitator for GDM testing.

1.b). Going for the test: Having the opportunity to go

Having decided to go for the test, women encountered the first 'doing' of the screening procedure: actually *going* for the test. This required they had the opportunity to go, which was influenced by several factors (Fig. 1 and Table 3).

The women's well-being during pregnancy was one such issue, which could delay going for the test. In interviews, some women from both areas mentioned that pregnant women were not supposed to travel since it could harm the fetus, and a few women explained that they had delayed the test because of vomiting or tiredness. A 28 year old woman, attending the urban centre for her first GDM screening test in the beginning of her third month, said:

> *"My gynaecologist told me to go [for the test] by the beginning of the second month. She said to go whenever I feel a little okay and when the nausea is all down and all that. But then it didn't seem to come down at all, and I was constantly throwing up and I was taking drips. There was no way I could come to this place [health centre] that early in the morning. It was impossible. So I had no chance of coming here for the diabetes test. But now, for the past two weeks, I was a little okay, so we just thought we will finish it off."* (Woman no. 10, urban area).

Another challenge was coordinating the test with job timings, especially for urban women with formal jobs. One informant, a 26 year old accountant pregnant for the first time, was working nightshifts in a US company in Chennai and said: *"If I have to go for a night shift, I can't do the test. I won't have sleep. From morning to the evening I have to sleep, and night I have to go for night shift. So, since I have taken leave, I am feeling relieved."* (Woman no. 12, urban area).

This woman had taken one week's unpaid leave in order to rest and finish the required 'doing' of pregnancy tests, including the GDM test. The urban centre was also open on Saturdays, and from observations and informal conversations it was clear that this helped many working pregnant women to come for the test (including woman no. 4 and woman no. 6 in this study).

Women without formal jobs had to coordinate testing attendance with household work and child care. Women living in joint households sometimes noted that their family had helped them free up time from household work to go for the test. A couple of women felt bad about asking for such help, and one woman noted that: *"To leave my child at home – I find it difficult."* (Woman no. 15, rural area). Some rural women therefore brought the child along with them to the health centre, which they were generally allowed to, but which could complicate completion of the second step of screening.

These factors were further aggravated by the fact that many women due to social norms needed to be accompanied by family members when travelling. This meant more coordination and potential delay. The need to have a person accompanying the pregnant woman was described by women as also being practical, e.g. securing transportation, social and for security, e.g. assistance if falling ill.

Difficulties with organising this were reported by a few women in the rural as well as urban settings. One 20-year old pregnant woman reported that it had taken her two months and a lot of arguing with her husband, from when she was advised to attend the test by her gynaecologist, till she could go to the test:

> *"I used to shout at him for not taking me. "When will you take me?" To take me here to check the sugar. When he came back from his native place I somehow told him to take me today. So [this] morning he brought me. I used to fight with him. "You take me to the doctor! Take me to the doctor!"."* (Woman no. 8, urban area).

A final reason not to undertake the test, according to HCPs, was the common Indian practice where women go to live in their parental home sometime during pregnancy. If the parental home was located in another health district, the women would not fall under the care of their usual health centre and could miss the screening notifications from their HCPs: *"Some of them would say that they have gone out of station [left their home], and that they could not do the test... I would tell them to do the test compulsory in the fourth month. Every month when they come for the test, I would check their notebook, and when I ask them why they didn't come in the fourth month, they would say that they had gone out of station."* (Government laboratory technician, rural health centre).

However, the interviewed women themselves mainly reported this as a reason why they did not collect the test results.

Step 2: Initiating, completing and getting the test report

In spite of the identified barriers, all interviewed women had managed to attend the health centre at least once for the GDM screening. Upon arrival at the health centre, the women had to meet other requirements for the sub-steps: 2.a being allowed to initiate the test, 2.b complete the test and 2.c getting the test report (Fig. 1).

2.a). Allowed to initiate the test: Attending at correct time and gestational age

Even if the pregnant women arrived at the health centre, particularly at the rural health centre, there were situations where the women were not allowed to take the test. Observations showed that in the urban centre and in the rural centre, when conducted by the private-non-profit laboratory technician, the test procedure was typically organised to be done early in the morning during a specific timeslot, with the women being fasting. Some women arrived too late and were therefore refused or at least strongly encouraged not do the test, and instead told to come back another day. Interviews provided more knowledge about why some women had problems complying with this aspect of 'doing' the test. A 25 year old woman from the rural area, who was first screened when six months pregnant, described how she had attended the test in her fourth month, but was refused the test:

> *"I came [for the GDM test], but they told me that "it has become late" and they told me that "we can't do the test". So I went back home. I travelled so far, and then when I came here I could not take the test since it was late. Because that day the bus came late."* (Woman no. 24, rural area).

Thus, transportation issues as well as not being aware of the test timings, and completing household work were other challenges mentioned by women for their inability to reach the centre in time.

One of the HCPs described how he was often faced with women coming too late: *"If they come for the test at 10 o'clock, the test would be over at 12 o'clock, so they have to wait till 12 o'clock. They would say that they will wait, but I can't wait, because I have to give the samples at the hospital. The other patients would have come at 8 o'clock, so then I need to speak to the patient and make her understand. At that moment the patient would be sad and upset. She would feel all her effort to come to take the test was in vain. So this is the problem that I face."* (Private-non-profit laboratory technician, rural primary health centre).

However, the women, who arrived in time for the test with the government employed laboratory technician, could still be turned down if they were not in the fourth, sixth or eight month of pregnancy. A 22 year old woman, five months pregnant with her second child, said she had been tested when pregnant with her first child. But in this pregnancy she had received contradicting advice from the HCPs about when to do the test: *"Last week a neighbour of mine did the test. They [the HCPs] told her that you have to do the sugar test in the fifth month... and [they] told me to go for the test".*

Arriving at the health centre, she was refused the test by the laboratory technician, who blamed her she had missed testing in the fourth month of pregnancy: *"He told me that only the sixth month women should do the test and not the fifth month women. It made me sad. If I don't take the test this month, I will have to come back the next month."* (Woman no. 21, rural area). The laboratory technician confirmed in an interview that he would assign new testing dates for all women coming for testing at incorrect gestational age. Thus, strict interpretations of guidelines and unaligned advice given by HCPs sometimes posed barriers for the pregnant women to initiate the test.

2.b). Completing the test: Drinking glucose solution, drawing of blood and waiting

Some women, who initiated the test, failed to complete it. For instance, if they vomited after drinking the glucose solution some women were told to go home and return for a new test another day. Furthermore, in practice, the test would take a whole day to complete with travelling, drinking the glucose solution, drawing of blood, waiting at least two hours for the test to be completed, and travelling back. Urban as well as rural women found the waiting time very long and arduous, and some rural women complained about the facilities at the health centre being crowded, dirty, and with too few and sometimes rude staff: *"They are doing it for our good only, but at times I think if I have to go in this hot sun for all these tests. I feel it hard. I would feel giddy. I would feel as of vomiting. I would start at 7 and there would be a big crowd of 50 women, who would be waiting to do the tests."* (Woman no. 18, rural area). For rural women, the test being free of charge was the main reason for attending the specific centre. In contrast, the urban women had few complaints about the physicality of the centre, but still found the waiting time long: *"I didn't know I would be dedicating a whole day for this, but it looks like I have."* (Woman no. 4, urban area).

2.c). Getting the test report and potential diagnosis in a timely manner: Awareness, waiting and returning

After completing the test, there was still some 'doing' left. At the rural government centre, the laboratory technicians would inform the pregnant women of the test results via phone, through their village health nurse, or more commonly tell the women to collect the test report at the next ANC visit, typically between a week to a month later. Being informed about the results meant being told if the test results 'were normal or not'. There was no mentioning of this in the government order, and one of the laboratory technicians described the procedure he followed:

> *"If the patients wait on the same day for the results it would become late... If it's an abnormal case [GDM] we would first inform the village health nurse to tell the woman to come, and we would then refer the woman to the General Hospital [in Chennai] on the same day... The other pregnant women would collect it when they come for the next check-up."* (Government laboratory technician, rural centre).

However, in a few cases it took longer before the women were informed. Among the reasons for this were that the women had not been informed about how and when to collect the report; wherefore they were not aware that they were supposed to return. Some women had been told to return to the health centre, but found it difficult to repeat all the required arrangements.

At the private centre the women would get a 3–5 min consultation with the doctor, who would inform the woman whether the results were high or not, give instructions for what to do next and answer any questions the woman or her accompanying family member would have. However, this required that the woman would stay at the health centre after the test and wait typically another 1.5–2 h for the blood samples to be analysed and for consultation with the doctor. It was observed that some women left the health centre after completing the test, without waiting for the report. Informal conversations during those observations indicated that they did so because they had to return to work or more often out of considerations for the accompanying person.

Discussion

The complex screening process

This study explored the factors that influence the GDM screening process in TN, India. Limited research has been conducted on the factors influencing GDM screening initiation and completion in low and middle resource settings [9], and to our knowledge this is the first study, which includes pregnant women's own perspectives.

Similarly to *Mol's* work, we have shown that the GDM screening process requires a substantial amount of 'doing' and navigation of the health system by pregnant women, who have to go through several phases and sub-steps, each of which is influenced by several factors within and outside the health system. Other studies of maternal health have proposed similar steps-based frameworks for understanding barriers to health services use. Thus, 'the three phases of delay' framework suggested by *Thaddeus and Maine,* to understand barriers for seeking 'institutionalised birth', [33] describes three delay-steps: (i) dealing with the decision-making process involved in seeking health care, (ii) reaching a health facility and (iii) receiving adequate care once at the facility.

Our study indicates that completion of GDM screening requires attendance of diverse services, at specific places at specific time points, including several repetitions, making it much more complex to successfully complete the screening procedure than the chronological 'delay model' suggest. These findings stress the importance of minimising and aligning the required 'doing' in screening and maternal health services. Complex and unaligned systems will surely fail to achieve the objective that all women should be tested for hyperglycaemia during pregnancy as stated by the International Federation of Obstetrics and Gynecology in their document on GDM [34].

The GDM diagnostic criteria currently being endorsed in TN by the Government do not require the women to be fasting and only requires one blood sample [16, 35]. It is, thus, a simpler process than many other existing criteria and screening approaches. Concerns about the feasibility of the main international guidelines in low and middle income countries have been raised by a number of groups [36–38], and this study further stresses the importance of guidelines and diagnostic criteria which are simple and feasible on the ground.

Women's perception of the screening process

In an earlier study from our group, challenges for GDM screening were investigated from the point of view of implementing partners of GDM projects in low and middle income countries [37]. Among the challenges identified were difficulties in screening women during the recommended time period, challenges in testing women in the fasting state, scarcity of test consumables, lack of equipment, and the screening procedure being too time consuming [37]. From our current study, it is clear that timing and waiting issues are considered problematic by both the pregnant women and HCPs. If the screening process cannot be shortened, it could be better utilised, e.g. by providing useful prenatal care. Also, the study showed the immense importance of HCPs' abilities to properly inform and communicate with women: discussion and dialogue between HCPs and women are very important facilitators for screening.

But equally important is the ability of women to activate and draw on social networks in order to complete the screening process. Social network and support as facilitators for health seeking have also been identified in studies focusing on other diseases and conditions [39–43]. The importance of this is further emphasised through our findings that 'fear' of not living up to social norms of being a good mother, with attached social stigma, was a central underlying motivating factor to attend the screening test. This can be corroborated by other studies from India, showing that women's inability to give birth to a healthy baby can be associated with stigmatisation [44–46]. Thus, a simple focus only on the behaviour, attitude etc. of the individual seems insufficient, and efforts should be made to further engage families and the local communities in ensuring the health of pregnant women and in combatting social stigma.

In this study, we showed how women across urban and rural divides in TN are highly motivated and make great efforts to complete the GDM screening test. But the findings also suggest that women with weak social networks, little family support and with poor access to the health centre are particularly vulnerable for not completing the process. This is much in line with evidence on factors influencing the use of general maternal health care in India (19;24–26). To ensure that these women are tested for GDM and receive treatment if needed, it is important that the identified barriers are addressed and facilitators are strengthened. This also requires actions within the health system, with the rural health system in particularly need of strengthening. It could among other things be considered to further consolidate the role of village health nurses, e.g. by equipping them with a glucometer to perform screening at the village level – literally at the women's doorstep, accompanying the pregnant women to the health centres, and further train them to communicate effectively with women, including delivering test results.

Study limitations

Our aim with this study was to explore how the process of GDM screening in TN is navigated and experienced, and what may cause or prevent delays or completion throughout the GDM screening and diagnosis process. We therefore sought to ensure maximum variation of women's living places, life circumstances, gestational age at screening, and experiences with the GDM screening process. All women interviewed had attended a health centre at least once for GDM screening and had, therefore, all been able to overcome the initial barriers for screening. We did not recruit any women who had not attempted to attend the test at all. These women are likely facing even more pronounced barriers than the ones reported here.

The study presents findings from an urban private diabetes centre and a rural government health centre. Time and resources did not allow for more diversity, such as urban government and rural private health centres; hence, we chose the two health care settings likely to illustrate the biggest contrasts for health seeking behaviour and systems resources.

Most interviews were conducted with the help of an interpreter, which inevitably introduces some challenges, though the translator can also act as a co-researcher, adding local knowledge and assisting the interpretation of data [47]. This was enhanced by careful training of the interpreter, discussions after each interview and of the verbatim transcriptions and translation of the Tamil language into English.

Conclusions

Our study investigated factors that influence the timely initiation and completion of the GDM screening process in an urban and a rural setting in TN. Factors both within and outside the health system were identified, including getting right information from HCPs, clinic timings, characteristics of the test, availability of transport, social network and support, and social norms and cultural practices. These factors should receive more attention in the future efforts to continue improving and expanding the GDM services in TN and the rest of India. Minimising and aligning complex stepwise processes of prenatal care and GDM screening delivery; mitigating barriers of waiting, timing and communication; and promoting social supportive facilitators for the screening process are important for further improving and expanding GDM screening – not only in TN but in other similar low and middle income settings as well.

Abbreviations

ANC: Antenatal care; DIPSI: Diabetes in Pregnancy Study Group India; GDM: Gestational diabetes mellitus; HCP: Health care provider; OGTT: Oral glucose tolerance test; TN: Tamil Nadu

Acknowledgements

Not applicable.

Funding

This research has been made possible due to the following grants: World Diabetes foundation, grant no.: WDF-I-12-606; worlddiabetesfoundation.org; recipient: KKN. Aase og Ejner Danielsens Fond, grant no.: 10–000876; http://www.danielsensfond.dk; recipient: KKN. Christian og Ottilia Brorsons Rejselegat for yngre videnskabsmænd- og kvinder; no grant number; http://www.brorsons-rejselegat.dk; recipient: KKN. Etly og Jørgen Stjerngreens fond; no grant number; http://samf.ku.dk/uddannelser/legater/stjerngrens; recipient: KKN.

Dr. Anil Kapur, Chairman of the World Diabetes Foundation is a co-author on this manuscript, but otherwise the funders did not have any role in the study design, data collection and analysis, decision to publish or preparation of the manuscript.

Authors' contributions

KKN, AK, and ICB contributed to the conception of the study. KKN, TR, AK, PD, VS, and ICB contributed to the design of the study. KKN collected the data. KKN performed the analyses with substantial inputs from TR. KKN wrote the first draft of the manuscript. All authors critically revised the manuscript for intellectual content, and have read and approved the final manuscript.

Ethics approval and consent to participate

The overall purpose of the study was described to the participants, and verbal informed consent obtained prior to the interview, including approval for audio recording the interview. Verbal consent was chosen over written consent as obtaining written consent was seen as counterproductive to the informal and comfortable atmosphere we were trying to create to facilitate rapport and building trust between the researchers and informants. The verbal informed consent was given in the presence of KKN and the research assistant. Ethical approval for the study, including the use of verbal informed consent, was given by the Institutional Ethics Committee at Dr. V. Seshiah Diabetes Research Institute and Dr. Balaji Diabetes Care Centre in Chennai.

Consent for publication

Not applicable.

Competing interests

This study was financially supported by the World Diabetes Foundation, which receives unrestricted grants from Novo Nordisk A/S. During the study, KKN was employed partly on a grant from the World Diabetes Foundation. AK is on the board of World Diabetes Foundation and holds shares in Novo Nordisk A/S. VS and AK are members of the executive board of the Diabetes in Pregnancy Study Group India.

Author details

[1]Department of Public Health, University of Copenhagen, Oester Farimagsgade 5, 1014 Copenhagen, Denmark. [2]Steno Diabetes Center Copenhagen, Niels Steensens Vej 6, 2820 Gentofte, Denmark. [3]World Diabetes Foundation, Brogaardsvej 70, 2820 Gentofte, Denmark. [4]Center for Pregnant Women with Diabetes, Department of Obstetrics, Rigshospitalet, The Institute of Clinical Medicine, Faculty of Health and Medical Sciences, University of Copenhagen, Blegdamsvej 9, 2100 Copenhagen, Denmark. [5]Dr. Seshiah Diabetes Research Institute and Dr. Balaji Diabetes Care Centre, 729 Poonamallee High Road, Aminjikarai, Chennai, Tamil Nadu 600029, India.

References

1. Black MH, Sacks DA, Xiang AH, Lawrence JM. Clinical outcomes of pregnancies complicated by mild gestational diabetes mellitus differ by combinations of abnormal oral glucose tolerance test values. Diabetes Care. 2010;33(12):2524–30.
2. Damm P. Future risk of diabetes in mother and child after gestational diabetes mellitus. Int J Gynaecol Obstet. 2009;104(Suppl 1):S25–6.
3. Kim C, Newton KM, Knopp RH. Gestational diabetes and the incidence of type 2 diabetes: a systematic review. Diabetes Care. 2002;25(10):1862–8.
4. Metzger BE, Lowe LP, Dyer AR, Trimble ER, Chaovarindr U, Coustan DR, et al. Hyperglycemia and adverse pregnancy outcomes. N Engl J Med. 2008;358(19):1991–2002.
5. International Diabetes Federation. IDF Diabetes Atlas. Sixth ed. Brussels: International Diabetes Federation; 2013.
6. McIntyre HD, Oats JJ, Zeck W, Seshiah V, Hod M. Matching diagnosis and management of diabetes in pregnancy to local priorities and resources: an international approach. Int J Gynaecol Obstet. 2011;115(Suppl 1):S26–9.
7. McIntyre HD, Colagiuri S, Roglic G, Hod M. Diagnosis of GDM: a suggested consensus. Best Pract Res Clin Obstet Gynaecol. 2015;29(2):194–205.
8. Nolan CJ. Controversies in gestational diabetes. Best Pract Res Clin Obstet Gynaecol. 2011;25(1):37–49.
9. Nielsen KK, Kapur A, Damm P, de Courten M, Bygbjerg IC. From screening to postpartum follow-up - the determinants and barriers for gestational diabetes mellitus (GDM) services, a systematic review. BMC Pregnancy Childbirth. 2014;14:41.
10. Mol A. Living with diabetes: care beyond choice and control. Lancet. 2009;373(9677):1756–7.
11. Mol A. What diagnostic devices do: the case of blood sugar measurement. Theoretical Medicine and Bioethics. 2000;21:9–22.
12. World Health Organization. Trends in Maternal Mortality: 1990 to 2010. WHO, UNICEF, UNFPA and The World Bank estimates. Geneva: World Health Organization; 2012.
13. Jain R, Pathak RR, Kotecha AA. Gestational diabetes: perinatal and maternal complication in 24-28 weeks. International Journal of Medical Science and Public Health. 2014;3(10):1283–8.

14. Rajput M, Bairwa M, Rajput R. Prevalence of gestational diabetes mellitus in rural Haryana: a community-based study. Indian J Endocrinol Metab. 2014; 18(3):350–4.
15. Seshiah V, Balaji V, Balaji MS, Paneerselvam A, Arthi T, Thamizharasi M, et al. Prevalence of gestational diabetes mellitus in South India (Tamil Nadu)–a community based study. J Assoc Physicians India. 2008;56:329–33.
16. Thiru VK. Subburaj. Screening of glucose intolerance during pregnancy to be made mandatory - instructions - issued. Secretary to Government, Tamil Nadu Health and Family Welfare Department: Chennai; 2007.
17. International Institute for Population Sciences (IIPS) and Macro International. National Family Health Survey (NFHS-3), India, 2005–06: Tamil Nadu. Mumbai: IIPS; 2008.
18. Nielsen BB, Hedegaard M, Thilsted SH, Joseph A, Liljestrand J. Does antenatal care influence postpartum health behaviour? Evidence from a community based cross-sectional study in rural Tamil Nadu, South India. Br J Obstet Gynaecol. 1998;105:697–703.
19. Griffiths P, Stephenson R. Understanding users' perspectives of barriers to maternal health care use in Maharashtra. India J Biosoc Sci. 2001;33(3): 339–59.
20. Baqui AH, Rosecrans AM, Williams EK, Agrawal PK, Ahmed S, Darmstadt GL, et al. NGO facilitation of a government community-based maternal and neonatal health programme in rural India: improvements in equity. Health Policy Plan. 2008;23(4):234–43.
21. Hazarika I. Women's reproductive health in slum populations in India: evidence from NFHS-3. J Urban Health. 2010;87(2):264–77.
22. Pathak PK, Singh A, Subramanian SV. Economic inequalities in maternal health care: prenatal care and skilled birth attendance in India, 1992-2006. PLoS One. 2010;5(10):e13593.
23. Nielsen BB, Liljestrand J, Thilsted SH, Joseph A, Hedegaard M. Characteristics of antenatal care attenders in a rural population in Tamil Nadu, South India: a community-based cross-sectional study. Health Soc Care Community. 2001;9(6):327–33.
24. Chattopadhyay A. Men in maternal care: evidence from India. J Biosoc Sci. 2012;44(2):129–53.
25. Khan Z, Mehnaz S, Siddiqui AR, Ansari A, Khalil S, Sachdeva S. All slums are not equal: maternal health conditions among two urban slum dwellers. Indian J Community Med. 2012;37(1):50–6.
26. Mistry R, Galal O, Lu M. Women's autonomy and pregnancy care in rural India: a contextual analysis. Soc Sci Med. 2009;69(6):926–33.
27. Balaji V, Balaji MS, Datta M, Rajendran R, Nielsen KK, Radhakrishnan R, et al. A cohort study of gestational diabetes mellitus and complimentary qualitative research: background, aims and design. BMC Pregnancy Childbirth. 2014;14(1):378.
28. Malterud K. Qualitative research: standards, challenges, and guidelines. Lancet. 2001;358(9280):483–8.
29. Tjørnhøj-Thomsen T, Whyte SR. Fieldwork and participant observation. In: Vallgårda S, Koch L, editors. Research methods in public health. Copenhagen: Gyldendal Akademisk; 2008.
30. Wiles R, Crow G, Charles V, Heath S. Informed Consent and the Research Process: Following Rules or Striking Balances? Sociol Res Online. 2007;12(2).
31. Pope C, Ziebland S, Mays N. Qualitative research in health care. Analysing qualitative data. BMJ. 2000;320(7227):114–6.
32. Graneheim UH, Lundman B. Qualitative content analysis in nursing research: concepts, procedures and measures to achieve trustworthiness. Nurse Educ Today. 2004;24(2):105–12.
33. Thaddeus S, Maine D. Too far to walk: maternal mortality in context. Soc Sci Med. 1994;38(8):1091–110.
34. Hod M, Kapur A, Sacks DA, Hadar E, Agarwal M, Di Renzo GC, et al. The International Federation of Gynecology and Obstetrics (FIGO) initiative on gestational diabetes mellitus: a pragmatic guide for diagnosis, management and care. Int J Gynecol Obstet. 2015;129(1):3–41.
35. Seshiah V, Sahay BK, Das AK, Balaji V, Shah S, Banerjee S, et al. Diagnosis and Management of Gestational Diabetes Mellitus: Indian guidelines. In: Muruganathan a, editor. Medicine update Vol. 23, 2013. Chennai: The Association of Physicians In India; 2013.
36. Colagiuri S, Falavigna M, Agarwal MM, Boulvain M, Coetzee E, Hod M, et al. Strategies for implementing the WHO diagnostic criteria and classification of hyperglycaemia first detected in pregnancy. Diabetes Res Clin Pract. 2014;103(3):364–72.
37. Nielsen KK, de Courten M, Kapur A. The urgent need for universally applicable simple screening procedures and diagnostic criteria for gestational diabetes mellitus - lessons from projects funded by the world diabetes foundation. Glob Health Action. 2012;5.
38. Utz B, Kolsteren P, De BV. Screening for gestational diabetes mellitus: are guidelines from high-income settings applicable to poorer countries. Clin Diabetes. 2015;33(3):152–8.
39. Mann JR, Mannan J, Quinones LA, Palmer AA, Torres M. Religion, spirituality, social support, and perceived stress in pregnant and postpartum Hispanic women. J Obstet Gynecol Neonatal Nurs. 2010;39(6):645–57.
40. Pereira M, Canavarro MC. Relational contexts in adjustment to pregnancy of HIV-positive women: relationships, social support and personal adjustment. AIDS Care. 2009;21(3):301–8.
41. Petraro P, Duggan C, Msamanga G, Peterson KE, Spiegelman D, Fawzi W. Predictors of breastfeeding cessation among HIV-infected women in Dar es salaam, Tanzania Matern Child Nutr. 2011;7(3):273–83.
42. Rauchfuss M, Fischer T, Bogner G, Maier B. Influence of so far neglected psychosomatic factors, BMI and smoking on pregnancy-induced hypertension (PIH). Pregnancy Hypertens. 2012;2(2):93–100.
43. Wado YD, Afework MF, Hindin MJ. Effects of maternal pregnancy intention, depressive symptoms and social support on risk of low birth weight: a prospective study from southwestern Ethiopia. PLoS One. 2014;9(5):e96304.
44. Bhattacharji S. Motherhood in Ancient India. In: Krishnaraj M, editor. Motherhood in India. Glorification without Empowerment? New Delhi: Routledge; 2010.
45. Riessman CK. "even if we Don't have children [we] can live". Stigma and infertility in South India. In: Mattingly C, Garro LC, editors. Narrative and the cultural construction of illness and healing. Berkeley and Los Angeles: University of California Press; 2000.
46. Riessman CK. Positioning gender identity in narratives of infertility. In: Inhorn MC, van Balen F, editors. Infertility around the globe. New thinking on childlessness, gender, and reproductive technologies. Berkeley and Los Angeles: University of California Press; 2002.
47. Edwards R. A critical examination of the use of interpreters in the qualitative research process. J Ethn Migr Stud. 1998;24(1):197–208.

13

The Gestational Diabetes Management System (GooDMomS): development, feasibility and lessons learned from a patient-informed, web-based pregnancy and postpartum lifestyle intervention

Wanda K. Nicholson[1,2,3,4,5*], A. Jenna Beckham[1], Karen Hatley[6,8], Molly Diamond[6,8], La-Shell Johnson[2], Sherri L. Green[5] and Deborah Tate[6,7,8]

Abstract

Background: Gestational diabetes mellitus (GDM) contributes to the epidemic of diabetes and obesity in mothers and their offspring. The primary objective of this pilot study was to: 1) refine the GDM Management System (GooDMomS), a web-based pregnancy and postpartum behavioral intervention and 2) assess the feasibility of the intervention.

Methods: In phase 1, ten semi-structured interviews were conducted with women experiencing current or recent GDM mellitus GDM to garner pilot data on the web based intervention interface, content, and to solicit recommendations from women about refinements to enhance the GooDMomS intervention site. Interviews were audiotaped, transcribed and independently reviewed to identify major themes with Atlas.ti v7.0. In phase 2, a single-arm feasibility study was conducted and 23 participants were enrolled in the GooDMomS program. Participants received web lessons, self-tracking of weight and glucose, automated feedback and access to a message board for peer support. The primary outcome was feasibility, including recruitment and retention and acceptability. Secondary outcomes included the proportion of women whose gestational weight gain (GWG) was within the Institute of Medicine (IOM) guidelines and who were able to return to their pre-pregnancy weight after delivery.

Results: Comments from semi-structured interviews focused on: 1) usability of the on-line self-monitoring diary and tracking system, 2) access to a safe, reliable social network for peer support and 3) ability of prenatal clinicians to access the on-line diary for clinical management. Overall, 21 (91 %) completed the pregnancy phase. 15/21 (71 %) of participants were within the Institute of Medicine (IOM) guidelines for GWG. Sixteen (70 %) completed the postpartum phase. 7/16 (43 %) and 9/16 (56 %) of participants returned to their pre-pregnancy weight at 6 and 30 weeks postpartum, respectively.

(Continued on next page)

* Correspondence: wknichol@med.unc.edu
[1]Department of Obstetrics and Gynecology, University of North Carolina School of Medicine, Chapel Hill, NC, USA
[2]Partnerships for Women's Endocrine and Reproductive Health (PoWER), University of North Carolina School of Medicine, Chapel Hill, NC, USA
Full list of author information is available at the end of the article

(Continued from previous page)

Conclusions: This study documents the feasibility of the GooDMomS program. The results can have implications for web technology in perinatal care and inform the current care paradigm for women with GDM. Findings are supportive of further research with recruitment of a larger sample of participants and comparison of the outcomes with the intervention and standard care.

Keywords: Gestational diabetes, Behavioral intervention, Web-based intervention, Pregnancy, Postpartum, uhealth, mhealth

Background

Gestational diabetes mellitus (GDM) is part of an endocrine and reproductive cycle that contributes to the epidemic of diabetes and obesity across generations. In utero alterations to fetal metabolism due to prolonged glycemic exposure have life-long consequences for the newborn; namely a 8-fold risk of diabetes as well as chronic obesity and its downstream sequelae. Also, the expectant mother with GDM is at greater risk for long-term obesity, overt diabetes [1,2] and the metabolic syndrome [3].

It may be possible to achieve weight and glucose control in women with GDM and reduce the risk factors for development of overt diabetes with behavioral modifications, but there is limited data on the effects of a combined pregnancy and postpartum behavioral intervention in women with GDM. Evidence from earlier studies of prenatal nutrition counseling [4], or late prenatal [5] or postpartum [5,6] curricula to prevent postpartum weight retention suggest that women with GDM can benefit from short-term interventions. The Diabetes Prevention Program (DPP) [7] included women with histories of GDM [8], but they were remote from diagnosis at the time of enrollment.

Women with GDM represent a unique population to test innovative methods to deliver theory-based behavioral interventions. First, women are not always fully aware of the effects of elevated glucose levels and excessive weight gain during pregnancy on their long-term health or the health of their offspring. Interventions tailored to address these specific gaps in knowledge are crucial to helping women make the lifestyle changes necessary for glucose and weight control. Despite the increased risk of type 2 diabetes, women with GDM often have competing demands of childcare, work and family commitments that make it difficult to adopt and maintain healthy lifestyle behaviors after delivery. Our goal was to use a mixed-methods approach to develop and test the feasibility of a patient-centered, web and text-based behavioral intervention to help women with GDM achieve weight and glucose control during pregnancy and postpartum. Alternative methods for delivering interventions, such as web-based technologies that are easily accessible to women with GDM and provide flexible contact patterns, should be considered.

We proposed a novel intervention that begins in pregnancy at the time of GDM diagnosis and extends seamlessly into the postpartum period and has both pregnancy and postpartum-specific maternal and fetal outcomes. A previous study examined the feasibility of a web-based intervention on increasing women's knowledge [9]. Our objective was to develop an intervention to change behavior and take advantage of an important "teachable moment" [10] and offers the possibility of affecting the life course of both the mother and her developing fetus. In phase 1, we developed and refined the GooDMomS intervention incorporating feedback received from semi-structured interviews and qualitative analysis. In phase 2, we conducted a pilot study of the web-based pregnancy and postpartum intervention. The primary outcome was to assess feasibility, including recruitment and retention. Secondary outcomes included the proportion of women with gestational weight gain within the Institute of Medicine (IOM) guidelines [11], weight retention at 6 weeks and 30 weeks postpartum. Other outcomes included weekly rate of gestational weight gain, change in HbA1c levels and insulin resistance, as measured by the Homeostatic Model Assessment [12]. Because the offspring of women with GDM have an increased risk of obesity and diabetes as young adults, we also examined the feasibility of collecting neonatal measures of infant body composition.

Methods

Phase 1: development and refinement of the GooDMomS intervention

Content

Our gal was to introduce a lifestyle program integrated seamlessly across two critical periods in the lifespan of both mother and child-the prenatal period with the diagnosis of GDM and metabolic alteration that occur and the early postpartum period where maternal behavioral modifications can impact the long-term health of the mother and her offspring. The intervention provides evidence-based recommendations for weight and glucose information control combined with current clinical practice guidelines. The University of North Carolina Institutional Review Board (IRB # 12–0782) approved the qualitative study in phase 1 and feasibility study in phase 2.

Web and text components

We emphasized two aspects of social cognitive theory (SCT) [13], self-efficacy and self-regulation, to guide intervention development. GooDMomS was developed to encourage self-management and the ability of women to modify their lifestyle behaviors through structured goal setting, automated feedback tailored to each individual's progress in weight, control, dietary intake and physical activity, self-monitoring and social support. GooDMomS was designed to promote self-management and self-regulation in weight and glucose control, including i) pregnancy and postpartum web lessons, ii) a web-based self-monitoring diary for participants to record their daily weight, exercise and glucose levels during pregnancy and weight, calories, and exercise during the postpartum period, iii) weekly healthy recipes and tips about maintaining a healthy lifestyle, iv) an online message board for peer support and to pose questions or concerns for the study's interventionist and v) weekly text messages.

Qualitative assessment

Design, recruitment, setting

We conducted 10 semi-structured interviews in English using a purposeful sample of women with current or recent GDM between January and April, 2012. We continued with interviews until saturation was achieved [14]. Participants had an average age of 33 years (range, 23–44 years). The racial composition of participants was four African Americans, four Caucasians and two Hispanic whites. All were attending university clinics for prenatal and postpartum care. Four participants were Medicaid recipients; seven participants were multiparous.

Procedure and analysis to assess ease of use and content

Participants attended a 30-min semi-structured interview. Interviews were conducted while women explored a computerized diabetes behavioral intervention. After obtaining written informed consent, each participant was asked a series of eight open-ended questions in English by a trained interviewer regarding the ease of use of the web components and suggestions were sought for recommended refinements. Question were posed to offer patient generated feedback regarding the most useful components and to suggest additions as they actively browsed the website and toggled back and forth to each of the components: 1) How easy was it to follow the layout of the web--based program, including font size, formatting of web lessons and clarity of the images, 2) Do the web lessons provide useful information, 3) Are there topics that we should add to the content of the web lessons, 4) How usable is the self-tracking page, 5) Is the personal progress report page useful?, 6) What are your thoughts about an online message board for communicating with other mothers with GDM, 7) What is the most useful section of the web-based program and 8) What is the least useful section of the program? The interviewer used reflective probes to encourage respondents to clarify and expand on their verbal comments. All interviews were audiotaped and reviewed independently by two reviewers (AJB, SLG) who coded each statement to identify salient themes. Additional codes for new and emerging concepts were based on a grounded theory approach [14] and organized into broad themes using Atlas.ti v6.2 (Berlin, Germany). A third investigator reconciled discrepancies. We continued to sample, conduct interviews, and analyze data until redundancy of information was obtained, at which time recruitment for interviews stopped.

Themes and representative quotes

Participant responses were categorized into 4 broad domains: 1) perceived ease of use of web components, 2) assessment of usefulness of web-based components, 3) attitudes about online peer support and 4) preferred components for a GDM clinical management program. Participants expressed interest in each of the website components.

Perceived ease of use Most participants ($n = 8$) thought the website was user-friendly and easy to access.

> "I thought it was concise. I mean, on the Web, me personally, you don't want to sit there reading pages and pages, so I think it was organized well. [It] had the bullet points broken out so you can get the gist of it pretty quickly."

Usefulness of web-based components Participants verbalized that the link to healthy recipes and the "tracking your progress" page to record daily weights, exercise and blood glucose levels were the most useful website component.

> "I will probably be using that every day,...*every day*, because it's, I guess it's quicker for me to jump on the computer and put it in than it is to write it in the book, because I'll forget it."

Attitudes about online peer support Women reported little to no experience with online discussion groups, but expressed a willingness to use a message board to communicate with other women with GDM

> "Using this program would probably...would be the first for me because I don't do the message boards and things of that nature, but I'm willing to give it a try, just, you know, because somebody may know something more than I do, and it never hurts to ask."

Preferred components of a web-based intervention
While each of the participants was pleased with the current features of the web program, they desired guidance for entrée selections at major restaurants so that they could maintain a healthy diet, while eating out.

> "Like, maybe some examples from a typical restaurant, things that might be good on a menu to order at a restaurant...... because, I don't know, I didn't feel like cooking when I was pregnant

Also, participants suggested modifying the site to allow their prenatal providers to have direct access to the site to view their glucose and weight information.

> It would be great if the doctors could actually have access to it or, you know, whoever [is] checking it for you."

Feedback and refinement of intervention website

Comments from the semi-structured interviews were presented to the research team and used to refine the web-based intervention. The final version of the website used in the feasibility study in Phase 2 (www.goodmoms.org) was comprised of multiple features grounded in social cognitive theory [15]. We integrated additional cooking tips and recipes into the website and expanded the self-tracking page to show graphic representation of fasting glucose levels and weekly weights. To promote the use of the message board, the importance of social support was integrated into the pregnancy and postpartum web lessons. The web-based intervention included a pregnancy site for the prenatal period and a postpartum site for after delivery. Access to the website was limited to active participants who were assigned a login/password combination and interventionists.

Further refinements included the development of four animated videos to 1) provide a better understanding of the effects of GDM on fetal growth, 2) demonstrate physical activities that could be safely performed in pregnancy and 3) emphasize strategies to promote healthy lifestyle behaviors, including exercise and breastfeeding after delivery and 4) promote compliance with postpartum glucose testing. Animation was used to explain biological pathways that contribute to the development of GDM and affect fetal growth. Each video had a structured script and was narrated by a professional narrator.

Phase 2: procedures for feasibility study

Study setting and design

We used a single arm, pretest-posttest study design in women diagnosed with GDM attending two university-based prenatal clinics and one community-based practice. One of the university-based clinics was located within the hospital and one was located within the surrounding community. The community office practice was located approximately 10 miles from the university. Each of the recruitment sites screens for GDM between 24 and 28 weeks of pregnancy using the two-step screening strategy recommended by American College of Obstetricians and Gynecologists which includes a 50 g, 1-h glucose challenge test, followed by a 100 g, 3-h oral glucose tolerance test in those with a 1-h value ≥ 140 mg/dl. An appointment with a nutritionist and diabetes educator are scheduled within one week of their diagnosis. Visits with their obstetricians usually occur at 2-week intervals. Glycemic targets are fasting levels < 95 mg/dl and 1-h levels < 140 mg/dl. If more than 40 % of the glycemic targets are not met in a given week, follow-up visits with the nutritionist and educator are arranged and women are placed on an insulin or oral agent.

Potential participants were referred for eligibility screening by the diabetes prenatal nurse at each of the recruitment sites. Per clinical protocol, the diabetes nurse contacts each patient by phone to inform them of their positive test results. Women who were diagnosed with GDM were provided with general information about the study during their calls with the diabetes nurses. If the patient expressed an interest in the study, her contact information was sent to the study recruiter who screened the participants for eligibility over the phone. If the participant was deemed eligible, the recruiter arranged to meet the potential participant at her next prenatal or nutrition/diabetes education visit to obtain informed consent, complete study enrollment and collect baseline data. We report this non-controlled intervention study using guidelines from Transparent Reporting of Evaluations with Non-Randomized Designs [16].

Study population

Women ages 21 years and older with newly diagnosed GDM were recruited between July, 2012 and April 2013. Additional inclusion criteria included women who were English speaking and had computer and internet access for personal use at least 8 h per week. Medical exclusion criteria included a history of chronic hypertension or pre-existing diabetes, recent epilepsy, cardiac event or stroke in last 6 months, and special nutritional needs (e.g. malignancy or other chronic disease).

Intervention

The GooDMomS intervention was comprised of two phases: prenatal and postpartum. The intervention incorporated three domains, including knowledge and perceptions of risk for the mother and the fetus/infant, behavioral challenges and strategies, and social support and lifestyle modifications.

Pregnancy phase

The pregnancy phase of the intervention began within 2 weeks of the diagnosis of GDM and continued until 36 weeks of pregnancy. After enrollment and baseline data collection, participants were provided with a unique login and password to gain access to the website. Within 48 h of enrollment, participants received an introductory call from the team's interventionist to address any technical problems, difficulties with login/password combinations and to respond to questions about the GooDMomS program. If a participant had not logged in within 1 week of enrollment, the interventionist called the participant to remind them to log into the program. During the first login of each program week, participants were posed a series of automated check-in questions that asked them to enter their weight and whether they had achieved their physical activity and dietary goals over the previous week. Current ACOG guidelines recommend at least 30 min or more of moderate exercise on most, if not all days of the week [17]. GooDMomS participants were encouraged to engage in 30 min of moderate exercise at least 5 times per week (150 min per week). If a participant did not achieve their goals, an additional question asked them to identify the barriers that may have contributed to not achieving the goal. The participant then received tailored readings to address the selected barriers.

In the pregnancy phase of the intervention, participants were given 6 web lessons (Appendix) presented over 6 weeks which were developed by the research team and informed by practice recommendations and clinical guidelines from the American College of Obstetricians and Gynecologists [18] and the American Diabetes Association [19]. We tailored the pregnancy phase of the intervention to the needs of women immediately following a diagnosis of GDM and centered on increasing women's understanding of the development of GDM, how maternal glucose levels can affect fetal growth and the role of diet and exercise in weight and glucose control during pregnancy. Participants were asked to login weekly to record their weight and fasting glucose levels, and to review web lesson, videos and health tips. Participants were also encouraged to post questions, concerns and successful weight or glucose control strategies on the program's message board. Participants were sent a weekly text message or email (based on their preference) that included a health tip or motivational phrase to help them achieve weight and glucose control. Participants were sent a text message congratulating them after delivery of the infant was confirmed through hospital records. During the 4th week after delivery, participants were sent a text message that included a health tip and a reminder that the study coordinator would be meeting them at their 6-week postpartum visit to begin the postpartum phase of the intervention. Each participant was contacted by the study coordinator via text, email or phone to confirm the day and time of their postpartum visit.

Postpartum phase

The goal of the postpartum phase of the intervention was to help women return to their pre-pregnancy weight or achieve a 5 % weight loss. The postpartum phase began with the 6-week postpartum visit and continued for 24 weeks. The program consisted of 24 web lessons (Appendix) adapted from the DPP [8] and previously delivered using web-based technology [20–23]. Many of the behavioral strategies used in DPP have parallels with the postpartum period, such as skills training in modeling healthy eating behaviors, and balancing time for infant care and family commitments with consistent physical activity. Web lessons were adapted to address some of the unique challenges faced by mothers in the early postpartum period, such as the challenging effects of newborn care on maternal sleep, how to exercise with an infant, and the importance of continuing healthy lifestyle behaviors after delivery to reduce the chances of developing postpartum insulin resistance and hyperglycemia. Participants' weights were displayed in graphic form by the program so that participants could view their progress over time. As with the pregnancy phase, participants received automated tailored feedback about their weight, physical activity and diet behaviors reported in the weekly website check-in questions. Participants also received weekly text messages and emails with health-related tips and strategies to further assist with reaching their goals. Physical activity goals were the same as those outlined for the pregnancy phase (30 min per week at least 5 times per week).

Webinars

Recognizing the need to balance the opportunity for peer support with the logistics of childcare, work and family commitments, we developed and conducted 4 live webinars (2 in the pregnancy phase and 2 in the postpartum) during the intervention. Webinars topics focused on eating habits and strategies to maintain healthy eating during social and work events. Additional topics included strategies for maintaining a regular exercise routine and how to cook healthy meals for their families and themselves. Webinars were led by trained interventionists and were semi-structured, allowing time for presentation of the topic, group interaction and problem solving barriers.

Measures

The primary outcome measure was feasibility, as determined by rates of recruitment and participant completion of the intervention. Socio-demographics and medical history were collected through self-report at baseline. Information on the use of oral diabetes medications or insulin was based on maternal self-report at the 6-week postpartum study visit. Women were asked to attend an enrollment visit and three follow-up study visits: the enrollment (first) visit occurred within 2 weeks of the diagnosis of GDM and baseline data was collected. The three follow-up study visits occurred at 36 weeks of pregnancy and 6 weeks and 30 weeks postpartum. Two trained research assistants collected baseline and follow-up data.

Clinical measures

Weight was measured at each study visit with a digital electronic scale. Gestational weight gain (GWG) was calculated as the difference between the weight at 36 weeks of pregnancy and the earliest first trimester weight. We used weight at 36 weeks as the final data collection time point rather than the weight at the time of maternity ward admission in order to minimize the variability in gestational age at the time of the final collection of weight. Earlier studies have used 36 or 37 weeks' gestation as the time for final weight measures. By using a similar endpoint, we are able to compare our outcome measures to other published data. To avoid the risk of bias in determining pre-pregnancy body mass index (BMI) category, we chose to use measured data from the earliest first trimester visit rather than a participant's self-reported pre-pregnancy weight. [24] The average weekly rate of weight gain during enrollment was calculated as the difference in weight between study enrollment and 36 weeks of pregnancy divided by the total number of weeks during this same time period. Postpartum weight retention was calculated as the difference in weight at 30 weeks postpartum and the earliest first trimester weight.

Other measures

Laboratory

Hemoglobin A1c (HbA1c) is emerging as a potential tool to predict development of GDM and a useful monitoring tool in pregnancy [25]. Maternal blood was collected in EDTA tubes, immediately inverted several times to prevent coagulation and transported to the institution's core lab. HbA1c was measured at baseline and at 36 weeks of pregnancy.

In the postpartum phase, fasting maternal blood was collected in serum separator tubes and transported on dry ice to the laboratory for analysis. Fasting glucose was measured with the UV-hexokinanse method on a glucose analyzer (Beckman Diagnostic) at 6 weeks and 30 weeks postpartum. Fasting insulin was measured via radioimmunoassay (Linco Research, Inc). Insulin resistance [26] was assessed, as measured by the homeostasis model of assessment-insulin resistance (HOMA-IR = insulin*glucose/405) [12].

Self-reported behaviors

We assessed the feasibility of administering questionnaires at baseline and at each of the 3 follow-up study visits. Self-efficacy in physical activity was assessed using a validated 5-item instrument [27]. min per day of walking in bouts of ≥ 10 min were determined using the Paffenberger questionnaire. Dietary intake was assessed with the Block Food Frequency Assessment [28]. Breastfeeding status was assessed using the infant feeding practices survey (http://www.cdc.gov/ifps/)

Infant measures

Because we conducted a multi-site study with different institutions for labor management and delivery, infant birth weight was based on maternal self-report. Infant weight at 6 weeks and 30 weeks after delivery was measured using a calibrated scale (Scale-Tronix, Wheaton, Ill) by study staff. Infant length obtained using an infant measuring board based on standard protocols. Harpenden calipers (British Indicators, Sussex, England) were used for triceps skinfold measurements [29]. Circumference of the head was measured using a measuring tape. Head circumference and skinfold thickness were measured twice and an average measurement was used in the analysis.

Acceptability A post-intervention focus group was used to explore the acceptability of the length and format of the intervention, timing of intervention delivery in relation to the diagnosis of GDM and initiation of the postpartum phase of the intervention after delivery.

Statistical analysis We conducted descriptive analyses (calculated means and frequencies) for socio-demographics, health variables, dietary intake and physical activity. The proportion of women whose gestational weight gain was within the IOM guidelines was assessed across BMI categories using the chi-square statistic. We calculated the change in postpartum weight based on all participants who completed both the 6-week and 30-week postpartum visits. We performed a sensitivity analysis, including all participants who had a 6 weeks postpartum weight, assuming that participant who did not have a 30-week follow-up weight remained at their 6 week postpartum weight. The proportion of participants who met or exceeded their postpartum weight loss goal at 6 weeks and 30 weeks postpartum was compared across BMI categories. Analysis of pre/post changes in minutes/week of moderate walking in bouts ≥ 10 min, A1c levels and HOMA-IR, was performed using paired t-tests. We also analyzed self-reported change in percent fat and fruit and vegetable score and self-efficacy in physical activity. Because depressive symptoms have been shown to affect eating behaviors, we also assessed depressive symptoms using the Edinburgh depression scale. All analyses were conducted using STATA statistical software, version 10.0 (Stata Corporation, College Station, TX).

Results

Feasibility

Of the 36 women who were screened for eligibility, 23 (64 %) were eligible, agreed to participate and completed baseline assessments (Fig. 1). Thirteen women were excluded because they were ineligible ($n = 2$), eligible, but declined to participate ($n = 10$) or did not complete the enrollment process (n-1). Retention was 91 % at the 36-week follow-up visit and 83 % and 70 % at 6 weeks and 30 weeks postpartum, respectively.

Website use

Website logins were recorded by the GooDMomS system. Sixty-five percent (15/23) of the participants logged into the website at least 3 times during the pregnancy phase of the intervention. Ten of the 16 participants (62 %) who completed the postpartum phase of the intervention logged into the system at least once during the postpartum period; six participants had 10 logins during the phase.

Demographics

Average maternal age at enrollment was 31.7 years (SD = 4.7). Of the 23 participants, 16 were Caucasian, 3 were African American, 3 Asian and 1 reported their race/ethnicity as "other" (Table 1). The racial distribution of the participants reflected the demographics of the two clinics included in the study. Most participants were married, had a college degree or attended some college, were

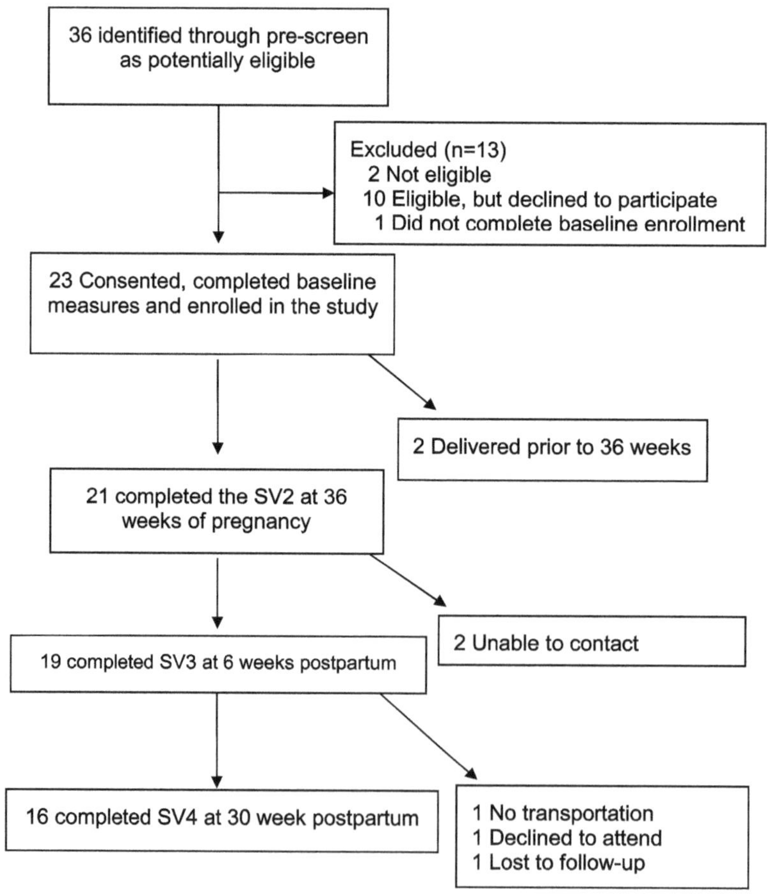

Fig. 1 Participant flow in GooDMoMs feasibility study

Table 1 Demographic and clinical characteristics of participants at baseline, $N = 23$

Socio-demographics	
Age, (yrs.), mean (SD)	31.5 (4.7)
Race	
White	16 (70)
African American	3 (13)
Asian	3 (13)
Other	1(4)
Hispanic	4 (17)
Education	
High school or less	5 (22)
Some college/complete college degree	12 (52)
Graduate/post graduate	6 (2.6)
Marital status	
Married	19 (83)
Single	4 (17)
Employed	14 (61)
Source of medical payment	
Commercial	18 (78)
Medicaid	2 (9)
Self-pay	2 (9)
Medicare	1 (4)
Parity, n, no prior delivery	11 (48)
1	5 (22)
2 or more	7 (30)
First-degree family history of diabetes	5 (22)
Smoking before pregnancy	23 (100)
Gestational age at baseline, (wks), mean (SD)	28.9 (3.4)
Pre-pregnancy BMI[a] (kg/m^2)	29.4 (11.2)
Normal (18.5–24.9)	9 (39)
Overweight (25.0–29.9)	4 (17)
Obese (30–34)	10 (43)
Earliest first trimester weight (kg), mean (SD)	71.7 (18.2)
Weight at enrollment, (kgs), mean (SD)	79 (18.8)
Gestational weight gain at enrollment (kgs), mean (SD)	7 (5)
Therapy during pregnancy after GDM diagnosis	
Diet	16 (70)
Glyburide or metformin	6 (26)
Insulin	1 (4)
Internet access at least 4 h per week	23 (100)
1-h 50-g glucose challenge test (mg/dl), mean (SD)	155 (10)
3-h, 100-g OGTT (mg/dl), mean (SD)	
Fasting	100 (5)
1-h	183 (30)
2-h	165 (25)
3-h	145 (15)
% dietary intake at baseline	
Percent fat (%), mean (SD)	36 (5)
Fruit and vegetable (servings/day), mean (SD)	3.2(1.6)
Moderate walking in bouts ≥ 10 min (minutes/week) mean (SD)	159 (185.7)

Kg kilograms; Data are reported as n (%) unless otherwise indicated
[a]Pre-pregnancy BMI is based on weight and height measured at earliest first trimester visit

employed at the time of enrollment, and had commercial insurance. Almost half of the participants were nulliparous. All participants reported internet access for at least 4 h per week. The median gestational age at enrollment was 28.9 weeks. Average first trimester BMI was 29.4 kg/m^2. Nine participants had a normal BMI, 4 were overweight and 10 were obese. Average weight at enrollment was 174.4 lb (SD = 41.4). There were no significant differences between women included in the study and women who were ineligible or declined to participate with regard to age, race/ethnicity, gestational age or parity. There was no difference in age, race or parity among women who completed study visits compared to those who did not complete the study.

Clinical outcomes

Gestational weight gain

Average gestational weight gain for all participants was 19.9 lbs ± 13.2. About three-quarters of participants were within the IOM guidelines for gestational weight gain at 36 weeks of pregnancy (Table 2). Fifty percent of women in the overweight or obese categories were within the IOM guidelines for weight gain. All of the participants with a normal BMI were within the IOM guidelines for weight. The average weekly rate of weight gain during the intervention period is summarized in Table 2. Half of the obese participants had an average weekly weight gain rate within the IOM guidelines; 78 % and 67 % of normal and overweight women, respectively, had a weekly rate of weight gain with the range recommended by the IOM.

Postpartum weight and weight retention

Participants achieved weight loss during the postpartum phase of the intervention (Table 3). Average weight loss between 6 and 30 weeks postpartum was 6.4 ± 52 lbs. Body mass index decreased by 2.6 kg/m^2 during the same time period. Average weight retention was 2.14 ± 15.2 and 0.9 ± 12 at 6 weeks and 30 weeks postpartum, respectively. Among participants with a normal pre-pregnancy BMI, 7/16 had met or exceeded their weight loss goal at 6 weeks postpartum; 9/16 had met or exceeded their weight loss goal by 30 weeks postpartum.

Table 2 Gestational weight gain of women with GDM and proportion meeting the IOM weight gain goals at 36 weeks of gestation

Weight gain variables	All participants N = 21	Pre-pregnancy BMI[1] Normal n = 9	Overweight n = 4	Obese n = 8
Total gestational weight gain, kgs, mean (SD)	9 (5.9)	10.3 (2.8)	7.7 (12)	6.9 (6.6)
Proportion with gestational weight gain within IOM[2] guidelines, n (%)	15 (71)	9 (100)	2 (50)	4 (50)
Gestational weight gain during GooDMomS intervention, lbs, mean (SD)	1.8 (2.1)	1.3 (1.9)	0.7(1.0)	2.4 (2.5)
Average number of weeks in intervention, mean (SD); range	6.6 (3) (2–12)	6.4(2.9) (2–11)	6 (2.0) (4–11)	7.1 (3.6) (2–12)
Average weekly rate of weight gain[3] during GooDMomS intervention	0.4(0.7) (−0.7, 2.7)	0.2 (0.4) (−0.7, 0.6)	0.2 (0.3) (−0.05,0.5)	0.6 (1.0) (−0.01, 3.2)
Proportion within 3rd trimester recommended weekly rate of weight gain during intervention, n(%)	13 (62)	7 (78)	2 (67)	4 (50)

GDM gestational diabetes mellitus, *IOM* Institute of Medicine. [1] Pre-pregnancy BMI categories (kg/m2) are based on weight measured at earliest first trimester prenatal visit: normal (18.5–24.9); overweight (25.0–29.9); obese (30 or greater)

[2]Gestational weight gain by IOM guidelines: normal BMI (11.3–15.9 kgs); overweight (6.8–11.3 kgs); obese (5–7.3 kgs)

[3]Weekly rate of weight gain (kg/week) by BMI category: normal [0.5 (0.4–0.5)]; overweight [0.3 (0.2–0.3)]; obese: [0.2 (0.2–0.3)]

Among overweight/obese participants, 6/8 (75 %) had returned to their pre-pregnancy weight at 6 weeks. At 30 weeks postpartum, 4/8 (50 %) overweight/obese participants met or exceeded their weight loss goal (percent change −25 %; $p = 0.3$). Two of the eight participants gained weight between the 6 weeks and 30 weeks postpartum visit.

Other outcomes

The majority of participants reported walking as their primary source of moderate physical activity. Participants reported an average of 159 ± 185.7 min of walking/week at baseline, 94 ± 83.4 min/week at 36 weeks, and 88.5 ± 153.3 min/week and 77.4 ± 123 min/week at 6 weeks and 30 weeks postpartum, respectively. There was no difference in self-efficacy scores for physical activity during pregnancy. However, scores were lower at 30 weeks postpartum compared to enrollment (mean change: −2.3; [−4.3, −0.2]; $p = 0.3$)

Daily fat intake decreased from baseline; fruit and vegetable consumption increased during the intervention period. Of the 16 participants that presented to the 6-week postpartum study visit, 12 participants were exclusively breastfeeding, one was partially breastfeeding and 3 were using formula. At 30 weeks postpartum, 10 participants were breastfeeding exclusively and 3 were partially breastfeeding. Two participants had depressive symptom scores above 12 (scores were 13 and 14) at baseline and were referred for counseling. Average depressive symptoms scores ranged from 5.9 ± 3.8 to 3.1 ± 3.7 at 30 weeks postpartum.

There was a small increase in mean A1C levels from baseline (5.08 ± 0.22) to 36 weeks' gestation (5.13 ± 0.16), but the change was not statistically significant (mean difference: 0.13; $p = 0.5$). Insulin resistance, as measured by

Table 3 Postpartum weight retention and proportion of women with GDM meeting or exceeding weight goals[1]

	6 weeks PP n = 16	30 weeks PP n = 16	Mean change,[2] p-value
Postpartum weight (kgs), mean ± sd	72.6 ± 18	69 ± 18.1	−2.9 ± 23.6 $p = 0.6$
Postpartum weight retention (kgs), mean ± sd	1.0 ± 6.9	0.4 ± 5.9	−0.5 ± 9.1; $p = 0.8$
Proportion meeting/exceeding weight goal[3], n (%)			Percent change,[3] p-value
All participants	7/16 (43 %)	9/16 (56 %)	13 %'; $p = 0.4$
Normal BMI (18.5–24.9 kg/m^2)	1/8 (12.5 %)	5/8 (62.5 %)	49 %; $p = 0.03$
Overweight/obese BMI (25–34 kg/m^2)	6/8 (75 %)	4/8 (50 %)	−25 %; $p = 0.3$

GDM gestational diabetes; kg = kilograms; sd = standard deviation; PP = postpartum

[1]Values are based on the 16 participants with complete weight data at 6 weeks and 30 weeks postpartum

[2]mean change represents the mean difference in weight retention at 6 weeks and 30 weeks postpartum

[3]postpartum weight goal was a return to the weight at the earliest first trimester visit or a 5 % weight loss, whichever was greater represents percentage change in the proportion of participants meeting or exceeding their weight loss goal

HOMA-IR increased between 6 weeks (2.3 ± 2.5) and 30 weeks (14.1 ± 21) postpartum period. Only 8 (50 %) of the 16 women participants who attended the 30 weeks postpartum visit were in a fasting state.

Infant measures

Of the 19 mothers presenting for the 6 week postpartum visit, 19 (100 %) infants were available for assessment at 6 weeks postpartum. Average weight at 6 weeks 4.0 ± 0.5 and triceps skinfold thickness was 8 ± 2.7 mm. Of the 16 participants presenting for the 30 week visit, nine (56 %) women also brought their infants for the newborn assessment. Average weight was 7.4 ± kg 1.2 and triceps skinfold thickness was 10.2 ± 3.7 mm.

Post-intervention focus group

We conducted a post-intervention focus group with 10 women who completed the intervention to gain feedback on 1) the usefulness of the intervention materials on the website, text messages and emails, 2) barriers to logging into the GooDMomS website and 3) perceived challenges to achieving their weight goals and glucose control. Participants thought that the intervention materials during pregnancy were useful and provided a better understanding of how gestational weight gain during pregnancy can affect the growth of the infant. The weekly emails and text messages during pregnancy and postpartum were well received by participants. In terms of intervention delivery, three themes emerged: 1) the need for a formal transition to the postpartum phase of the intervention with an emphasis on postpartum goals and objectives, 2) modifications to the website to notify participants when someone has posted a question or message on the message board to promote better interaction among participants, and 3) transition to a mobile application. Women expressed that logging into the system using a desktop or laptop computer during the postpartum phase was challenging due to the demands of childcare and that a mobile phone accessible intervention would enhance their ability to login consistently.

Discussion with lessons learned

In Phase 1, we were able to engage women with current or recent GDM to inform refinements to the GooDMomS intervention for the feasibility study in Phase 2. Our results show that a web-based, pregnancy and postpartum behavioral intervention for women with GDM is feasible. We were able to adapt ACOG [18] and ADA [19] guidelines for glucose and weight management during pregnancy and the DPP lifestyle intervention [8] to develop a pregnancy and postpartum intervention for women with GDM and their offspring. Our overall retention rate of 70 % at 6 months postpartum is acceptable. Collection of self-reported lifestyle behaviors using standardized questionnaires was also feasible. Of the participants who completed the study visits, we were able to collect questionnaires on 100 % (enrollment, visit 1), 80 % at visit 2, and 87 % and 81 %, respectively, at study visits 3 and 4. The Block Food Frequency questionnaire [28] required additional time during study visits and was burdensome to some participants.

During the pregnancy phase, the majority of participants were able to stay within the IOM guidelines for gestational weight gain. The intervention helped women to meet their postpartum weight loss goals by reducing postpartum weight retention in normal weight women and helping overweight and obese women lose weight. It is possible that postpartum weight loss was greater than 6.4lbs, as we used a fairly conservative sensitivity analysis to assess postpartum weight that included only those participants with weight data at both 6 weeks and 30 weeks after delivery.

It was challenging for participants to reach the physical activity goal outlined in the intervention. Despite web lessons that focused on the benefits of moderate physical activity, there was a decline in moderate walking during pregnancy and postpartum. It may be that some participants had lingering concerns about the risks of exercise during pregnancy, although none of the participants had contraindications to physical activity. Further refinements to the web lessons to emphasize the safety of exercise in pregnancy and postpartum may improve participants' ability to reach their physical activity goals.

This study contributes to the care of women with GDM in several important ways. First, we refined and introduced an intensive web-based lifestyle intervention integrated seamlessly across two critical periods in the lifespan of both mother and child – the prenatal period following the diagnosis of GDM and the metabolic alterations that occur in women and their offspring in the postpartum period. Prior studies of behavioral interventions in women with GDM have largely been confined to the pregnancy/delivery period [4], the postpartum timeframe alone [6,30], or on early childhood growth following delivery [31–33]. Ferrara and colleagues [5] assessed pregnancy and postpartum intervention, that was conducted using in-person sessions and telephone contacts. To our knowledge, GooDMomS is one of the first pregnancy and postpartum interventions delivered via web-based technologies. Second, this study adds to the literature on behavioral interventions that can be successfully delivered to pregnant and postpartum women, as the feedback from the post study focus group indicated that the intervention interface and content was both accessible and useful [34]. National studies and investigations within our institution [35] confirm access to and use of web-based technologies among pregnant women. Third, this study represents one of the first efforts to measure the preliminary effects of a web-supported behavioral intervention that begins with the diagnosis of GDM, continues through pregnancy and postpartum and include weight and body composition measures of the offspring.

Strengths of this study include our mix-methods approach. We used qualitative methods to refine the intervention in phase 1 and quantitative methods to test feasibility in phase 2. We also engaged women who had participated in the feasibility study in meaningful conversations to gain feedback and insights on the GooDMomS intervention. Participants reported that the intervention was acceptable and useful during the pregnancy and postpartum phases of the program. With the functionality of the system, we were able to directly assess logins rates rather than relying on participant self-report as a measure of utilization. Further refinements to GooDMomS that facilitate its use on smartphones or as a mobile app may improve utilization.

There are limitations to our findings. The small sample size and pre/post design in phase 2 was appropriate to assess feasibility, but a larger scale controlled study is needed to determine effect sizes and confirm the results. This feasibility study helped to inform specific refinements to the intervention that can help to improve acceptability by future participants. Also we were able to confirm the viability of our recruitment strategies as well as the identification and enrollment of participants. Participants represented a convenience sample of women attending a tertiary care prenatal care clinic, which limits generalizability of the findings to women obtaining care in other types of health care settings.

Several lessons were learned from this feasibility study. The follow-up rate at the 30-week postpartum study visit (70 %) was lower than expected. Limited transportation and work commitments were barriers to follow-up at the 30-week visit. Additionally, participants faced some difficulties in transporting their newborns to the 30-week visit and then back to their place of childcare. In future studies, it may be more effective to schedule postpartum follow-up visits to correlate with well child visits and arrange for data collection to take place within the pediatrician's office. As such, we may be able to improve long-term retention and enhance data collection. It was also challenging for women to present in a fasting state at the postpartum visits. Our study experience was similar to reports that have documented the low rates of compliance with postpartum glucose testing in women with recent GDM. Providing an opportunity for participants to complete the postpartum testing on a weekend may improve compliance. Regarding the intervention, postpartum login rates were lower than in the pregnancy phase of the study. Additional text messages to remind participants to log into GooDMomS as well as a re-introduction to the goals and objectives of the postpartum phase of the program at the 6 weeks postpartum study visit could enhance postpartum login rates. Family commitments and the demands of infant care were verbalized by participants in the post-intervention focus groups as contributing to the lower login rates and less adherence to the study protocol. Further work is needed to determine the best methods to promote consistency in healthy behaviors and website logins after delivery. Behavioral interventions that promote lifestyle change are critical to reducing perinatal obesity, hyperglycemia and the risk of type 2 diabetes.

Conclusions

Our study suggests that a web-based behavioral intervention combined with text messages and emails and tailored to the needs of women with GDM is feasible and well received by participants. Study results show that GooDMomS can help women stay within the IOM guidelines for gestational weight gain and achieve their postpartum weight loss goals. GooDMomS can potentially play an important role in changing the current paradigm of pregnancy care for women with GDM. More importantly, the program may serve to fill an important gap in care after delivery, particularly with regard to physical activity and postpartum weight loss. Further study is needed in a larger sample of participants with short and long-term clinical outcome measures in mothers and infants.

Appendix

Table 4 Gestational Diabetes Management Systems Web Lessons

Pregnancy Web Lessons and videos	Postpartum Web Lessons
1. Gestational Diabetes – The Basics	1. Getting Started
2. Video Lesson #1: How did I get Gestational Diabetes	
3. Treating Your Gestational Diabetes (Part A)	2. Energy Balance
4. The Benefits of Exercise for Women with Gestational Diabetes	3. Daily Weighing

Table 4 Gestational Diabetes Management Systems Web Lessons *(Continued)*

5. Video Lesson #2: Benefits of Exercise for you and your baby	4. Becoming More Active
6. Treating Your Gestational Diabetes (Part B)	5. Incorporating Physical Activity into Your Everyday Life
7. Benefits of Breastfeeding for You and Your Baby	6. Be a Fat Detective
8. Preparing for postpartum Glucose Testing	7. Eating Out on a Calorie Budget
9. Video Lesson #3: Getting ready for your postpartum visit and glucose testing	8. Feeding Your Family
	9. Social Support
	10. Take Charge of What's Around You
	11. Cues for Activity
	12. Simple Ways to Control Calories
	13. Recipe Modification
	14. Emotional Overeating
	15. Barriers to Diet and Exercise - Fatigue
	16. Time Management
	17. Problem Solving
	18. Meal Planning
	19. Stress Management
	20. Eating Patterns
	21. Thoughts and Weight Control
	22. Maintaining Motivation
	23. Staying in Control of Your Weight
	24. Becoming a Weight Control Expert

Abbreviations
GDM: GDM; GooDMomS: GDM system; HbA1c: glycosylated hemoglobin

Acknowledgements
We acknowledge the women who participated in the GooDMomS development phase and the feasibility study. We also want to thank Ziya Glizice for his advice regarding the final statistical analysis.
This study was presented, in part, at the 77th Annual Meeting of the American Diabetes Association, Chicago Illinois, June 24, 2013.

Funding
This research was supported by the National Institute of Diabetes and Digestive and Kidney Diseases (5R21DK9518901A1) and the Nutrition Obesity Research Center (P50DK056350). Its contents are solely the responsibility of the authors and do not necessarily represent the official views of the National Institutes of Health.

Authors' contributions
WN was involved in the conceptual framework of the study. She developed the study design, conducted the statistical analysis and was a primary writer. AJB contributed to the conceptual framework, conducted the semi-structured interviews and qualitative analysis and revised portions of the manuscript. KH, MD and SLG, and LJ assisted in the interpretation of the analyses and reviewed portions of the manuscript. DT contributed to the interpretation of the study results and provided revisions to the text of the manuscript. All authors read and approved the final manuscript.

Competing interests
The authors declare that they have no competing interests.

Consent for publication
Not applicable.

Animal studies
Not applicable.

Author details
[1]Department of Obstetrics and Gynecology, University of North Carolina School of Medicine, Chapel Hill, NC, USA. [2]Partnerships for Women's Endocrine and Reproductive Health (PoWER), University of North Carolina School of Medicine, Chapel Hill, NC, USA. [3]Diabetes and Obesity Core, Center for Women's Health Research, University of North Carolina School of Medicine, Chapel Hill, NC, USA. [4]The Diabetes Center, University of North Carolina School of Medicine, Chapel Hill, USA. [5]Cecil G. Sheps Center for Health Services Research, University of North Carolina School of Medicine, Chapel Hill, NC, USA. [6]Department of Nutrition, University of North Carolina School of Medicine, Chapel Hill, USA. [7]Department of Health Behavior, University of North Carolina Gillings Global School of Public Health, Chapel Hill, USA. [8]Program on Obesity Treatment, University of North Carolina Gillings Global School of Public Health, Chapel Hill, NC, USA.

References

1. Kim C, Newton KM, Knopp RH. GDM and the incidence of type 2 diabetes: a systematic review. Diabetes Care. 2002;25(10):1862–8.
2. Bellamy L, Casas JP, Hingorani AD, Williams D. Type 2 diabetes mellitus after GDM: a systematic review and meta-analysis. Lancet. 2009;373(9677):1773–9.
3. Damm P. Future risk of diabetes in mother and child after GDM mellitus. Int J Gynaecol Obstet. 2009;104 Suppl 1:S25–6.
4. Landon MB, Spong CY, Thom E, Carpenter MW, Ramin SM, Casey B, Wapner RJ, Varner MW, Rouse DJ, Thorp Jr JM, Sciscione A, Catalano P, Harper M, Saade G, Lain KY, Sorokin Y, Peaceman AM, Tolosa JE, Anderson GB. A multicenter, randomized trial of treatment for mild GDM. N Engl J Med. 2009;361(14):1339–48.
5. Ferrara A, Hedderson MM, Albright CL, Ehrlich SF, Quesenberry Jr CP, Peng T, Feng J, Ching J, Crites Y. A Pregnancy and Postpartum Lifestyle Intervention in Women With GDM Mellitus Reduces Diabetes Risk Factors: A feasibility randomized control trial. Diabetes Care. 2011.
6. Nicklas JM, Zera CA, England LJ, Rosner BA, Horton E, Levkoff SE, Seely EW. A web-based lifestyle intervention for women with recent GDM mellitus: a randomized controlled trial. Obstet Gynecol. 2014;124(3):563–70.
7. Knowler WC, Barrett-Connor E, Fowler SE, Hamman RF, Lachin JM, Walker EA, Nathan DM. Reduction in the incidence of type 2 diabetes with lifestyle intervention or metformin. N Engl J Med. 2002;346(6):393–403.
8. Ratner RE, Christophi CA, Metzger BE, Dabelea D, Bennett PH, Pi-Sunyer X, Fowler S, Kahn SE. Prevention of diabetes in women with a history of GDM: effects of metformin and lifestyle interventions. J Clin Endocrinol Metab. 2008;93(12):4774–9.
9. Carolan-Olah M, Steele C, Krenzin G. Development and initial testing of a GDM information website for multi-ethnic women with GDM. BMC Pregnancy Childbirth. 2015;15:145.
10. McBride CM, Emmons KM, Lipkus IM. Understanding the potential of teachable moments: the case of smoking cessation. Health Educ Res. 2003;18(2):156–70.
11. Council IMNR. Weight gain during pregnancy: reexamining the guidelines. Washington, DC: The National Academies Press; 2009.
12. Matthews DR, Hosker JP, Rudenski AS, Naylor BA, Treacher DF, Turner RC. Homeostasis model assessment: insulin resistance and beta-cell function from fasting plasma glucose and insulin concentrations in man. Diabetologia. 1985;28(7):412–9.
13. Bandura A. Social foundations of thought and action: a social cognitive theory. Englewood Cliffs; 1986.
14. Crabtree BF MW. Doing qualitative research, vol. No. 18. Newbury Park: Sage Publications; 1992.
15. Bandura A. Social foundations of thought and action: a social cognitive theory. Englewood Cliffs: Prentice-Hall; 1986.
16. Des Jarlais DC, Lyles C, Crepaz N. Improving the reporting quality of nonrandomized evaluations of behavioral and public health interventions: the TREND statement. Am J Public Health. 2004;94(3):361–6.
17. Gynecologists ACoOa. Exercise during pregnancy and postpartum, Number 30 (Replaces Committee Opinion). Obstet Gynecol. 2002; Reaffirmed 2009.
18. bulletin ACoOaGP. Management of GDM, #137. Obstetrics and Gynecology. 2013.
19. Association AD. Standards of Medical Care in Diabetes. Diabetes Care. 2011;34(Suppl):S11–61.
20. Tate DF, Jackvony EH, Wing RR. Effects of Internet behavioral counseling on weight loss in adults at risk for type 2 diabetes: a randomized trial. JAMA. 2003;289(14):1833–6.
21. Tate DF, Jackvony EH, Wing RR. A randomized trial comparing human e-mail counseling, computer-automated tailored counseling, and no counseling in an Internet weight loss program. Arch Intern Med. 2006;166(15):1620–5.
22. Tate DF, Wing RR, Winett RA. Using Internet technology to deliver a behavioral weight loss program. JAMA. 2001;285(9):1172–7.
23. Tate DF, LaRose JG, Griffin LP, Erickson KE, Robichaud EF, Perdue L, Espeland MA, Wing RR. Recruitment of young adults into a randomized controlled trial of weight gain prevention: message development, methods, and cost. Trials. 2014;15(1):326.
24. Shin D, Chung H, Weatherspoon L, Song WO. Validity of prepregnancy weight status estimated from self-reported height and weight. Matern Child Health J. 2014;18(7):1667–74.
25. Jovanovic L, Savas H, Mehta M, Trujillo A, Pettitt DJ. Frequent monitoring of A1C during pregnancy as a treatment tool to guide therapy. Diabetes Care. 2011;34(1):53–4.
26. Retnakaran R, Qi Y, Sermer M, Connelly PW, Hanley AJ, Zinman B. Beta-cell function declines within the first year postpartum in women with recent glucose intolerance in pregnancy. Diabetes Care. 2010;33(8):1798–804.
27. Marcus BSVNR, Rossi JS. Self-efficacy and the states of exercise behavior change. Res Q Exerc Sport. 1992;63:60–6.
28. Block GGC, Rosenbaum EH, Jenson C. A rapid food screener to assess fat and fruit and vegetable intake. Am J Prev Med. 2000;18:284–8.
29. Catalano PM, Thomas AJ, Avallone DA, Amini SB. Anthropometric estimation of neonatal body composition. Am J Obstet Gynecol. 1995;173(4):1176–81.
30. Rautio N, Jokelainen J, Korpi-Hyovalti E, Oksa H, Saaristo T, Peltonen M, Moilanen L, Vanhala M, Uusitupa M, Tuomilehto J, Keinanen-Kiukaanniemi S. Lifestyle intervention in prevention of type 2 diabetes in women with a history of GDM mellitus: one-year results of the FIN-D2D project. J Womens Health (Larchmt). 2014;23(6):506–12.
31. Daniels LA, Magarey A, Battistutta D, Nicholson JM, Farrell A, Davidson G, Cleghorn G. The NOURISH randomised control trial: positive feeding practices and food preferences in early childhood - a primary prevention program for childhood obesity. BMC Public Health. 2009;9:387.
32. McCallum Z, Wake M, Gerner B, Baur LA, Gibbons K, Gold L, Gunn J, Harris C, Naughton G, Riess C, Sanci L, Sheehan J, Ukoumunne OC, Waters E. Outcome data from the LEAP (Live, Eat and Play) trial: a randomized controlled trial of a primary care intervention for childhood overweight/mild obesity. Int J Obes (Lond). 2007;31(4):630–6.
33. Wen LM, Baur LA, Rissel C, Wardle K, Alperstein G, Simpson JM. Early intervention of multiple home visits to prevent childhood obesity in a disadvantaged population: a home-based randomised controlled trial (Healthy Beginnings Trial). BMC Public Health. 2007;7:76.
34. Berger AA, Peragallo-Urrutia R, Nicholson WK. Systematic review of the effect of individual and combined nutrition and exercise interventions on weight, adiposity and metabolic outcomes after delivery: evidence for developing behavioral guidelines for post-partum weight control. BMC Pregnancy Childbirth. 2014;14:319.
35. Peragallo Urrutia R, Berger AA, Ivins AA, Beckham AJ, Thorp Jr JM, Nicholson WK. Internet Use and Access Among Pregnant Women via Computer and Mobile Phone: Implications for Delivery of Perinatal Care. JMIR Mhealth Uhealth. 2015;3(1):e25.

14

"Why screen if we cannot follow-up and manage?" Challenges for gestational diabetes screening and management in low and lower-middle income countries: results of a cross-sectional survey

Bettina Utz* and Vincent De Brouwere

Abstract

Background: The prevalence of gestational diabetes (GDM) in low and lower middle income countries (LLMIC) is increasing. Despite its associated short and long term complications for mothers and their newborns, there is a lack of knowledge about how to detect and manage GDM. The objective of our study was to identify the challenges that first line healthcare providers in LLMIC face in screening and management of GDM.

Methods: We conducted a cross-sectional survey of key informants from 40 low and lower-middle income countries in Africa, South-Asia and Latin-America by sending out questionnaires to 182 gynecologists, endocrinologists and medical doctors. Sixty-seven respondents from 26 LLMIC provided information on the challenges they encounter. Data was thematically analyzed and revealed eight overarching themes, including guidelines; human resources; access; costs; availability of services, equipment and drugs; patient and community factors; and collaboration and communication.

Results: Unavailability of guidelines combined with lack of knowledge about GDM on the part of both providers and patients poses a substantial barrier to detection and management of GDM, leading to deficiencies in screening and counseling. Limited access to regular monitoring and follow-up care as a result of distance and costs, in particular with respect to additional expenses related to specific tests and changes in diet were identified as important challenges. Services were not available at all levels nor was adequate testing equipment. Patient factors included lack of motivation and compliance with the recommended therapy. Respondents also highlighted the lack of communication and collaboration between different specialists and treatment delays as a result of patients being seen by multiple providers.

Conclusions: Providers from LLMIC face various challenges related to screening and managing GDM. Policy makers need to address these challenges by strengthening their health care system as a whole and by assuring that non-communicable diseases are better integrated into the existing packages of free or subsidized maternal health care.

Keywords: Gestational diabetes mellitus, Maternal health, Maternal morbidity, Neonatal health, Non-communicable diseases, Health systems, Low and lower-middle income countries

* Correspondence: Butz@itg.be
Public Health Department, Institute of Tropical Medicine (ITM), Nationalestraat 155, 2000 Antwerp, Belgium

Background

Global prevalence of diabetes mellitus in women of reproductive age is steadily increasing [1]. Similarly, the incidence of hyperglycemia diagnosed for the first time during pregnancy is on the rise and has reached nearly 17 % worldwide [1, 2]. The proportion of women with gestational diabetes (GDM) has not yet been assessed in many low and lower-middle income countries (LLMIC). However, the few studies conducted in Sub-Saharan Africa reveal prevalence rates in pregnant women ranging from 2 % to 14 % in Sub-Saharan Africa [3–5], and up to 18 % in South Asia [6, 7].

These numbers are worrying, as GDM is associated with a range of immediate and long term complications for both mothers and their newborns. Babies of affected mothers are at higher risk of being delivered preterm, of being macrosomic or suffering from hypoglycemia, jaundice or respiratory distress. Mothers have an increased risk of developing pregnancy-induced hypertension or pre-eclampsia, of experiencing a shoulder dystocia or a postpartum hemorrhage and are more likely to deliver by caesarean section [8]. Maternal diabetes is also a known condition associated with stillbirths [9], 10 % of which are attributable to non-communicable diseases [10]. In the long term, GDM affected women and their newborns are more prone to developing manifest diabetes mellitus [8, 11].

Although guidelines from high income settings on GDM screening and management are available and freely downloadable from the internet [12, 13], there is a lack of knowledge about the extent to which guidelines developed in high income settings are appropriate for use in less developed countries, where resources are scarce and access to care is limited [14].

The objective of our survey was therefore to identify existing challenges for first line health care providers in LLMIC regarding the detection and management of GDM and to use the findings to inform leaders of professional associations and policy makers involved in maternal and newborn health programmes. By identifying these challenges, the study aimed to contribute to the development of strategies for improving detection and management of GDM.

Methods

We conducted a cross-sectional survey in 40 out of the 56 LLMIC in Africa, South-Asia and Latin- America eligible for World Bank funding [15] to assess clinical practices used in detection and management of GDM and to explore existing challenges. To identify key informants, such as representatives of national professional societies or leading gynecologists in low and lower middle income settings we contacted members of our institutional networks in the respective countries. Identified key contacts were invited to participate in the survey. We then used snowball sampling, asking these key contacts to identify additional health care professionals in their respective countries, including gynecologists, endocrinologists and medical doctors working in the public and/or private sector at all levels of the health care system and involved in providing care to pregnant women and in screening and management of GDM. The survey tool, a self-administered semi-structured questionnaire containing a mixture of multiple choice and open-ended questions, was available in four languages (English, French, Spanish or Portuguese) and was sent out by email to a total of 182 gynecologists, endocrinologists and medical doctors in 40 LLMIC. Questionnaires were not sent to countries that were either affected by crisis or war (5) or where we failed to identify a key informant (11). Returning the completed questionnaire was considered as consent to participate in the study. A total of 77 respondents from 27 LLMIC returned the questionnaires and 67 respondents from 26 countries answered the open ended questions on challenges they encountered with GDM screening and management (Fig. 1). All data was handled anonymously with profession and country as sole identifiers and double entered into SPSS Version 21. All open responses were copied into an excel file and thematically analyzed. After sorting and grouping the data, eight thematic areas were identified. These included guidelines, human resources, access, costs, availability of services, of equipment and drugs, patient and community factors as well as collaboration and communication. Ethical approval for the study was granted by the Institutional Review Board of the Institute of Tropical Medicine, Antwerp, Belgium.

Results

Various challenges regarding GDM detection and management were highlighted by 67 survey respondents, including 59 gynecologists, five endocrinologists and three general practitioners from 26 LLMIC. 61.2 % of the respondents providing information on challenges were from Africa, 37.3 % from South-Asia and 1.5 % from Latin-America. 22.4 % of them were representatives at national level, 49.3 % were working in the public sector, 23.9 % in private facilities (including faith-based and non-governmental) and 4.5 % in both the public and private sector.

Guidelines

Several respondents highlighted problems concerning guidelines in their countries. Some informants complained that no standard protocols were available in their settings. In countries where protocols were available, these were sometimes not adequately disseminated, not

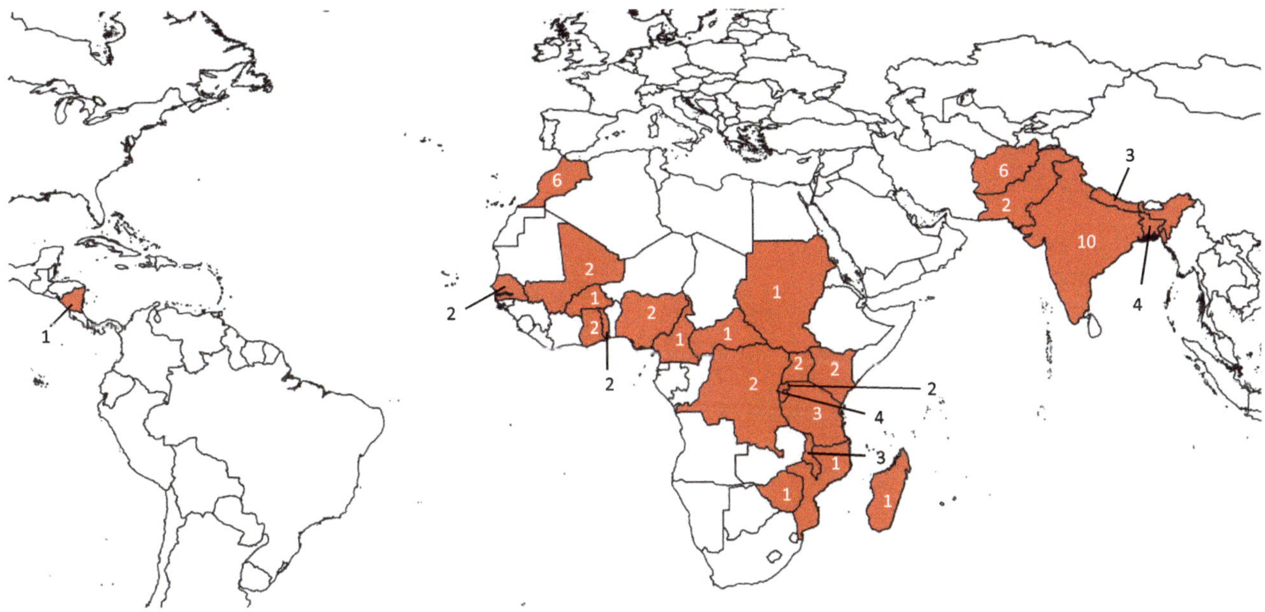

Fig. 1 Map depicting location of respondents

easily comprehensible or not used by the health care providers (Table 1a).

Human resources

Regarding health care providers' knowledge, survey respondents indicated that providers lack the required knowledge to screen for GDM and/or manage affected patients. In many settings, no particular training in GDM is provided, partly due to a lack of financial resources. Providers complained that updates are not available, which, coupled with limited internet access, restricts their ability to obtain latest practice updates. Many providers also indicated that general awareness of GDM is low due to lack of knowledge regarding GDM prevalence in their countries. One respondent stated that interest in GDM is limited, even among specialists.

Respondents also mentioned that counselling by providers is inadequate. One informant highlighted a lack of midwifes trained to provide counselling on GDM risks in the communities.

Respondents stated that despite the call for universal screening, some health care providers only screen women with risk factors. Others do not even screen when risk factors are present. Furthermore, is was reported that few lab technicians know about specific tests to detect GDM, such as the O'Sullivan glucose challenge test (Table 1b).

Access

Access to care was mentioned as a challenge for screening and management. In countries, in which antenatal care (ANC) coverage is low, some patients attend ANC either late in pregnancy or deliver without having attended any ANC consultation. In some settings, only 15 % of women attend public facilities. According to one respondent this can pose problems, particularly because harmonization of practices with the often unregulated private sector is challenging.

Transport can be an obstacle, especially for women receiving insulin. Difficulties in ensuring regular monitoring and follow-up of patients were highlighted by various respondents as major challenges. The complexity of the care system and the need to consult different health care providers also makes access for pregnant women difficult (Table 1c).

Costs

Financial access to care and the ability to pay for transport and treatment were identified as major barriers to adequate management of GDM. Costs are not only related to accessing health care facilities, but include expenses for specific screening tests, for repeat testing and for other investigations such as obstetric ultrasound scans. Patients diagnosed with GDM often face additional costs of purchasing testing equipment such as glucometers and testing-strips for self-monitoring their blood glucose, as well as for medication and hospitalization. Respondents highlighted that some examinations, such as the O'Sullivan test or obstetric ultrasound scans, are only performed in private laboratories or practices. In addition, costs related to diet play an equally important role. In many low resource settings women are accustomed to a traditional carbohydrate rich diet. Proteins, fruits and vegetables, all ingredients of a balanced

Table 1 Reported challenges with GDM screening and management grouped by thematic area

a. Guidelines	b. Human resources	c. Access & follow-up	d. Costs	e. Service availability	f. Equipment & drugs	g. Community & patients	h. Collaboration & coordination
Lack of national guidelines/ standard protocols	Not enough awareness of problem as no prevalence studies/poor knowledge about GDM	Access (travel)/ access to care	Patients have to pay, not affordable to screen and manage/socioeconomic status does not allow to test all women, even those with high risk	No government facility for screening/ screening not in all government facilities	No screening reagents/limited resources to test/to have sufficient lab supplies for measurements of GDM	Lack of knowledge in population/ low community information/low patient awareness/lack of knowledge of women about diabetes risk and its frequency	No multidisciplinary team with endocrinologist and nutritionist
Limited guidelines for screening/ management	Lack of provider sensitization	15 % women attend public facilities only	Hard for poor to get repeated test done and hard to convince them	GDM only screened and managed at tertiary and private level	Stock-out of screening material and test strips/stock out lab equipment and reagents	Ignorance and false belief about diabetes development/ignorance about diabetes and its consequences in pregnancy/	Multidisciplinary collaboration challenge because few endocrinologists and neonatologists
Guidelines not properly disseminated and used	Lack of capacity/technical competency/no capacity building/training/few lab technicians know to do O'Sullivan test	ANC coverage low	Costs of lab tests and ultrasound/costs of treatment and tests/costs for travel, investigations, medication, hospitalization	Laboratory not available 24/7	Unavailability of test strips and sometimes glucometers	Get patient to understand complications of diabetes/ spending a lot of time convincing them about long term problems and also have to ring and remind about follow-up visits	Pregnancy not managed together by endocrinologist and obstetrician
Policy guidelines not well articulated	Most providers screen in case of risk factors only/ screening not even done when risk factors present or when previous obstetric history would indicate	Late presentation for ANC/late booking/ emergency deliveries, women were not follow-up before	No insurance coverage for most, so cannot afford cost of follow-up	Shortage of laboratories in the public sector/good labs only urban	Sometimes glucose strips not available/ screening not routinely as no dipsticks	Low compliance to ANC and testing/in first trimester not able to do test in patient with vomiting/ some patients easily nauseated and may throw up after anhydrous glucose/2nd and 3rd trimester: some patients are not willing to wait for two hours	Laboratory service not fast and patient has to wait for result
Limited access to internet	Inadequate counselling/If proper counselling mothers very cooperative/no educated midwives who can counsel women in community	Patient without fridge needs to go to close center for treatment but with the problem of transport	Long hospitalization to balance glucose levels/ patients requested to get glucometer even while admitted	No screening because of technical problems of lab	Many difficulties in the lab to do correctly O'Sullivan test and HbA1C, primarily due to lack of reagents and organizational issues	Frequent pricking and venous puncture/SMBG cumbersome/ difficulty of self-monitoring blood glucose/many patients illiterate and cannot use rapid test/rare that women have a private glucometer	Result seen after 1 week by doctor/ late detection by gynecologists
No forum for updates	Few specialists interested in GDM/not enough endocrinologists/ nutritionist may not be around/no nutritionists	Majority of pregnant women not followed-up correctly/poor monitoring of patients	Patients have to pay for additional exams and drugs: therefore many women are not screened-treated/financial access limit the demand for specific tests	Glycaemia not regularly checked at lower level of care	Glucose availability/ getting anhydrous glucose for tests	Some patients do not undergo screening at recommended times/ patient does not come at advised delivery date/patients only come when complication	Patient has to consult several doctors for management

Table 1 Reported challenges with GDM screening and management grouped by thematic area *(Continued)*

	Surveillance problem (glycaemia, lab, US, CTG) to best plan delivery	OGTT requested at clinic and patients do it at lab when they have money for it/O'Sullivan test too expensive and often not done in public labs	No routine blood tests	Calibration of glucometers not checked against lab standards	Patients don't always follow management instructions/non-compliance with investigations, diet control/deficient compliance, needs husband cooperation, convince for prevention	Crowding in maternity does not allow to screen routinely and follow-up
	Women lost to follow up/ Mothers are not returning for postnatal follow-up	Ultrasound often expensive and done in private facilities	No general screening so most cases are picked up late	Difficult to get charts for glucose surveillance	GDM complex, needs close supervision while patient has domestic commitments/no gym, only brisk walking as exercise possible	Two hours blood sample needs to be taken to lab in time otherwise result error/organization for OGTT is a challenge
	Glucose not well monitored after discharge	Costs for medication affect patient compliance/ difficulties to buy insulin/ expensive glucose strips for home monitoring	Non availability of O' Sullivan test and OGTT/for OGTT patient sent to secondary level/O'Sullivan test often not done in public labs	Shortage of drugs to treat GDM in the public sector	Adherence to nutrition/adherence to diet/discontinuation of diet, exercise and drugs/Inadequate control of glucose by diet and exercise (lack of motivation)/ getting patients to follow diet and to take insulin if required/difficulty for women to keep their sugar level balanced/very difficult to commence a diet, difficult to change dietary habits	Patients don't know where to go for screening and follow-up/complex care system for women
		Low income makes diet control difficult as proteins expensive, they eat much carbs/cannot adhere to diet because expensive	Ultrasound often done in private facilities- in the public sector difficult to get appointment	Use of oral agents not very popular with most health care providers	Glucose not well monitored after discharge/getting them to continue physical exercise and diet even after delivery/screening after delivery is systematically prescribed but not always realized by the patient/mothers not returning for postnatal follow-up	
		No financial resources for training of providers	HBA1C hardly performed/Cannot check surfactant levels	Accessibility of insulin analogues/insulin during labor as no infusion pumps	Some fear about insulin/side effects of insulin/women reluctant or irregular to take insulin/difficult to store insulin	

carbohydrate restricted diet, are expensive and therefore adhering to such a diet is difficult, especially for poorer women with GDM (Table 1d).

Availability

Services

Service availability plays an important role in the detection and management of GDM. In addition to limited availability of screening services in public facilities of different levels, informants indicated that laboratories often pose a challenge. Technical problems were mentioned, as well as a shortage of laboratories in the public sector. Respondents stated that laboratories do not provide services 24/7 and certain tests, such as the O'Sullivan test, the oral glucose tolerance test (OGTT) and the glycosylated hemoglobin analysis (HbA1C) are not always done. One respondent mentioned that laboratories performing such specific tests are often located in urban areas. Due to difficulties getting these tests done in the public sector, women have to turn to private facilities. Furthermore, there is a shortage of specific health care providers, such as endocrinologists and nutritionists, to provide expert advice in many low income settings (Table 1e).

Equipment and drugs

When it comes to equipment, a shortage of laboratory supplies and screening reagents including anhydrous glucose, urine dipsticks and capillary test-strips was mentioned. The regular calibration of glucometers against laboratory standards was considered a technical challenge for ensuring adequate management.

Drug availability was identified as yet another constraint, particularly availability of insulin analogues. Difficulties for patients buying insulin (market availability as well as costs), and challenges for health care providers administering insulin during labour without having infusion pumps at their disposal, were also identified as obstacles (Table 1f).

Patient/community factors

Survey respondents indicated that patient and community related factors are key barriers. They reported a lack of awareness of diabetes in pregnancy, ignorance of the potential risks and false perceptions regarding GDM. Convincing patients of the need to commence and adhere to a specific diet, to check glucose levels regularly and to attend regular follow-up visits were listed as substantial challenges for health care providers. These challenges were compounded in settings in which the husband's approval is essential to women's ability to seek healthcare. Furthermore, adherence to a diet, treatment and regular monitoring may interfere with the domestic responsibilities of affected women.

Discontinuation of diet and treatment were also mentioned and partly explained by lack of motivation. Respondents reported a reluctance to comply with insulin management due to fears related to the administration of insulin and to its side effects. Regarding physical exercise, limited options and the unavailability of dedicated locations (e.g. gyms) where women can exercise often restrict recommendations to brisk walking. Self-monitoring of blood glucose was pointed out as a challenge by several respondents. Illiteracy and the difficulty of acquiring a private glucometer were considered reasons for women's inability to self-monitor glucose.

Women often do not comply with the recommended diet during pregnancy and discontinue glucose monitoring, their diet and exercise after delivery. Many women would not return for a re-test post-partum, despite having been advised to do so. Other reported patient related factors regarding screening include vomiting after glucose ingestion, particularly when given in the first trimester. It was also highlighted that some women are not willing to wait for two hours to get their blood tested (Table 1g).

Collaboration and coordination

Inadequate collaboration between different specialists might negatively impact efficient management of GDM, particularly in settings in which additional logistical hurdles exist. Respondents mentioned that collaboration between different professionals is often difficult. Similarly, the lack of multidisciplinary teams was reported. Good coordination is essential, as patients have to circulate between different services and might even have to consult various specialists. Informants mentioned delays in care because patients have to undergo requested tests at the laboratory and then have to revisit the doctor with the results. In case of delays during this process, women are subject to extensive waiting times and this might increase the risk of drop outs. Furthermore, time lags between taking blood and its final analysis in the laboratory could cause measurement errors. Sometimes services are overcrowded, which negatively impacts on health care providers' capacity to screen patients. Similarly, lack of sufficient patient information in terms of where to go for screening and follow-up might cause further delays and result in loss to follow-up (Table 1h).

Limitations

The collected challenges present individual views of key informants, mainly of obstetricians from the different countries. As such, these challenges are indicative of problems in individual health care services and might therefore not be generalizable. However, the similarity of the challenges reported by various key respondents would suggest that comparable problems are encountered in several low and lower-middle income countries.

The fact that we only collected information from health care providers and did not include the views of patients represents another limitation of this study.

Discussion

Our study reveals that providers in LLMIC face various challenges related to screening and management of GDM. General availability of guidelines and provision of specific training on GDM is one of the repeatedly mentioned obstacles. Some of these problems have been presented in a recent study conducted in Tanzania, where guidelines on diabetes were only available in 13 % of all facilities and only a third of doctors felt comfortable with the management of diabetes [16].

According to our findings, costs associated with GDM screening and management represent one of the major reasons for which GDM is not adequately addressed in LLMIC. Financial constraints have also been highlighted in a study on diabetes care in Tunisia, where costs related to travel, medication and testing presented serious constraints [17]. Costs of detection and management of GDM are not necessarily part of the packages of care that are offered to pregnant women and these often exclude specific laboratory tests, additional ultrasound investigations or equipment for self-testing such as glucometers and test strips. Furthermore, expenses related to hospitalization in LLMIC have shown to have detrimental effects on families, as these not only involve direct but also substantial indirect costs [18].

However, costs are only one of many factors that hamper adequate management of GDM in LLMIC. Even if costs could be reduced, issues such as compliance and motivation of patients to follow recommendations would persist. Studies have shown that patients who are involved in decision making have better health outcomes [19]. But this would require that patients are informed about their condition. Our findings reveal a lack of knowledge about GDM and its associated risks, as well as false beliefs that may threaten the benefits that can be expected from screening [20]. Good communication between patients and providers, as well as between providers themselves, could ensure that patients feel well informed and, as a consequence, comply with medical advice.

The role of community health workers in diabetes care is not a new concept and their potentially beneficial role in coaching can result in improved compliance and better outcomes [21, 22]. Nevertheless, their role in providing supportive care for GDM affected patients remains to be assessed. To reduce costs and improve monitoring, some innovative ideas have been reported from Kenya, where former GDM patients trained women in self-monitoring of their blood glucose levels and healthcare providers offered backup management support in the form of weekly mobile telephone follow-ups [23].

Several challenges highlighted in our study are related to resources both in terms of staff requirements and regarding equipment and drugs. Solving these problems would require improved overall health care organization that better integrates non-communicable diseases into the existing packages of care. In many LLMIC, maternal and perinatal mortality is still high and there is a persisting need to improve access to and provision of emergency obstetric and neonatal care. However, the parallel emergence of non-communicable diseases affecting maternal and newborn health in these settings will gradually place a double burden on existing health systems [24]. To increase awareness and improve universal detection of GDM in pregnancy, delegation of tasks to mid-or lower level health care providers could represent one potential solution and has already been initiated in India where, according to the latest national guidelines GDM screening now takes place at the first level of care [25]. Required health system related adjustments of GDM detection and management practices target clinical information systems, decision support through evidence based guidelines, redesign of health care delivery systems, self-management support and the use of community resources and are in line with the elements reflected in the chronic care model conceptualized by Wagner [26].

The long list of challenges regarding patient and community related factors mentioned by care givers indicates a need for critical reflection on the reasons for which health care providers face such difficulties in managing patients with GDM in their settings. Are we using patient related obstacles as a scapegoat for our failure to provide adequate care and follow-up? To enable patients to follow medical advice, we need to invest more in sensitizing women and their families about GDM and to tailor our interventions and recommendations to their needs and potential - not vice versa. Uniform GDM guidelines are an important first step but more needs to be done to avoid dissatisfaction on the part of both providers and clients. Otherwise the question asked by one respondent "*Why screen if we cannot follow-up and manage? Only to put pressure on the woman or on the care team?*" will not be satisfactorily addressed.

Conclusion

Providers from LLMIC face various challenges related to screening for and management of GDM. Policy makers need to address these challenges by strengthening their respective health care system as a whole and by ensuring that non-communicable diseases are better integrated into existing packages of free or subsidized maternal health care.

Abbreviations
ANC: Antenatal care; GDM: Gestational diabetes mellitus; HbA1C: Glycosylated hemoglobin; LLMIC: Low and lower middle income countries; OGTT: Oral glucose tolerance test; SMBG: Self-monitoring of blood glucose

Acknowledgements
We would like to sincerely thank all survey participants who provided information on their clinical practice and the challenges they encounter and thus contributed to a better understanding of the obstacles and problems they are facing when screening and managing women with gestational diabetes. We are grateful to all our network members who supported us and established contact with informants in their respective countries. We thank Juan Sabater, Felipe Rochas Lopez, Valeria Campos Da Silveira and Loubna Belaid for their assistance translating the questionnaires and Sarah Shelmerdine for copyediting the manuscript.

Funding
No funding was received for this study.

Authors' contributions
BU designed the study, performed the analysis and drafted the manuscript. VDB commented and edited the manuscript. Both authors read and approved the final manuscript.

Competing interests
The authors declare that they have no competing interests.

References
1. International Diabetes Federation. Diabetes Atlas. 7th Edition. 2015. http://www.idf.org/diabetesatlas. Accessed 5 Nov 2016.
2. Reece EA, Leguizamón G, Wiznitzer A. Gestational diabetes: the need for a common ground. Lancet. 2009;373(9677):1789–97.
3. Kuti MA, Abbiyesuku FM, Akinlade KS, Akinosun OM, Adedapo KS, Adeleye JO, Adesina OA. Oral glucose tolerance testing outcomes among women at high risk for gestational diabetes mellitus. J Clin Pathol. 2011;64(8):718–21.
4. Mwanri AW, Kinabo J, Ramaiya K, Feskens EJ. Prevalence of gestational diabetes mellitus in urban and rural Tanzania. Diabetes Res Clin Pract. 2013; 103(1):71–8.
5. Mwanri AW, Kinabo J, Ramaiya K, Feskens EJ. Gestational diabetes mellitus in sub-Saharan Africa: systematic review and metaregression on prevalence and risk factors. Trop Med Int Health. 2015;20(8):983–1002.
6. Jesmin S, Akter S, Akashi H, Al-Mamun A, Rahman MA, Islam MM, Sohael F, Okazaki O, Moroi M, Kawano S. Screening for gestational diabetes mellitus and its prevalence in Bangladesh. Diabetes Res Clin Pract. 2014;103(1):57–62.
7. Seshiah V, Balaji V, Balaji MS, Paneerselvam A, Arthi T, Thamizharasi M, Datta M. Prevalence of gestational diabetes mellitus in South India (Tamil Nadu)–a community based study. JAPI. 2008;56:329–33.
8. Wang Z, Kanguru L, Hussein J, Fitzmaurice A, Ritchie K. Incidence of adverse outcomes associated with gestational diabetes mellitus in low-and middle-income countries. Int J Gynaecol Obstet. 2013;121(1):14–9.
9. Aminu M, Unkels R, Mdegela M, Utz B, Adaji S, van den Broek N. Causes of and factors associated with stillbirth in low- and middle-income countries: a systematic literature review. BJOG. 2014;121 Suppl 4:141–53.
10. Lawn JE, Blencowe H, Waiswa P, Amouzou A, Mathers C, Hogan D, Flenady V, Froen JF, Qureshi ZU, Calderwood C, et al. Stillbirths: Rates, risk factors, and acceleration towards 2030. Lancet. 2016;387(10018):587–603.
11. Bellamy L, Casas J-P, Hingorani AD, Williams D. Type 2 diabetes mellitus after gestational diabetes: a systematic review and meta-analysis. Lancet. 2009;373(9677):1773–9.
12. NICE. Diabetes in pregnancy: management of diabetes and its complications from preconception to the postnatal period. http://www.nice.org.uk/guidance/ng3. 2015. Accessed 15 Jun 2015.
13. ADA. Standards of medical care in diabetes 2014. Diabetes Care. 2014;37 Suppl 1:S14–80.
14. Utz B, Kolsteren P, De Brouwere V. Screening for Gestational Diabetes Mellitus: Are Guidelines From High-Income Settings Applicable to Poorer Countries? Clin Diabetes. 2015;33(3):152–8.
15. The World Bank Group. IDA-The World Bank's Fund for the Poorest. http://www.ida.worldbank.org/financing/ida-financing. 2016. Accessed 29 Jun 2016.
16. Peck R, Mghamba J, Vanobberghen F, Kavishe B, Rugarabamu V, Smeeth L, Hayes R, Grosskurth H, Kapiga S. Preparedness of Tanzanian health facilities for outpatient primary care of hypertension and diabetes: a cross-sectional survey. Lancet Glob Health. 2014;2(5):e285–92.
17. Alberti H, Boudriga N, Nabli M. Primary care management of diabetes in a low/middle income country: a multi-method, qualitative study of barriers and facilitators to care. BMC Fam Pract. 2007;8(1):63.
18. McIntyre D, Thiede M, Dahlgren G, Whitehead M. What are the economic consequences for households of illness and of paying for health care in low-and middle-income country contexts? Soc Sci Med. 2006;62(4):858–65.
19. Guadagnoli E, Ward P. Patient participation in decision-making. Soc Sci Med. 1998;47(3):329–39.
20. Hirst JE, Tran TS, Do MAT, Rowena F, Morris JM, Jeffery HE. Women with gestational diabetes in Vietnam: a qualitative study to determine attitudes and health behaviours. BMC Pregnancy Childbirth. 2012;12(1):81.
21. Shah M, Kaselitz E, Heisler M. The role of community health workers in diabetes: update on current literature. Curr Diab Rep. 2013;13(2):163–71.
22. Farzadfar F, Murray CJ, Gakidou E, Bossert T, Namdaritabar H, Alikhani S, Moradi G, Delavari A, Jamshidi H, Ezzati M. Effectiveness of diabetes and hypertension management by rural primary health-care workers (Behvarz workers) in Iran: a nationally representative observational study. Lancet. 2012;379(9810):47–54.
23. Pastakia S, Ajwang'Onyango B, Ouma M, Christoffersen-Deb A, Cherop C. Addressing the challenge of GDM in the developing world: perspectives from rural Western Kenya. Diabetes Voice. 2014;59(1):51–4.
24. Ashwal E, Hadar E, Hod M. Diabetes in low-resourced countries. Best Pract Res Clin Obstet Gynaecol. 2015;29(1):91–101.
25. MoHFW. National Guidelines for Diagnosis & Management of Gestational Diabetes Mellitus. New Delhi: Ministry of Health and Family Welfare India; 2014. http://www.nrhmorissa.gov.in/writereaddata/Upload/Documents/National%20Guidelines%20for%20Diagnosis%20&%20Management%20of%20Gestational%20Diabetes%20Mellitus.pdf. Accessed 29 June 2016.
26. Wagner EH. Chronic disease management: what will it take to improve care for chronic illness? Eff Clin Pract. 1997;1(1):2–4.

15

Primary prevention of gestational diabetes mellitus through nutritional factors

Mikel Donazar-Ezcurra[1*], Cristina López-del Burgo[1,2,3] and Maira Bes-Rastrollo[1,2,4]

Abstract

Background: Gestational diabetes mellitus (GDM), defined as any degree of glucose intolerance with onset during pregnancy, is increasing worldwide, mostly because obesity among women of reproductive age is continuously escalating. GDM is associated with adverse maternal and fetal outcomes. The aim of this article was to systematically review literature on the effectiveness of nutritional factors before or during pregnancy to prevent GDM.

Methods: We assessed the primary prevention of GDM through nutritional factors, as diet and supplements. We searched on PubMed, Cochrane Databases and ClinicalTrials.gov from inception to June 2016. Clinical trials and adjusted prospective cohort studies were included.

Results: Eight clinical trials and twenty observational studies assessing the association between dietary factors and primary prevention of GDM were included. Furthermore, six clinical trials and two observational studies related to supplements were also added. Only two nutritional interventions were found to significantly reduce the incidence of GDM, besides the supplements. However, the observational studies showed that a higher adherence to a healthier dietary pattern can prevent the incidence of GDM, especially in high risk population before getting pregnant.

Conclusions: The results indicate that there may be some benefits of some nutritional factors to prevent GDM. However, better-designed studies are required to generate higher quality evidence. At the moment, no strong conclusions can be drawn with regard to the best intervention for the prevention of GDM.

Keywords: Gestational Diabetes Mellitus, Primary prevention, Nutritional factors, Diet and dietary supplements

Background

Gestational diabetes mellitus (GDM), defined as any degree of glucose intolerance with onset during pregnancy, is increasing worldwide. In fact, prevalence has increased by 10–100% in the last 20 years [1]. More mothers entering pregnancy as obese and of advanced maternal age has contributed to the escalation of GDM cases. Several risk factors are known for GDM; advanced maternal age, obesity, physical inactivity, parity, ethnicity, family history of type type 2 diabetes (T2D), history of macrosomic babies, and a previous history of GDM [2, 3].

GDM is associated with adverse maternal and fetal outcomes during pregnancy and long term health [4]. In order to prevent these adverse outcomes, such as T2D, it is imperative to understand the hormonal changes and altered glucose metabolism that are associated with the development of GDM during pregnancy [5]. GDM occurs when insulin receptors are not able to respond adequately to control blood sugar levels due to hormones produced in pregnancy, such as human placental lactogen, which impacts susceptible insulin receptors. This in turn causes inappropriately high levels of blood sugar. Due to the similarities in the underlying pathophysiology and risk factors of GDM and T2D, it is probable that the factors that are effective in the prevention of T2D may be successful in the prevention of GDM as well. These factors include dietary pattern, physical activity, a decrease in rates of obesity and gestational weight gain. It is important to identify population factors to reduce the increasing rates of GDM as it

* Correspondence: mikeldoez@gmail.com
[1]Department of Preventive Medicine and Public Health, University of Navarra, C/Irunlarrea1, 31008 Pamplona, Navarra, Spain

is doing for T2D. The aim of the researchers was to systematically review literature on clinical trials and prospective cohort studies focusing on the effectiveness of nutritional factors (diet and supplements) before or during pregnancy to prevent GDM.

The study protocol is available as a supplementary file in this article.

Methods

We undertook this systematic review following a protocol in accordance with the current recommendations of PRISMA and MOOSE guidelines [6, 7].

No ethical approval is required for this research project.

Search strategy

Articles were researched in the following databases: PubMed, Cochrane Databases and ClinicalTrials.gov from inception to June 2016. The keywords used for the search were: "gestational diabetes", "diet" and "nutrition". Another search was done for the keywords of "supplement" and "gestational diabetes". The search strategy was done independently by two researchers, and both extracted the relevant studies to be included in this systematic review. The disagreement between the researchers was resolved consulting a third researcher in order to reach an accord. We restricted publications to English, French and Spanish languages. All the researchers have an advanced level in these three languages. The selection process of the articles began from reading the titles. After this initial phase, the selected papers were reviewed by reading their abstracts. At that time, these selected studies were separated for further analysis to identify relevant publications, according to the inclusion/exclusion criteria. For the selection of studies, inclusion criteria were adopted such as: clinical trials or adjusted prospective cohort studies, originals, and primary prevention of GDM through nutritional factors. Due to inherent limitations other epidemiological studies were excluded. Exclusion criteria were: presence of diabetes mellitus type 1 or 2 prior to pregnancy, presence of diseases prior to pregnancy requiring dietary treatment, evaluation of diet as a treatment for patients with GDM, only physical activity for prevention of GDM and research on animals. Additional articles were identified from the reference lists of relevant studies and reviews.

Results and discussion

Study selection

Our initial research in the aforementioned electronic databases produced 1992 citations. Eighty-five articles were identified as potential articles for further full text review. After the next exclusion process, 28 articles were included and another seven were added from reference lists. The most important reason for exclusion was that diet or supplements were evaluated as a treatment for GDM, not as a primary prevention. We identified a total of 35 relevant articles (Fig. 1. Legend; Flow-chart of prospective cohort studies and clinical trials included in the systematic review. The search used the following combinations of terms: "diet" or "nutrition" and "gestational diabetes mellitus". A second search was done with the terms "supplement" and "gestational diabetes mellitus". Filters; Human; languages: English, French and Spanish; date: up to June 30, 2016). Twenty-eight were related to diet and primary prevention of GDM, eight were clinical trials (Additional file 1: Table S1) and 20 were prospective cohort studies (Additional file 2: Table S2). There were eight articles related to supplements and primary prevention of GDM, six clinical trials (Additional file 3: Table S3) and two prospective cohort studies (Additional file 4: Table S4). Lastly, there was one article [8] that studied whether dietary and supplemental iron were related to the occurrence of GDM (Additional file 2: Tables S2 and Additional file 4: Table S4).

Quality of the included studies

Of the 14 clinical trials included, only one was not randomized [9]. All women were pregnant when intervention had begun in the clinical trials. The diagnosis of GDM was based on the Oral Glucose Tolerance Test (OGTT), although the measurements of the OGTT was not the same in all articles, some considered the fasting glucose level abnormal when ≥ 5.3 mmol/l [9–11], but others consider it to be abnormal when ≥ 4.8 mmol/l [12], ≥5.1 mmol/l [13, 14] or ≥5.5 mmol/l [15]. Furthermore, the glucose level readings at 1 h and at 2 h were also

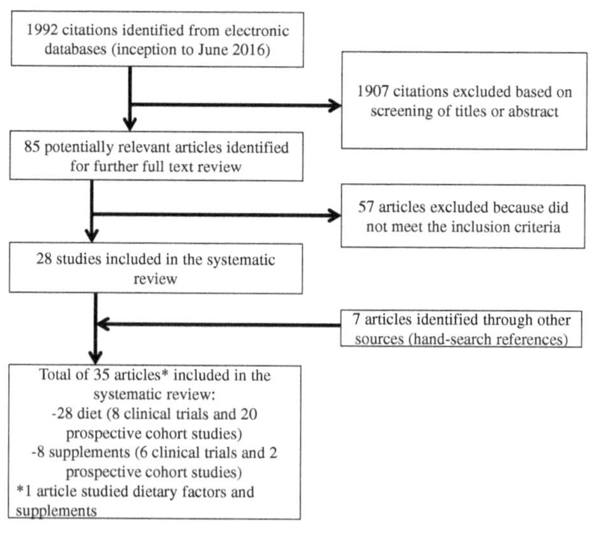

Fig. 1 Flow-chart of prospective cohort studies and clinical trials included in the systematic review

different. One article studied GDM incidence as a secondary outcome [16] and another one does not give a definition of GDM, although they studied glucose blood levels during the pregnancy of the participants [17].

The observational studies were adjusted for the most important variables (such as age, parity, tobacco products, BMI, physical activity, family history of diabetes, alcohol, ethnicity, total calories consumed). Twelve of these articles [8, 18–28] were based on the Nurses' Health Study II cohort, which includes more than 13,000 women who reported a singleton pregnancy. In this cohort, GDM cases were identified through self-reported information. The principal measures estimated in these studies were Risk Ratios (RR) and differences in means of GDM incidence.

Main findings

On one hand, no diet intervention was found to significantly reduce the incidence of GDM except for the intervention of the non-randomized controlled pragmatic trial [11] and the intervention on lifestyle (including diet) of Koivusalo et al. [10], (see Additional file 1: Table S1). Wolff et al. [17] found that an intensive intervention reduces the deterioration of glucose metabolism in obese pregnant women, though they did not report any incidence of GDM. Only two supplement interventions with probiotics and myo-inositol during pregnancy showed a decrease in the rates of GDM compared with a placebo. Luoto et al. [12] intervention showed that probiotics (Lactobacillus Rhamnosus GG and Bifidobacterium Lactis Bb12) reduced the incidence of GDM; 13% (diet/probiotics) versus 36% (diet/placebo) and 34% (control), $p = 0.003$. Luoto et al. [12] explain in their article that probiotic consumption may protect against GDM because these microorganisms can modify intestinal microbiota, altering the fermentation of dietary polysaccharides and improving intestinal barrier function. They also mentioned the importance of the capability of probiotics to regulate the inflammatory pathways. It is understandable that the protection against GDM provided by probiotics, could be mediated through immunomodulatory pathways and polysaccharide fermentation. Moreover, myo-inositol supplements were found to reduce the incidence of GDM in pregnant women (Matarrelli et al. [14]: RR = 0.127; 95% CI, 0.032–0.502; $p = 0.001$ and D'Anna et al. [13]: OR = 0.34; 95% CI, 0.17–0.68; $p = 0.001$) and appear to be an insulin sensitizer. It was reported to reduce plasma glucose levels in insulin resistant conditions such as polycystic ovary syndrome and during the third trimester of GDM pregnancies [29]. The subjacent mechanism of myo-inositol on metabolic benefits is not defined at the moment. It may produce an intracellular effect directly on the activation of acetil CoA carboxylase stimulating lipogenesis. Another theory says that it is a precursor of D-chiro-inositol, which contains inositol phosphoglycan in the extracellular matrix of the cells. It has been proposed that the binding of insulin to specific receptors stimulates D-chiro-inositol, facilitating the transport to the inside of the cell [30]. This explains how myo-inositol interacts in the insulin-signaling cascade [31].

On the other hand, the observational studies collected in Table S2 (Additional file 2) showed that achieving a healthier dietary pattern [25], such a Mediterranean dietary pattern, and lowering the intake of foods with high heme iron content, sugar sweetened cola, potatoes, fatty foods and sweets, can reduce the incidence of GDM, especially among the high-risk population and before getting pregnant [8, 21–23, 32–34].

Known evidence indicates that women who develop GDM have altered functions of β-cells and insulin resistance, limiting their capacity to cope with the metabolic challenges of pregnancy [35]. Similarly, it is known that iron is a redox-active transitional metal, a strong pro-oxidant which promotes the creation of hydroxyl radicals, increasing oxidative stress. The pancreatic β-cell is particularly sensitive to this type of stress due to weak antioxidant protection [36]. Nevertheless, adherence to healthy diets, such as the Mediterranean one, may reduce GDM risk by minimizing such susceptibilities before pregnancy. Common components of these dietary patterns include fruits and vegetables, relatively small amounts of red and processed meats, and high quality carbohydrates. Fruits and vegetables in particular have many antioxidant properties, in addition to providing fiber and micronutrients such as magnesium and vitamin C. The combination of all these factors may protect against metabolic deterioration counteracting free radicals and improving systemic oxidative stress [37].

Limitations

It is possible that a publication bias may have occurred as there is a limited amount of publications related to the study of primary intervention of GDM through diet, and absorption of supplements, probiotics and other minerals. In addition, the researchers are not discounting the existence of other articles in databases that were not used for this study.

Clinical applications

In this systematic review we found that the majority of the interventions done during pregnancy are not effective in preventing GDM, and although there were cases where supplements proved to be beneficial, the evidence is very scarce. However, dietary patterns prior to pregnancy seem to reduce the risk of GDM. Programs encouraging young women to achieve a healthy dietary pattern before getting pregnant seem to be the best way to prevent GDM. Measures adopted during pregnancy seem to be ineffective because they require more time to properly curb the development of GDM, especially among the high-risk population.

Implications for future research

There is a strong need for additional research on this topic. Although some prospective cohort studies have found an association between some nutrients or dietary patterns and the incidence of GDM, the existence of consistency of the results in other populations should be very desirable to prove causal associations between nutritional factors and the risk of GDM. We did not find any controlled trial that evaluated the intervention in dietary pattern before patients get pregnant and the incidence of GDM. Nevertheless, there is an ongoing European multicenter randomized controlled trial in overweight and obese pregnant women on lifestyle intervention and/or vitamin D supplementation [38]. Researchers have recently published the results of the pilot study finding that a healthy eating has a preventive impact on the risk of GDM [39]. Final results of the trial will be published in the near future.

Conclusions

Overall, since there is evidence that some dietary patterns, such as the Mediterranean diet, seem to lower the risk of developing GDM, and since it has also been shown to prevent other diseases (T2D, metabolic syndrome, cardiovascular diseases), the advice to adhere to this type of dietary pattern could be the best way at present to prevent GDM. Furthermore, it can be a good way to prevent other pregnancy related diseases, such as, hypertension and growth restriction. However, better designed prospective and intervention studies, providing high-quality data are required before conclusions can be drawn about the best intervention for the prevention of GDM.

Additional files

Additional file 1: Table S1. Characteristics of clinical trials for the primary prevention of Gestational Diabetes Mellitus through dietary factors [9–11, 15–17, 40, 41].

Additional file 2: Table S2. Characteristics of prospective cohort studies for the primary prevention of Gestational Diabetes Mellitus through dietary factors [8, 18–28, 32–34, 42–46].

Additional file 3: Table S3. Characteristics of clinical trials for the primary prevention of Gestational Diabetes Mellitus through supplements [12–14, 47–49].

Additional file 4: Table S4. Characteristics of prospective cohort studies for the primary prevention of Gestational Diabetes Mellitus through supplements [8, 50].

Abbreviations

GDM: Gestational diabetes mellitus; OGTT: Oral glucose tolerance test; T2D: Type 2 diabetes

Acknowledgements

The authors thank the library of the University of Navarra for the cooperation in achieving the data required as well for the technical support

Funding

CIBERobn Physiopathology of Obesity and Nutrition, Spanish Government Instituto de Salud Carlos III and the European Regional Development Fund (FEDER). Grants: PI13/00615, PI14/01668, the Navarra Regional Government (122/2014) and the University of Navarra.

Authors' contributions

MDE, CLB and MBR designed research; MDE and MBR conducted the literature search and extracted the data and this was analysed and interpreted by CLB and MBR. MDE drafted the manuscript. This was critically reviewed by CLB and MBR for important intellectual content and subsequent revisions to the paper were undertaken by MDE as a result. All authors approved the final manuscript.

Competing interests

The authors declare that they have no competing interests.

Consent for publication

Not applicable.

Author details

[1]Department of Preventive Medicine and Public Health, University of Navarra, C/Irunlarrea1, 31008 Pamplona, Navarra, Spain. [2]IDISNA, Navarra's Health Research Institute, Pamplona, Navarra, Spain. [3]Institute for Culture and Society, University of Navarra, Pamplona, Navarra, Spain. [4]CIBERobn, Instituto de Salud Carlos III, Madrid, Spain.

References

1. Ferrara A. Increasing prevalence of gestational diabetes mellitus: A public health perspective. Diabetes Care. 2007;30:141–6.
2. Chasan-Taber L, Schmidt MD, Pekow P, et al. Physical Activity and Gestational Diabetes Mellitus among Hispanic Women. J Womens Health. 2008;17:999–1008.
3. Teh WT, Teede HJ, Paul E, Harrison CL, Wallace EM, Allan C. Risk factors for gestational diabetes mellitus: Implications for the application of screening guidelines. Aust NZ J Obstet Gynaecol. 2011;51:26–30.
4. Jovanovic L, Pettitt DJ. Gestational Diabetes Mellitus. JAMA. 2001;286:2516–8.
5. Ramírez-Torres MA. The importance of gestational diabetes beyond pregnancy. Nutr Rev. 2013;71:37–41.
6. Moher D, Liberati A, Tetzlaff J. Altman DG and the PRISMA Group. Preferred Reporting Items for Systematic Reviews and Meta-Analyses: The PRISMA Statement Plos Medicine. 2009;6, e1000097.
7. Stroup DF, Berlin JA, Morton SC, et al. Meta-Analysis of Observational studies in Epidemiology. A proposal for reporting. JAMA. 2000;283:2008–12.
8. Bowers K, Yeung E, Williams M, et al. A prospective study of prepregnancy dietary iron intake and risk for Gestational Diabetes Mellitus. Diabetes Care. 2011;34:1557–63.
9. Luoto R, Kinnunen TI, Aittasalo MI. Primary prevention of gestational diabetes mellitus and large-for-gestational-age newborns by lifestyle counseling: a cluster-randomized controlled trial. PLoS Med. 2011;8, e1001036.
10. Koivusalo SB, Rönö K, Klemetti MM, Roine RP, Lindström J, Erkkola M, et al. Gestational diabetes mellitus can be prevented by lifestyle intervention: the Finnish Gestational Diabetes Prevention Study (RADIEL): a randomized controlled trial. Diabetes Care. 2016;39:24–30.
11. Mustila T, Raitanen J, Keskinen P, Saari A, Luoto R. Pragmatic controlled trial to prevent childhood obesity in maternity and child health care clinics: pregnancy and infant weight outcomes (the VACOPP study). BMC Pediatr. 2013;13:80.

12. Luoto R, Laitinen K, Nermes M, Isolauri E. Impact of maternal probiotic-supplemented dietary counselling on pregnancy outcome and prenatal and postnatal growth: a double-blind, placebo-controlled study. Brit J Nutr. 2010;103:1792–9.
13. D'Anna R, Di Benedetto A, Scilipoti A, Santamaria A, Interdonato ML, Petrella E, et al. Myo-inositol Supplementation for Prevention of Gestational Diabetes in Obese Pregnant Women: A Randomized Controlled Trial. Obstet Gynecol. 2015;126:310–5.
14. Matarrelli B, Vitacolonna E, D'Angelo M, et al. Effect of dietary myo-inositol supplementation in pregnancy on the incidence of maternal gestational diabetes mellitus and fetal outcomes: a randomized controlled trial. J Matern Fetal Neonatal Med. 2013;26:967–72.
15. Markovic TP, Muirhead R, Overs S, Ross GP, Louie JC, Kizirian N, et al. Randomized Controlled Trial investigating the effects of a Low-Glycemic Index Diet on pregnancy outcomes inwomen at high risk of Gestational Diabetes Mellitus: The GI Baby 3 Study. Diabetes Care. 2016;39:31–8.
16. Asbee SM, Jenkins TR, Butler JR, White J, Elliot M, Rutledge A. Preventing excessive weight gain during pregnancy through dietary and lifestyle Counseling. Obstet Gynecol. 2009;113:305–12.
17. Wolff S, Legarth J, Vangsgaard K, Toubro S, Astrup A. A randomized trial of the effects of dietary counseling on gestational weight gain and glucose metabolism in obese pregnant women. Int J Obes (Lond). 2008; 32:495–501.
18. Bao W, Bowers K, Tobias DK, Hu FB, Zhang C. Prepregnancy dietary protein intake, major dietary protein sources, and the risk of Gestational Diabetes Mellitus. Diabetes Care. 2013;36:2001–8.
19. Bao W, Tobias DK, Olsen SF, Zhang C. Pre-pregnancy fried food consumption and the risk of gestational diabetes mellitus: a prospective cohort study. Diabetologia. 2014;57:2485–91.
20. Bao W, Bowers K, Tobias DK, et al. Prepregnancy low-carbohydrate dietary pattern and risk of gestational diabetes mellitus: a prospective cohort study. Am J Clin Nutr. 2014;99:1378–84.
21. Bao W, Tobias DK, Hu FB, Chavarro JE, Zhang C. Pre-pregnancy potato consumption and risk of gestational diabetes mellitus: prospective cohort study. BMJ. 2016;12:352. h6898.
22. Bowers K, Tobias DK, Yeung E, Hu FB, Zhang C. A prospective study of prepregnancy dietary fat intake and risk of gestational diabetes. Am J Clin Nutr. 2012;95:446–53.
23. Chen L, Hu FB, Yeung E, Willett W, Zhang C. Prospective study of pre-gravid sugar sweetened beverage consumption and the risk of gestational diabetes mellitus. Diabetes Care. 2009;32:2236–41.
24. Chen L, Hu FB, Yeung E, Tobias DK, Willett WC, Zhang C. Prepregnancy consumption of fruits and fruit juices and the risk of Gestational Diabetes Mellitus. Diabetes Care. 2012;35:1079–82.
25. Tobias DK, Zhang C, Chavarro J, et al. Prepregnancy adherence to dietary patterns and lower risk of gestational diabetes mellitus. Am J Clin Nutr. 2012;96:289–95.
26. Zhang C, Schulze MB, Solomon CG, Hu FB. A prospective study of dietary patterns, meat intake and the risk of gestational diabetes mellitus. Diabetologia. 2006;49:2604–13.
27. Zhang C, Liu S, Solomon CG, Hu FB. Dietary fiber intake, dietary glycemic load, and the risk for gestational diabetes mellitus. Diabetes Care. 2006; 29:2223–30.
28. Zhang C, Tobias DK, Chavarro JE. Adherence to healthy lifestyle and risk of gestational diabetes mellitus: prospective cohort study. BMJ. 2014;349:g5450.
29. Corrado F, D'Anna R, Di Vieste G, et al. The effect of myo-inositol supplementation on insulin resistance in patients with gestational diabetes. Diabet Med. 2011;28:972–5.
30. Baillargeon JP, Iuorno MJ, Apridonidze T, Nestler JE. Uncoupling between insulin and release of a D-chiro-inositol-containing inositolphosphoglycan mediator of insulin action in obese women with polycystic ovary syndrome. Metab Syndr Relat Disord. 2010;8:127–36.
31. Saltier AR. Second messenger of insulin action. Diabetes Care. 1990;13:244–56.
32. He JR, Yuan MY, Chen NN, et al. Maternal dietary patterns and gestational diabetes mellitus: a large prospective cohort study in China. Brit J Nutr. 2015;113:1292–300.
33. Qiu C, Frederick IO, Zhang C, Sorensen TK, Enquobahrie DA, Williams MA. Risk of gestational diabetes mellitus in relation to maternal egg and cholesterol intake. Am J Epidemiol. 2011;173:649–58.
34. Qiu C, Zhang C, Gelaye B, Enquobahrie DA, Frederick IO, Williams MA. Gestational diabetes mellitus in relation to maternal dietary heme iron and non heme iron intake. Diabetes Care. 2011;34:1564–9.
35. Buchanan TA. Pancreatic B-cell defects in gestational diabetes: implications for the pathogenesis and prevention of type 2 diabetes. J Clin Endocrinol Metab. 2001;86:989–93.
36. Buchanan TA, Xiang A, Kjos SL, Watanabe R. What is gestational diabetes? Diabetes Care. 2007;30:105–11.
37. Hamer M, Chida Y. Intake of fruit, vegetables, and antioxidants and risk of type 2 diabetes: systematic review and meta-analysis. J Hypertens. 2007; 25:2361–9.
38. Jelsma JG, Van Poppel MN, Galjaard S, et al. DALI: Vitamin D and lifestyle intervention for gestational diabetes mellitus (GDM) prevention: an European multicentre, randomised trial-study protocol. BMC Pregnancy Childbirth. 2013;13:142.
39. Simmons D, Jelsma JGM, Galjaard S, Devlieger R, Assche A, Jans G. Results from a European multicenter randomized trial of physical activity and/or healthy eating to reduce the risk of Gestational Diabetes Mellitus: The DALI Lifestyle Pilot. Diabetes Care. 2015;38:1650–6.
40. Thornton YS, Smarkola C, Kopacz SM, Ishoof SB. Perinatal outcomes in nutritionally monitored obese pregnant women: A randomized clinical trial. J Natl Med Assoc. 2009;101:569–71.
41. Vinter CA, Jensen DM, Ovesen P, Bech-Nielsen H, Jorgensen JS. TheLiP (LifestyleinPregnancy) Study. A randomized controlled trial of lifestyle intervention in 360 obese pregnant women. Diabetes Care. 2011;34:2502–7.
42. Karamanos B, Thanopoulou A, Anastasiou E, et al. Relation of the Mediterranean diet with the incidence of gestational diabetes. Eur J Clin Nutr. 2014;68:8–13.
43. Radesky JS, Okena E, Rifas-Shimana SL, Kleinmana KP, RichEdwards JW, Gillmana M. Diet during early pregnancy and development of gestational diabetes. Paediatr Perinat Epidemiol. 2008;22:47–59.
44. Saldana TM, Siega-Riz AM, Adair LS. Effect of macronutrient intake on the development of glucose intolerance during pregnancy. Am J Clin Nutr. 2004;79:479–86.
45. Wang Y, Storlien LH, Jenkins AB. Dietary variables and glucose tolerance in pregnancy. Diabetes Care. 2000;23:460–4.
46. Zhang C, Williams MA, Sorensen TK. Maternal plasma ascorbic acid (vitamin C) and risk of gestational diabetes mellitus. Epidemiology. 2004;15:597–604.
47. Chan K, Chan B, Lam K, Tam S, Lao T. Iron supplement in pregnancy and development of gestational diabetes-a randomised placebo-controlled trial. BJOG. 2009;116:789–98.
48. Kinnunen TI, Luoto R, Helin A, Hemminki E. Supplemental iron intake and the risk of glucose intolerance in pregnancy: re-analysis of a randomised controlled trial in Finland. Matern Child Nutr. 2014 [epub ahead of print].
49. Zhou SJ, Yelland L, McPhee AJ, Quinlivan J, Gibson RA, Makride M. Fish-oil supplementation in pregnancy does not reduce the risk of gestational diabetes or preeclampsia. Am J Clin Nutr. 2012;95:1378–84.
50. Helin A, Kinnunen TI, Raitanen J, et al. Iron intake, haemoglobin and risk of gestational diabetes: a prospective cohort study. BMJ Open. 2012;2, e001730.

16

Prevalence of gestational diabetes mellitus based on various screening strategies in western Kenya: a prospective comparison of point of care diagnostic methods

Sonak D. Pastakia[1*], Benson Njuguna[2], Beryl Ajwang' Onyango[2], Sierra Washington[3], Astrid Christoffersen-Deb[4], Wycliffe K Kosgei[5] and Ponnusamy Saravanan[6,7]

Abstract

Background: Early diagnosis of gestational diabetes mellitus (GDM) is crucial to prevent short term delivery risks and long term effects such as cardiovascular and metabolic diseases in the mother and infant. Diagnosing GDM in Sub-Saharan Africa (SSA) however, remains sub-optimal due to associated logistical and cost barriers for resource-constrained populations. A cost-effective strategy to screen for GDM in such settings are therefore urgently required. We conducted this study to determine the prevalence of gestational diabetes mellitus (GDM) and assess utility of various GDM point of care (POC) screening strategies in a resource-constrained setting.

Methods: Eligible women aged ≥18 years, and between 24 and 32 weeks of a singleton pregnancy, prospectively underwent testing over two days. On day 1, a POC 1-h 50 g glucose challenge test (GCT) and a POC glycated hemoglobin (HbA1c) was assessed. On day 2, fasting blood glucose, 1-h and 2-h 75 g oral glucose tolerance test (OGTT) were determined using both venous and POC tests, along with a venous HbA1c. The International Association of Diabetes in Pregnancy Study Group (IADPSG) criteria was used to diagnose GDM. GDM prevalence was reported with 95% confidence interval (CI). Specificity, sensitivity, positive predictive value, and negative predictive value of the various POC testing strategies were determined using IADPSG testing as the standard reference.

Results: Six hundred-sixteen eligible women completed testing procedures. GDM was diagnosed in 18 women, a prevalence of 2.9% (95% CI, 1.57% - 4.23%). Compared to IADPSG testing, POC IADPSG had a sensitivity and specificity of 55.6% and 90.6% respectively while that of POC 1-h 50 g GCT (using a diagnostic cut-off of ≥7.2 mmol/L [129.6 mg/dL]) was 55.6% and 63.9%. All other POC tests assessed showed poor sensitivity.

Conclusions: POC screening strategies though feasible, showed poor sensitivity for GDM detection in our resource-constrained population of low GDM prevalence. Studies to identify sensitive and specific POC GDM screening strategies using adverse pregnancy outcomes as end points are required.

Trials registration: Clinical trials.gov: NCT02978807, Registered 29 November 2016.

Keywords: Gestational diabetes mellitus, Screening, Prevalence, Diagnosis, Low middle income

* Correspondence: spastaki@gmail.com
[1]Department of Pharmacy Practice, Purdue Kenya Partnership, PO Box 5760, Eldoret 30100, Kenya
Full list of author information is available at the end of the article

Background

Gestational diabetes mellitus (GDM) is associated with adverse maternal and fetal outcomes which include macrosomia and subsequent delivery risks such as birth trauma and increased need for caesarian delivery in the short term [1, 2]. Long term, mothers with GDM and their offspring are at an elevated risk for obesity, type 2 diabetes mellitus (T2DM) and other cardiovascular diseases [3–6]. Prompt diagnosis of GDM is the first step towards effective management and prevention of adverse outcomes. GDM case detection in Sub-Saharan Africa (SSA) however, remains sub-standard [7, 8].

The World Health Organization (WHO) adopted criteria developed by the International Association of Diabetes and Pregnancy Study Group (IADPSG) in 2013 for the diagnosis of GDM [9, 10]. This approach however, has certain limitations that limit its applicability in regular diabetes screening in SSA. Firstly, it requires women to come in fasting for an antenatal clinic (ANC) visit between weeks 24–28, posing logistical obstacles such as long distance to clinic and associated transport costs [11, 12]. Furthermore, women who aren't informed during an earlier visit or forget to come in fasting, require a subsequent visit. Secondly, quality lab infrastructure and reagents for venous glucose testing are not readily available in most SSA health facilities and where available, require operation by skilled and trained personnel who may be unavailable [13–16]. Thirdly, multiple samples required for testing are cumbersome to obtain, both for the woman and healthcare personnel [15]. Finally, associated costs for IADPSG testing are high and may be unaffordable to a majority of low-income patients [14, 17].

Practical and scalable GDM screening and diagnostic tools are urgently required in SSA [18]. Ideal tools to overcome the above limitations should be: accurate in the non-fasting state, avoid need for multiple venous samples, require minimal training to operate, and be cost-effective [15]. Point of care (POC) testing devices possess these characteristics and therefore may be practical tools for GDM screening in a rural/semi-urban SSA setting with limited resources and patient follow-up.

Our study evaluated the accuracy of various POC testing modalities for the diagnosis of GDM compared to the recommended IADPSG testing. We also determined the prevalence of GDM in a previously unstudied rural/semi-urban setting of Western Kenya.

Methods

Our prospective study enrolled pregnant women from any of three ANC clinics namely: the Moi Teaching and Referral Hospital (MTRH), the Uasin Gishu District Hospital (UGDH), and Mediheal hospital. MTRH is one of only two national referral hospitals in Kenya and serves a varied demography of patients from both rural and urban Western Kenya. UGDH is a small public hospital which primarily serves patients from Eldoret town (semi-urban) and its environs (rural). Mediheal is a private institution primarily serving patients of higher income status from urban Eldoret compared to the other two facilities.

All pregnant women at 24–32 weeks of gestation with singleton pregnancies were eligible for inclusion. We extended the gestational age beyond the recommended 24–28 weeks to provide flexibility for women who did not precisely recall the date of their last normal menstrual period. Gestational age was confirmed using Naegele's rule and compared to the pregnant woman's fundal height. Any observed discrepancy of ≥3 weeks was resolved with evaluation by ultrasound. Women were excluded if they had a pre-existing diagnosis of diabetes, were less than 18 years old, were on medications that affect glucose control, or were unable or unwillling to provide informed consent.

Full approval from the Moi University and MTRH institutional research ethics committee (approval number – IREC/2012/66) and the Indiana University-Purdue University institutional review board were acquired prior to study initiation. Written informed consent was obtained from all participants. Baseline demographic and clinical information was obtained for all women using a structured questionnaire administered on enrollment.

Testing procedures were completed over 2 days. Day 1 tests were conducted on the day of enrollment in a non-fasting state. A capillary blood sample was obtained to perform a POC random blood glucose (RBG) test (Optium H®, Abbott Diabetes Care) and glycated hemoglobin (HbA1c) (A1C Now®, PTS Diagnostics). An unexpected stockout necessitated the switch to the desktop DCA Vantage (Siemens®) for HbA1c for 76% of the women. A 50 g glucose load was then administered as a solution from a commercially available glucose product and capillary blood samples were collected at 1-h for POC measurement.

All participants were then expected to return the next day (or within 1 week for those unable to follow-up immediately) after having fasted overnight for ≥8 h. If a patient had a POC 1-h glucose post-50 g load ≥7.78 mmol/L (140 mg/dL) however, they were notified that their result met the threshold for a positive screening and were informed of their need to confirm their diagnosis on their own if they were unable to come back for day 2 testing as part of the study.

Day 2 testing procedures included recommended IADPSG testing alongside the analogous POC tests (Fig. 1). Capillary and venous blood samples for measurement of POC and venous fasting blood glucose (FBG) (COBAS® analyzer, Roche Diagnostics), venous HbA1c and a complete blood count with differential was performed. A

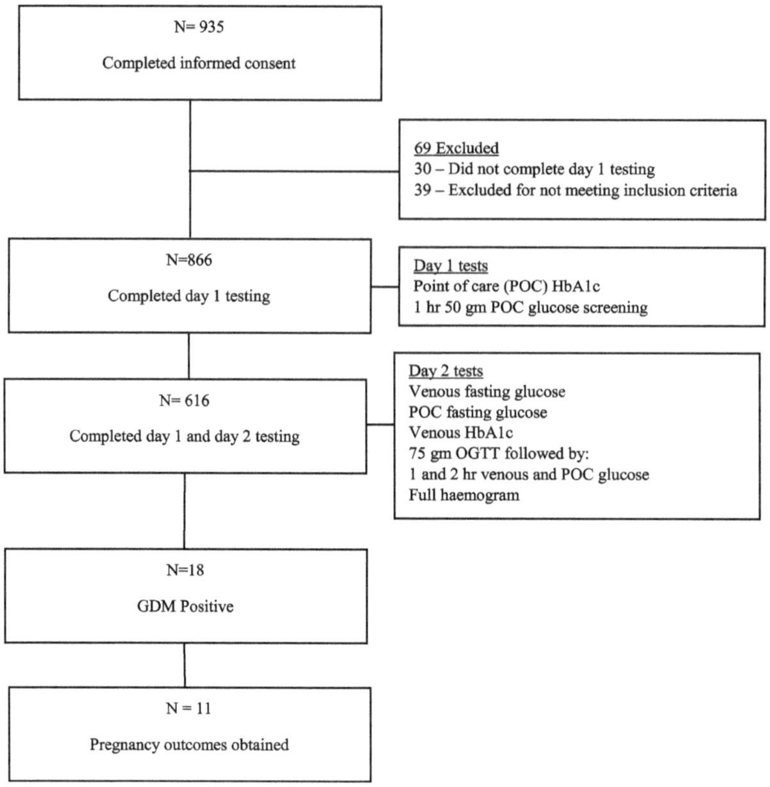

Fig. 1 Study schema and patient flow

75 g glucose load was then administered with capillary and venous blood samples collected at 1-h and 2-h for measurement of POC and venous glucose levels.

All study participants received standard antenatal care offered at the ANC clinics. Pregnant women who were diagnosed with GDM using IADPSG criteria were referred to a home-based glucose monitoring program for care of GDM [19]. GDM positive mothers were also called at least 6 weeks after they had delivered to return to clinic for a fasting blood glucose test to assess whether they had progressed to diabetes, and provide information on their delivery.

For fasting, 1-h and 2-h glucose testing following a 75 g oral glucose tolerance test (OGTT), we utilised glucose cut-offs consistent with IADPSG criteria to define GDM, [20] that is, venous fasting blood glucose (FBG) >5.1 mmol/L (92 mg/dL), or 1-h glucose >10 mmol/L (180.0 mg/dL), or 2-h glucose >8.5 mmol/L (153.0 mg/dL).

We also defined HbA1c values ≥6.5% and RBG ≥ 11.1 mmol/L (199.8 mg/dL) as meeting criteria for GDM diagnosis based on their use as cutpoints for overt diabetes, however, only patients who met IADPSG GDM diagnostic criteria for the OGTT were informed of having a GDM diagnosis and were managed as having GDM [20, 21].

The primary outcomes assessed were the prevalence of GDM determined by IADPSG testing and the sensitivity, specificity, negative predictive value (NPV) and positive predictive value (PPV) of different potential screening strategies when compared to the gold standard 75 g OGTT venous testing recommended by IADPSG. Secondary outcomes includedthe association between POC and corresponding venous testing results, assessed by calculating the mean absolute relative difference (MARD), correlation coefficient, and constructing Bland-Altman graphs for each comparable glucose value. In addition, obstetric outcomes were assessed by contacting all women diagnosed with GDM via phone and completing a standard data collection form which specifically assessed the presence of common GDM related complications. All outcomes were assessed by an independent Obstetrics and Gynaecology specialist to assess the potential association with GDM. Every woman was specifically assessed for fetopelvic disproportion, perineal trauma, preeclampsia, shoulder dystocia, birth injury for baby, congenital malformation, neonatal hypoglycemia, and admission to the neonatal intensive care unit, polycythemia, or hyperbilirubinemia.

The sensitivity, specificity, NPV and PPV of each screening strategy was determined using 2 by 2 matrices with the IADPSG criteria as the gold standard reference. Based on data from prior trials, we structured our sample size calculation to identify a screening strategy that maintained a specificity of 80% and sensitivity of 70% for the three screening strategies we employed. Prior estimates of GDM in SSA are widely distributed with prevalence estimates as low as 0% in some rural regions and as high as 13.9% among high-risk women in urban areas. [8] Considering this wide variability, we conservatively estimated that the prevalence in our semi-urban cohort would be 7%. Based on this assumption, and anticipating a 30% loss-to-follow up, we needed to screen 667 pregnant women to identify 36 cases with GDM between 24 and 32 weeks gestation for a sensitivity precision of 0.15 and indirectly, a specificity precision of 0.034. Through the recruitment of 667 women, we would be able to generate a precise ±2% confidence interval around the estimated GDM prevalence. All analyses were conducted using Stata Statistical software package (StataCorp, College Station, TX).

Results and discussion

Results

We exceeded our recruitment target by recruiting 935 eligible pregnant women between July 2013 and August 2015, of whom 886 completed day 1 testing (Fig. 1). Baseline characteristics for all enrolled women are presented in Table 1. 250 (28.9%) enrolled participants did not come back for the day 2 return visit which required fasting, while 616 (71.1%) completed day 1 and day 2 testing. There were no significant differences in demographic characteristics between women who only completed day 1 testing and those who completed both days.

Among women who completed day 1 and day 2 testing, the mean age was 26.1 years and mean gestational age was 28.3 weeks. 94 (15.3%) reported a family history of diabetes while 37 (6%) had a systolic and/or diastolic blood pressure above the cut-off for hypertension diagnosis. No patients reported a known history of GDM.

Among women who completed day 1 and day 2 testing, the mean venous fasting glucose was 4 mmol/L (72.0 mg/dL) and mean venous HbA1c was 5.2% (33 mmol/mol). Mean values for the 1 h and 2 h venous glucose were 5.9 mmol/L (106.2 mg/dL) and 5.55 mmol/L (99.9 mg/dL) respectively. Means for the rest of the glucose testing procedures are presented in Table 2.

Eighteen women met IADPSG GDM diagnostic criteria, resulting in an overall GDM prevalence of 2.9% (95% CI, 1.57% - 4.23%) when including only the women who completed day 1 and day 2 testing in our analysis. The majority of GDM patients were diagnosed through a venous FBG whereby 12 of the women met criteria for venous FBG 5.1 mmol/L (91.8 mg/dL) but not 1 h- or 2-h 75 g OGTT cut-off values. 2-h OGTT venous glucose ≥10 mmol/L (180.0 mg/dL) and 1-h OGTT venous glucose ≥8.5 mmol/L (153.0 mg/dL) solely identified an additional 3 and 1 patients respectively. The remaining 2 women were positive on all three IADPSG GDM criteria. These 18 GDM positive women had a median weight of 72.3 kg, median age of 28 years, median gestational age of 28 weeks, 5.5% (N = 1) with a family history of diabetes, median systolic blood pressure of 117 mmHg, and median diastolic blood pressure of 70 mmHg. Statistical evaluation of the significance of differences between the GDM positive population and non-GDM population was limited by the small sample of GDM positive women.

The sensitivity, specificity, NPV and PPV of the various screening strategies are shown in Table 3. POC screening

Table 1 Characteristics of women who attended non-fasting and fasting visit

	Completed Only Day 1 testing (N = 250)	Completed Day 1 and 2 testing (N = 616)
Study Location		
MTRH	145	283
UGDH	105	326
Mediheal	0	7
Age (years) (SD)	25.8 (±4.8)	26.1 (±5.1)
Estimated Gestational Age (weeks) (SD)	28.2 (±2.8)	28.3 (±2.6)
Weight (kg) (SD)	61.6 (±10.5)	68.9 (±12.2)
Average SBP (mm/Hg) (SD)	115.8 (±13.5)	112.6 (±18.1)
Average DBP (mm/Hg) (SD)	72.5 (±9.9)	70.8 (±12.9)
SBP ≥ 140 mmHg and/or DBP ≥90 mmHg N(%)	14 (5.6%)	37 (6.0%)
Family history of DM N(%)	38 (15.2%)	94 (15.3%)
Known history of GDM N (%)	0 (0%)	0 (0%)
Average Haemoglobin	N/A	12 (±1.5)
Haemoglobin < 8 N (%)	N/A	14 (2.3%)

MTRH Moi Teaching and Referral Hospital, *UGDH* Uasin Gishu District Hospital, *SBP* Systolic Blood Pressure, *DBP* Diastolic Blood Pressure, *DM* Diabetes mellitus, *GDM* Gestational Diabetes Mellitus

Table 2 GDM Prevalence and blood glucose results

	Completed Only Day 1 testing (*N* = 250)	Completed Day 1 and 2 testing (*N* = 616)
Number (%) diagnosed with GDM based on venous 75 g OGTT IADPSG criteria		18 (2.9%)
Average POC RBG (SD)	4.7 (±1.0)	4.8 (±1.0)
Average POC result after 50 g glucose load (SD)	6.6 (±1.4)	6.9 (±1.4)
Average POC FBG (SD)	N/A	4.2 (±0.6)
Average venous FBG (SD)	N/A	4.0 (±0.5)
Average POC HbA1c (SD)	5.1 (±0.8)	5.2 (±0.5)
Average venous HbA1c (SD)	N/A	5.2 (±0.5)
Average POC 1 h blood glucose post 75 g (SD)	N/A	6.9 (±1.4)
Average venous blood glucose 1 h post 75 g (SD)	N/A	5.9 (±1.4)
Average POC blood glucose 2 h post 75 g (SD)	N/A	6.1 (±1.2)
Average venous blood glucose 2 h post 75 g (SD)	N/A	5.5 (±1.1)

MTRH Moi Teaching and Referral Hospital, *UGDH* Uasin Gishu District Hospital, *SBP* Systolic Blood Pressure, *DBP* Diastolic Blood Pressure, *DM* Diabetes mellitus, *GDM* Gestational Diabetes Mellitus, *POC* point of care, *RBG* Random blood glucose, *FBG* Fasting blood glucose; All blood glucose results presented are in mmol/L, hemoglobin presented in g/dl

Table 3 Performance of various screening strategies

	Sensitivity TP/(TP + FN) 95% CI	Specificity TN/(TN + FP) 95% CI	Negative Predictive Value TN/(TN + FN)	Negative likelihood ratio Point estimate 95% CI	Positive Predictive Value TP/(TP + FP)	Positive likelihood ratio Point estimate 95% CI
Venous 75 g OGTT[a]	1 18/(18 + 0) (0.82–1)	1 598/(598 + 0) (0.99–1)	1 598/(598 + 0)	n/a	1 (18/18 + 0)	n/a
POC RBG ≥ 7 mmol/L (126.0 mg/dL)	0.17 3/(3 + 15) (0.06–0.39)	0.97 581/(581 + 17) (0. 95–98)	0.97 581/(581 + 15)	0.86 (0.70–1.1)	0.15 3/(3 + 17)	5.86 (1.89–18.23)
POC 1 h 50 g ≥ 7.8 mmol/L (140.4 mg/dL)	0.44 8/(8 + 10) (0.25–0.66)	0.79 470/(470 + 128) (0.75–0.82)	0.98 470/(470 + 10)	0.71 (0.47–1.07)	0.06 8/(8 + 128)	2.08 (1.21–3.56)
POC 1 h 50 g ≥ 7.2 mmol/L (129.6 mg/dL)	0.56 10/(10 + 8) (0.34–0.75)	0.64 382/(382 + 216) (0.60–0.67)	0.98 382/(382 + 8)	0.70 (0.41–1.17)	0.04 10/(10 + 216)	1.54 (1.00–2.36)
Venous FBG ≥ 5.1 (91.8 mg/dL)	0.78 14/(14 + 4) (0.55–0.91)	1 598/(598 + 0) (.99–1)	0.99 598/(598 + 4)	n/a	1 14/(14 + 0)	0.22 (0.09–0.53)
POC FBG ≥ 5.1 mmol/L (91.8 mg/dL)	0.33 6/(6 + 12) (0.16–0.56)	0.95 567/(567 + 31) (0.93–0.96)	0.98 567/(567 + 12)	0.70 (0.51–0.98)	0.16 6/(6 + 31)	6.43 (3.08–13.45)
POC 75 g OGTT	0.56 10/(10 + 8) (0.34–0.75)	0.91 542/(542 + 56) (0.88–0.93)	0.99 542/(542 + 8)	0.49 (0.29–0.82)	0.15 10/(10 + 56)	5.93 (3.66–9.61)
POC HbA1c ≥ 6.5%	0.22 4/(4 + 14) (0.09–0.45)	0.99 592/(592 + 6) (0.98–0.99)	0.98 592/(592 + 14)	0.79 (0.61–1.01)	0.4 4/(4 + 6)	22.15 (6.84–71.72)
Venous HbA1c ≥ 6.5%	0.11 2/(2 + 16) (0.03–0.33)	0.99 591/(591 + 7) (0.98–0.99)	0.97 591/(591 + 16)	0.90 (0.76–1.06)	0.22 2/(2 + 7)	9.49 (2.12–42.54)

TP true positives, *FN* false negatives, *TN* true negatives, *FP* false positives, *HbAlc* glycated hemoglobin, *OGTT* oral glucose tolerance test, *POC* point of care, *RBG* random blood glucose, *FBG* fasting blood glucose

[a]All results were compared to the venous 75 g oral glucose tolerance test to demonstrate diagnostic accuracy

strategies showed low sensitivity with the POC 75 g OGTT strategy ('POC IADPSG') having the highest sensitivity of 56% and a specificity of 91%. The 1-h post 50 g glucose load POC had a sensitivity of 44% when utilising a cut-off of 7.8 mmol/L (140.4 mg/dL) which increased to 56% on adjusting the cut-off to 7.2 mmol/L (129.6 mg/dL). The specificity of this lower cut-off however dropped from 79% to 64%. Of the non-POC strategies, venous FBS was the most accurate with a sensitivity of 77% and specificity of 100%. When applying the venous HbA1c diagnostic criteria of ≥6.5%, 10 women were identified as GDM positive, however only 30% of these women were positive via the venous 75 g OGTT. The POC HbA1c also demonstrated limited value for identifying women who would be positive on the venous 75 g HbA1c as it was found to have a sensitivity of only 22% despite having a specificity of 99%.

We found a MARD in the test results between POC testing and the corresponding venous testing method of 9.3%,19.4%, 16.0%, and 7.7% for fasting, 1-h, 2-h, and HbA1c testing respectively. The correlation coefficients and p-values for the fasting, 1-h, 2-h, and HbA1c values were 0.56 ($p < 0.001$), 0.72 ($p < 0.001$), 0.69 ($p < 0.001$), and 0.49 ($p < 0.001$) respectively. Fasting glucose had the best performance in terms of the MARD despite having the lowest correlation coefficient of the three. This was attributed to the larger impact small variations had on the correlation coefficient at lower glucose values as seen in the Bland Altman plot of the fasting results (Fig. 2a), where the y-axis measurements shows a relatively smaller difference between the two methods of glucose measurement. The unpredictability of the variability is also illustrated in Fig. 2a-d, as the results are scattered above and below zero on all four of the plots illustrating that POC results could be higher or lower than venous results.

Among the 18 women who were positive for GDM based on IADPSG OGTT criteria, 5 (26.3%) were able and willing to provide details on their delivery and return for a follow-up fasting glucose at least six weeks after delivery. None of these women were found to have diabetes upon repeat screening. An additional 6 (31.6%) women were contacted only by phone with the remaining 7 (42.1%) women being completely unreachable. The average birth weight for the 11 women providing data was 3.4 kg with one woman having a macrosomic infant weighing 4.9 kg without any other complications. An additional 2 women underwent Cesarean delivery with one of the babies requiring neonatal intensive care unit admission for an unspecified reason. There was 1 woman who suffered from an intrauterine fetal death which was thought to be unrelated to GDM. Perineal trauma was experienced by 3 additional women without any other clinical sequelae.

Discussion

We found the prevalence of GDM among pregnant women receiving care in Western Kenya to be 2.9%. We used the IADPSG diagnostic criteria to determine prevalence, a strategy associated with a 2.4 times higher case detection compared to older methods [22]. Our low prevalence may be due to several factors. Firstly, we employed a universal screening strategy among pregnant women regardless of pre-existing risk factors. Secondly, among enrolees, risk factors such as previous GDM, advanced maternal age and elevated blood pressure were low, although, family history of DM was reported in 15.3% of women. Thirdly, our study population represented a mixed population of urban and rural women. GDM risk factors in urban populations include overweight and obese body mass index (BMI), sedentary lifestyle and poor dietary habits. Malnutrition during pregnancy, on the other hand, may be a risk factor for GDM in rural patients [23]. The majority of our enrollees were recruited from two public hospitals which predominatly serve a rural population from farming communities who are less likely to be obese and more likely to be active. We therefore posit that such risk factors were less likely in our study population although complete socio-economic evaluation and determination of BMI are required for firm conclusions to be made.

POC GDM screening strategies performed poorly when trying to approximate the women who would be GDM positive based on the venous 75 g OGTT recommended by IADPSG. The venous 50 g glucose challenge test (GCT) is extensively used as a screening strategy for GDM [24]. We conducted a POC version of the 50 g GCT and found a 56% sensitivity and 64% specificity at a glucose cut-off of ≥7.2 mmol/L (129.6 mg/dL). In contrast, Coustan and colleagues found that the conventional venous 50 g GCT at a glucose cut-off of 6.9 mmol/L (124.2 mg/dL) had a 79% sensitivity and 87% specificity [25]. The POC version of the 50 g GCT may be used as a screening test to identify patients who require furthur testing but its low sensitivity limits its utility. A POC 75 g OGTT strategy had a sensitivity of 56.6% with a specificity of 90.6%. This method may therefore provide reasonable accuracy if a POC strategy is required. However, since this strategy requires for patients to come in fasting, a venous fasting test alone would be a superior approach despite the need for venipuncture as this alone had a 77.7% sensitivity and 100% specificity in our study. For field testing in populations unable to access health facilities regularly however, the POC 75 g OGTT may be used to identify patients who requiring further testing.

POC fasting capillary glucose (FCG) testing using a glucose cut-off of ≥5.1 mmol/L (91.8 mg/dL) in our study had a very low sensitivity of 33.3%. Fadl and colleagues found a slightly higher sensitivity of 47% using

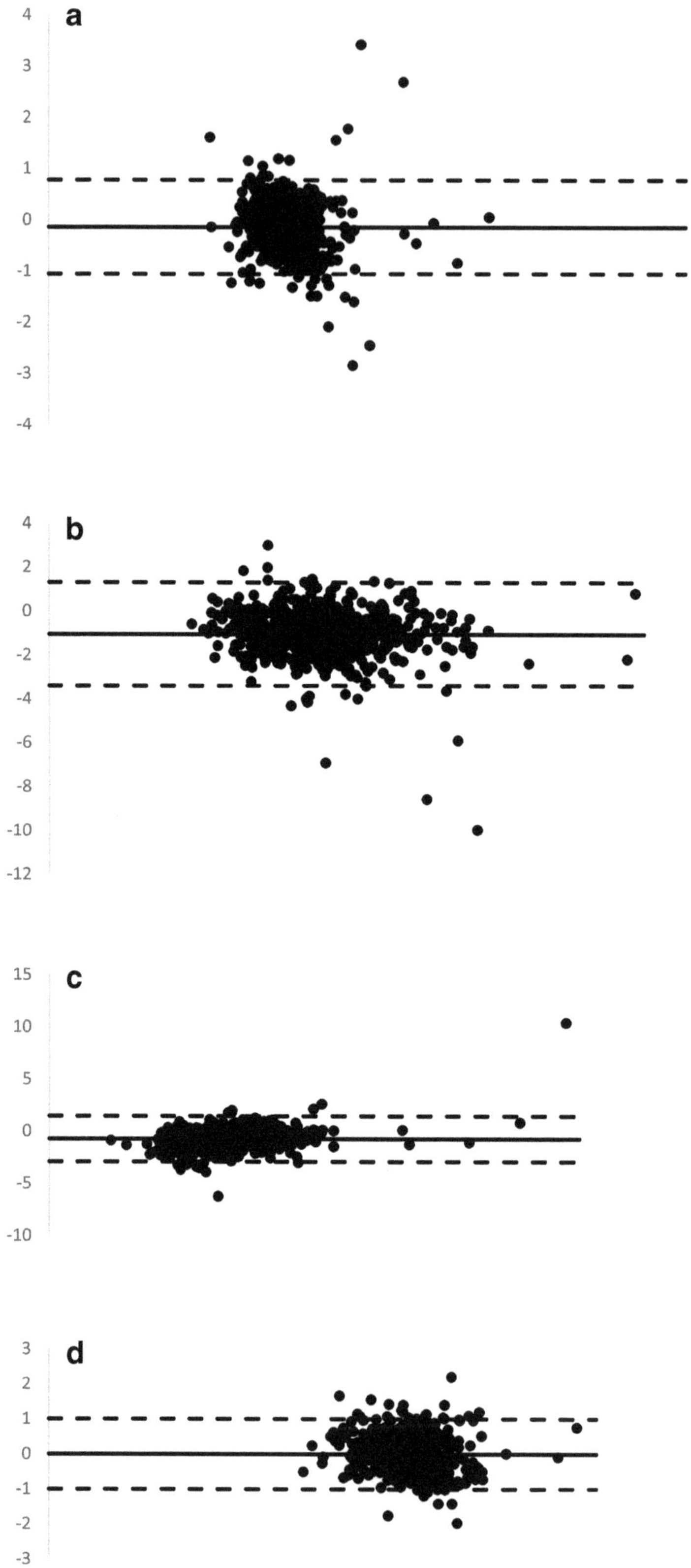

Fig. 2 Bland Altman Plots of the Venous and POC Testing Strategies Utilized in this Study. **a** - Fasting Blood Glucose, Venous vs. POC, Correlation coefficient 0.56, $p < 0.001$. **b** - 1 h post 75 g glucose load, Venous vs. POC, correlation coeffiecient = 0.72, $p < 0.001$. **c** - 2 h post 75 g glucose load, Venous vs. POC, correlation coefficient = 0.6910, $p < 0.001$. **d** - HbA1c, Venous vs. POC, correlation coefficient = 0.49, $p < 0.001$

an FCG cut-off of ≥5 mmol/L (90.0 mg/dL) among a population at low-risk for GDM [26]. Contralily, Agarwal and colleagues reported a sensitivity of 71.9% and specificity of 76.8% using a FCG cut-off of ≥5.0 mmol/L (90.0 mg/dL) [27]. Their study however, was conducted in a setting with a high prevalence (13.4%) of GDM which may explain the difference in findings.

Additional investigation is required to identify more accurate POC screening strategies for low-risk GDM populations such as ours. Capacity for portable field testing is desirable so as to reach pregnant women unable to access facilities with adequate lab testing resources. Additionally, future evaluation of a feasible screening strategy should also incorporate the study of pregnancy outcomes for all screened women in order to assess the clinical significance of various glucose cut-offs and testing strategies within the context of low and middle-income countries (LMICs). The hyperglycemia and adverse pregnancy outcomes (HAPO) study used this approach to demonstrate that adverse outcomes increase continously from fasting venous glucose values as low as 4.2 mmol/L (75.6 mg/dL) [2]. A similar approach in low-resource populations not included in the HAPO study may be a more accurate method of establishing a feasible and clinically significant screening strategy for GDM. Such an effort would potentially establish population specific cut-off points and contextual testing strategies based directly on pregnancy outcomes within such populations.

Our study has several limitations. Firstly, our low GDM prevalence limited our ability to evaluate different glucose cut-off points for POC testing to establish a clinically useful cut-off with good sensitivity and specificity. We increased the sample size to factor in this unexpectedly low GDM prevalence, we were nevertheless unable to identify the number of cases necessary to meet our prespecified threshold. However, based on the limited concordance found between the various POC strategies tested and the reference IADPSG criteria, the results of our investigation are unlikely to change. Secondly, we found considerable variability between POC test results and corresponding venous test results. This variability increased when patients were tested in non-fasting conditions although we could not find a predictable factor in this variation which we could use to adjust the POC values. Consequently, this may have further limited our ability to draw firm conclusions as far as POC screening strategies were concerned. This study was conducted in a setting that is 2100–2700 m (7000–9000 ft) above sea level, where the high altitude may affect the accuracy of POC glucose testing [28]. Lastly, we were unable to follow up the pregnancy outcomes for all screened mothers, a strategy that may more accurately identify glucose cut-off points with significant clinical outcomes [2]. Because of this limitation and the desire to obtain pregnancy outcomes related to GDM in SSA, we are currently undertaking a larger scale study where we hope to identify Kenyan specific risk thresholds related to glucose screening cutpoints as done within the HAPO study.

Conclusion

We found a low prevalence of GDM (2.9%) in our setting of Eldoret, Western Kenya. The POC GDM screening strategies we evaluated, although feasible for the universal GDM screening of pregnant women in low resource settings, were found to have a low sensitivity in our study population. Amongst the venous tests evaluated, the majority of GDM positive patients (77.8%) were identified by FBG testing. Further investigations are required to identify accurate POC GDM screening strategies with an emphasis on adverse pregnancy outcomes as an endpoint.

Abbreviations

ANC: Antenatal clinic; FBG: Fasting blood glucose; FCG: Fasting capillary glucose; FN: False negatives; FP: False positives; GCT: Glucose challenge test; GDM: Gestational diabetes mellitus; HAPO: Hyperglycemia and adverse pregnancy outcomes; HbA1c: Glycated hemoglobin; IADPSG: International association of diabetes and pregnancy study group; LMIC: Low and middle income countries; MARD: Mean absolute relative difference; MTRH: Moi Teaching and Referral Hospital; NPV: Negative predictive value; OGTT: Oral glucose tolerance test; POC: Point of care; PPV: Positive predictive value; RBG: Random blood glucose; SD: Standard deviation; SSA: Sub-Saharan Africa; T2DM: Type 2 diabetes mellitus; TN: True negatives; TP: True positives; UGDH: Uasin Gishu District Hospital; WHO: World Health Organisation

Acknowledgements

We would like to acknowledge the efforts of Carolyne Cherop, Mercy Nabwire Ouma, James Kamadi and Benson Kiragu who collected data for this study. The authors thank Abbott Diabetes Care for providing glucose testing supplies and the Abbott Fund for providing financial support for this effort. They also thank Eli Lilly and Company for donating insulin and providing seed funding to support the authors' overarching work in diabetes.

Funding

This research was supported by the President's Emergency Plan for AIDS Relief through the U.S. Agency for International Development under the terms of Cooperative Agreement No. AID-623-A-12-0001. The contents of this article are the sole responsibility of AMPATH and do not necessarily reflect the views of USAID or the U.S. government. This publication was also made possible by the Indiana Clinical and Translational Sciences Institute, funded in part by grant UL1 TR001108 from the National Institutes of Health, National Center for Advancing Translational Sciences, Clinical and Translational Sciences Award.

Authors' contributions

SDP oversaw all aspects of this study including conceptualization, implementation, analysis, and manuscript preparation. BN was the major contributor in writing of the manuscript. BA assisted with the implementation of the study and manuscript preparation. SW assisted with the initial conceptualization of the project and manuscript preparation. ACD assisted with the implementation of the study and manuscript preparation. WK assisted with the implementation of the study, clinical oversight, and manuscript preparation. PS assisted with the interpretation of data and manuscript preparation. All authors read and approved the final manuscript

Competing interests

Donations of insulin were received from Eli Lilly and Company and donated point of care glucose testing supplies were received from Abbott Diabetes Care.

Sonak Pastakia has previously served as a consultant for Abbott Diabetes Care but the work presented here is unrelated to those efforts. The other authors have no conflict of interest to declare

Author details
[1]Department of Pharmacy Practice, Purdue Kenya Partnership, PO Box 5760, Eldoret 30100, Kenya. [2]Department of Pharmacy, Moi Teaching and Referral Hospital, PO Box 3, Eldoret 30100, Kenya. [3]Department of Reproductive Medicine, University of California, San Diego, CA 92103, USA. [4]Department of Obstetrics & Gyneacology, University of Toronto, Toronto, ON M5G 1E2, Canada. [5]Division of Reproductive Health, Moi Teaching and Referral Hospital, PO Box 3, Eldoret 30100, Kenya. [6]Department of Diabetes, Endocrinology & Metabolism, Warwick Medical School, University of Warwick, Coventry CV4 7AL, UK. [7]Diabetes and Endocrine Centre, George Eliot Hospital, Nuneaton CV107DJ, UK.

References

1. Crowther CA, Hiller JE, Moss JR, McPhee AJ, Jeffries WS, Robinson JS. Effect of treatment of gestational diabetes mellitus on pregnancy outcomes. N Engl J Med. 2005;352(24):2477–86.
2. Metzger BE, Lowe LP, Dyer AR, Trimble ER, Chaovarindr U, Coustan DR, Hadden DR, McCance DR, Hod M, McIntyre HD, et al. Hyperglycemia and adverse pregnancy outcomes. N Engl J Med. 2008;358(19):1991–2002.
3. Bellamy L, Casas JP, Hingorani AD, Williams D. Type 2 diabetes mellitus after gestational diabetes: a systematic review and meta-analysis. Lancet (London, England). 2009;373(9677):1773–9.
4. Metzger BE. Long-term outcomes in mothers diagnosed with gestational diabetes mellitus and their offspring. Clin Obstet Gynecol. 2007;50(4):972–9.
5. Vrachnis N, Antonakopoulos N, Iliodromiti Z, Dafopoulos K, Siristatidis C, Pappa KI, Deligeoroglou E, Vitoratos N. Impact of maternal diabetes on epigenetic modifications leading to diseases in the offspring. Exp Diabetes Res. 2012;2012:538474.
6. Dabelea D, Crume T. Maternal environment and the transgenerational cycle of obesity and diabetes. Diabetes. 2011;60(7):1849–55.
7. Macaulay S, Dunger DB, Norris SA. Gestational diabetes mellitus in Africa: a systematic review. PLoS One. 2014;9(6):e97871.
8. Mwanri AW, Kinabo J, Ramaiya K, Feskens EJ. Gestational diabetes mellitus in sub-Saharan Africa: systematic review and metaregression on prevalence and risk factors. Trop Med Int Health. 2015;20(8):983–1002.
9. Topp SM, Chipukuma JM, Chiko MM, Matongo E, Bolton-Moore C, Reid SE. Integrating HIV treatment with primary care outpatient services: opportunities and challenges from a scaled-up model in Zambia. Health Policy Plan. 2013;28(4):347–57.
10. Metzger BE, Gabbe SG, Persson B, Buchanan TA, Catalano PA, Damm P, Dyer AR, Leiva A, Hod M, Kitzmiler JL, et al. International association of diabetes and pregnancy study groups recommendations on the diagnosis and classification of hyperglycemia in pregnancy. Diabetes Care. 2010;33(3):676–82.
11. Asundep NN, Carson AP, Turpin CA, Tameru B, Agidi AT, Zhang K, Jolly PE. Determinants of access to antenatal care and birth outcomes in Kumasi, Ghana. J Epidemiol Global Health. 2013;3(4):279–88.
12. Mrisho M, Obrist B, Schellenberg JA, Haws RA, Mushi AK, Mshinda H, Tanner M, Schellenberg D: The use of antenatal and postnatal care: perspectives and experiences of women and health care providers in rural southern Tanzania. BMC Pregnancy Childbirth 2009, 9:10-10.
13. McIntyre HD, Oats JJ, Zeck W, Seshiah V, Hod M. Matching diagnosis and management of diabetes in pregnancy to local priorities and resources: an international approach. Int J Gynaecol Obstet. 2011;115(Suppl 1):S26–9.
14. Zeck W, McIntyre HD. Gestational diabetes in rural East Africa: a call to action. J Women's Health (2002). 2008;17(3):403–11.
15. Agarwal MM, Weigl B, Hod M. Gestational diabetes screening: the low-cost algorithm. Int J Gynecol Obstet. 2011;115(Supplement 1):S30–3.
16. McIntyre HD, Oats JJN, Zeck W, Seshiah V, Hod M. Matching diagnosis and management of diabetes in pregnancy to local priorities and resources: an international approach. Int J Gynecol Obstet. 2011;115(Supplement 1):S26–9.
17. Seshiah V, Balaji V, Shah SN, Joshi S, Das AK, Sahay BK, Banerjee S, Zargar AH, Balaji M. Diagnosis of gestational diabetes mellitus in the community. J Assoc Physicians India. 2012;60:15–7.
18. Pastakia SD, Onyango BA, Ouma MN, Christofferson-Deb A, Cherop C. Addressing the challenge of GDM in the developing world: perspectives from rural western Kenya. Diabetes Voice. 2014;59:51-4.
19. Pastakia SD, Cheng SY, Kirui NK, Kamano JH. Dynamics, impact, and feasibility of self-monitoring of blood glucose in the rural, resource-constrained setting of western Kenya. Clin Diabetes. 2015;33(3):136–43.
20. Diabetes IAo, Panel PSGC. International Association of Diabetes and Pregnancy Study Groups Recommendations on the diagnosis and classification of hyperglycemia in pregnancy. Diabetes Care. 2010;33(3):676–82.
21. American Diabetes Association. Classification and diagnosis of diabetes. Diabetes Care. 2016;39(Supplement 1):S13–22.
22. Jenum AK, Morkrid K, Sletner L, Vangen S, Torper JL, Nakstad B, Voldner N, Rognerud-Jensen OH, Berntsen S, Mosdol A, et al. Impact of ethnicity on gestational diabetes identified with the WHO and the modified International Association of Diabetes and Pregnancy Study Groups criteria: a population-based cohort study. Eur J Endocrinol. 2012;166(2):317–24.
23. Harder T, Rodekamp E, Schellong K, Dudenhausen JW, Plagemann A. Birth weight and subsequent risk of type 2 diabetes: a meta-analysis. Am J Epidemiol. 2007;165(8):849–57.
24. Committee on Practice Bulletins-Obstetrics. Practice bulletin no. 137: gestational diabetes mellitus. Obstet Gynecol. 2013;122(2 Pt 1):406–16.
25. Coustan DR, Nelson C, Carpenter MW, Carr SR, Rotondo L, Widness JA. Maternal age and screening for gestational diabetes: a population-based study. Obstet Gynecol. 1989;73(4):557–61.
26. Fadl H, Ostlund I, Nilsson K, Hanson U. Fasting capillary glucose as a screening test for gestational diabetes mellitus. BJOG. 2006;113(9):1067–71.
27. Agarwal MM, Dhatt GS, Othman Y, Gupta R. Gestational diabetes: fasting capillary glucose as a screening test in a multi-ethnic, high-risk population. Diabet Med. 2009;26(8):760–5.
28. Fink KS, Christensen DB, Ellsworth A. Effect of high altitude on blood glucose meter performance. Diabetes Technol Ther. 2002;4(5):627–35.

17

Does charge-free screening improve detection of gestational diabetes in women from deprived areas

Andreas Beyerlein[1,2*], Daniela Koller[3], Anette-Gabriele Ziegler[1,2,4,5], Nicholas Lack[6] and Werner Maier[5,7]

Abstract

Background: Gestational diabetes mellitus (GDM) occurs in 2–6 % of all pregnancies. We investigated whether area level deprivation is associated with a higher risk for GDM and whether GDM detection rates in deprived regions changed after the introduction of charge-free GDM screening in Germany in 2012.

Methods: We analyzed population-based data from Bavaria, Germany, comprising *n* = 587,621 deliveries in obstetric units between 2008 and 2014. Area level deprivation was assessed municipality-based using the Bavarian Index of Multiple Deprivation (BIMD), divided into quintiles and assigned to each mother based on her residential address. We estimated annual odds ratios (ORs) for GDM diagnosis by BIMD quintile with adjustment for maternal obesity, maternal age, migration background and single mother status.

Results: Women from the most deprived regions were less likely to be diagnosed with GDM before introduction of charge-free GDM screening (OR = 0.76 [95 % confidence interval: 0.66, 0.86] compared to least deprived areas), in 2008. In contrast, high area level deprivation was associated with significantly increased risk of GDM diagnosis in 2013 (OR [95 % confidence interval] = 1.15 [1.02, 1.29]). The OR was also elevated, although not significantly, in 2014 (OR [95 % confidence interval] = 1.05 [0.93, 1.18]).

Conclusions: The prevalence of GDM seems to have been underreported in women from highly deprived areas before introduction of the charge-free GDM screening in Germany. In fact, women living in deprived regions seem to have an increased risk for GDM and may profit from access to charge-free GDM screening.

Keywords: Gestational diabetes mellitus, Area level deprivation, Bavarian index of multiple deprivation, Charge-free screening

Background

Gestational diabetes mellitus (GDM) occurs in 2–6 % of all pregnancies in industrialized countries [1] with an increasing prevalence in recent years [2, 3]. In 2010, the World Health Organization (WHO) presented new diagnostic criteria for the classification of GDM [4] which Germany adopted in 2011. Based on the new criteria GDM was diagnosed if at least one of the values for fasting, 1-h, and 2-h plasma glucose concentration as measured in a 75-g oral glucose tolerance test exceeded diagnostic thresholds, while at least two elevated values were required for GDM diagnosis before 2011. Apart from that, every pregnant woman in Germany without pre-existing diabetes has been offered a charge-free GDM screening since 2012, whereas formerly the optional test had to be paid for by the mother.

Maternal obesity is the major risk factor for GDM [5] but there are also other potential determinants such as gestational weight gain, maternal age, parity, family history of diabetes, ethnicity or life-style habits [6–10]. At an area level, it was reported that living in neighbourhoods with a high prevalence of fast food restaurants was significantly associated with an increased risk of GDM [11]. Maternal socioeconomic status (SES) might be another potential risk factor. In general, SES can be assessed either at individual

* Correspondence: andreas.beyerlein@helmholtz-muenchen.de
[1]Institute of Diabetes Research, Helmholtz Zentrum München, Neuherberg, Germany
[2]Forschergruppe Diabetes der Technischen Universität München, Munich, Germany

level (e. g. based on educational level) or from area-based socioeconomic measures such as deprivation indices. There have been a number of studies on the association between individual level SES and GDM, yielding inconsistent results [12]. The association of area level deprivation and GDM has been rarely investigated, however, and the sparse literature provided rather inconsistent results. While neighbourhood deprivation was not found to be associated with GDM risk in data from Southwest England, higher glucose values at GDM diagnosis were observed in Canadian women living in highly deprived areas [13, 14].

Interestingly, high area level deprivation has already been found to be associated with increased risk for obesity [15] and type 2 diabetes [16, 17], particularly in women [18].

Here, we had the opportunity to analyze a large population-based dataset from Bavaria, Germany, which allowed investigating the association between area level deprivation and GDM risk. Additionally, we were able to assess the impact of the introduction of a charge-free GDM screening [19] on this association.

Methods

Data were extracted from a standard dataset regularly collected for national benchmarking of obstetric units in terms of clinical performance. The BAQ (Bayerische Arbeitsgemeinschaft für Qualitätssicherung - Bavarian Institute for Quality Assurance in hospital care) conducts corresponding regional evaluations for Bavaria, Germany. Data are transferred electronically to the BAQ office after personally identifying characteristics have been removed and replaced by an anonymous unique reference number. Amongst others, these data contain information on maternal age, weight and height, postal code of the mother's residential address, GDM, and pre-gestational diabetes as previously described [20, 21]. GDM was diagnosed by the women's gynaecologists who are assumed to follow the official guidelines from the German Diabetes Association. These guidelines were revised in 2011 following the WHO's new diagnostic criteria [4]. Information on maternal weight and gestational age at first prenatal care visit was extracted by midwives and nurses from the mother's pregnancy booklet (issued to every pregnant woman in Germany for complete documentation of all antenatal care visits) and augmented with additional information upon hospital admission. Mother's height and weight recorded at first visit (median gestational age: 8 completed weeks) were used to derive her body mass index (BMI). The BAQ data do not contain variables on individual level SES apart from fairly rough surrogates such as smoking during pregnancy or migration background.

We assessed area level deprivation using the Bavarian Index of Multiple Deprivation (BIMD) [22] derived from official statistics and methods used in the UK for assessment of regional deprivation [23]. The BIMD including seven subdomains of deprivation (income, employment, education, municipal revenue, social capital, environment, security) was computed for all 2,056 Bavarian municipalities. We categorized the municipalities by BIMD quintiles, with the first quintile designating the least deprived and the fifth quintile the most deprived municipalities. Assignment of BIMD quintile to each mother was done based on postal code of her residential address.

According to current German maternity guidelines established in 2012, every pregnant woman without preexisting diabetes is offered a glucose-challenge test between the 24th and 27th gestational week. In a second step, women with increased glucose values in the glucose-challenge test will be tested by an oral glucose tolerance test for diagnosis of GDM. The charges of this two-step procedure are now fully covered by the women's health insurance, whereas formerly the test had to be paid for by the mother. To compare periods before and after its introduction we considered the data of all deliveries in Bavarian obstetric units from 2008 to 2014 ($n = 645,774$). Of these, 4,564 women with known pre-gestational diabetes were excluded. The BIMD could not be assigned to a further 53,589 women because the postal codes of their residential addresses referred to a location outside Bavaria or were missing, thus leaving a final sample size of $n = 587,621$. We used logistic regression to estimate odds ratios (ORs) and corresponding 95 % confidence intervals (CIs) with GDM as the outcome variable and BIMD quintiles as the explanatory variable (lowest deprivation as reference) separately for each year from 2008 to 2014. All models were calculated both crude and adjusted for maternal obesity (BMI ≥ 30 kg/m^2) at first visit, maternal age (<35 compared to ≥ 35 years), migration background and single mother status, as these were significant predictors in unadjusted analyses. Likewise we assessed associations between GDM and all subdomains of the BIMD (as a continuous variable).

Statistical analyses were performed with SAS (version 9.3, SAS Institute Inc., Cary, NC, USA) and R (version 3.0.3, https://cran.r-project.org).

Results

The proportion of women with a diagnosis of GDM increased from 3.4 % in 2008 to 4.0 % in 2014 (Table 1), resulting in a relative increase in prevalence of about 17 %. Maternal obesity, age, migration background and single mother status were significantly associated with GDM in both 2008 and 2014 ($p < 0.05$), while smoking during pregnancy and parity (multiparous compared to primiparous) were not (data not shown). In contrast to GDM, the relative increase in prevalence for any of these factors was 11 % (as observed for obesity) or lower.

The rate of GDM diagnosis increased in 2011, when the new definition was established in Germany, in all BIMD

Table 1 Description of the study population in 2008 and 2014

	Year 2008 (n = 81,129)	Year 2014 (n = 92,589)
Gestational diabetes mellitus	n = 2,745 (3.4 %)	n = 3,682 (4.0 %)
Obese (BMI > 30 kg/m^2)	n = 8,819 (10.9 %)	n = 11,169 (12.1 %)
Age > 35 years	n = 21,163 (26.1 %)	n = 25,615 (27.7 %)
Migration background	n = 14,401 (17.8 %)	n = 17,772 (19.2 %)
Single mother	n = 7,731 (9.9 %)	n = 6,864 (8.2 %)
Multiparous woman	n = 40,635 (50.1 %)	n = 45,219 (48.8 %)
Smoking during pregnancy	n = 5,457 (6.7 %)	n = 4,262 (4.6 %)
BIMD quintile 1 (least deprived)	n = 10,306 (12.7 %)	n = 12,716 (13.7 %)
BIMD quintile 2	n = 9,679 (11.9 %)	n = 10,329 (11.2 %)
BIMD quintile 3	n = 23,948 (29.5 %)	n = 27,831 (30.1 %)
BIMD quintile 4	n = 13,198 (16.3 %)	n = 14,829 (16.0 %)
BIMD quintile 5 (most deprived)	n = 23,998 (29.6 %)	n = 26,884 (29.0 %)

BIMD Bavarian Index of Multiple Deprivation

quintiles and dropped slightly in 2012 when the universal two-step GDM screening was introduced (Fig. 1). However, the GDM prevalence remained at a considerably higher level compared to before 2011 in women from deprived areas, but not in women from regions with low level deprivation. Women from the most deprived areas were less likely to be diagnosed with GDM in 2008 (OR [95 % CI] = 0.76 [0.66, 0.86] for the fifth quintile compared to the first quintile in adjusted analyses, Table 2). In contrast, a higher area level deprivation was significantly associated with increased risk of GDM diagnosis in 2013 (OR [95 % CI] = 1.15 [1.02, 1.29] for the fifth quintile compared to the first quintile). The OR was also elevated, although not significantly, in 2014 (OR [95 % CI] = 1.05 [0.93, 1.18]). Further analyses suggested that these trends over time were at least partly based on changes in areas with low employment rates, as employment deprivation was the only BIMD subdomain associated with both lower GDM risk by trend in 2008 (OR [95 % CI] = 0.98 [0.94, 1.02]) and significantly higher risk in 2014 (OR [95 % CI] = 1.05 [1.02, 1.09], Table 3).

Discussion

Our data show that area level deprivation is associated with GDM prevalence in a subtle way: Women from highly deprived areas were less likely to be diagnosed with GDM than women from less deprived regions before introduction of the charge-free GDM screening, but vice versa after 2012.

Hence, it appears likely that GDM was largely underreported in women from deprived areas before 2012. We therefore assume that living in deprived regions, especially with high unemployment rates, is indeed associated with a slightly increased risk for GDM as observed in our data from 2013 (significantly) and 2014 (not significantly). This is in accordance with previous studies related to type 2 diabetes [16–18]. Our findings further indicate that particularly women from deprived areas may profit from charge-free GDM screening.

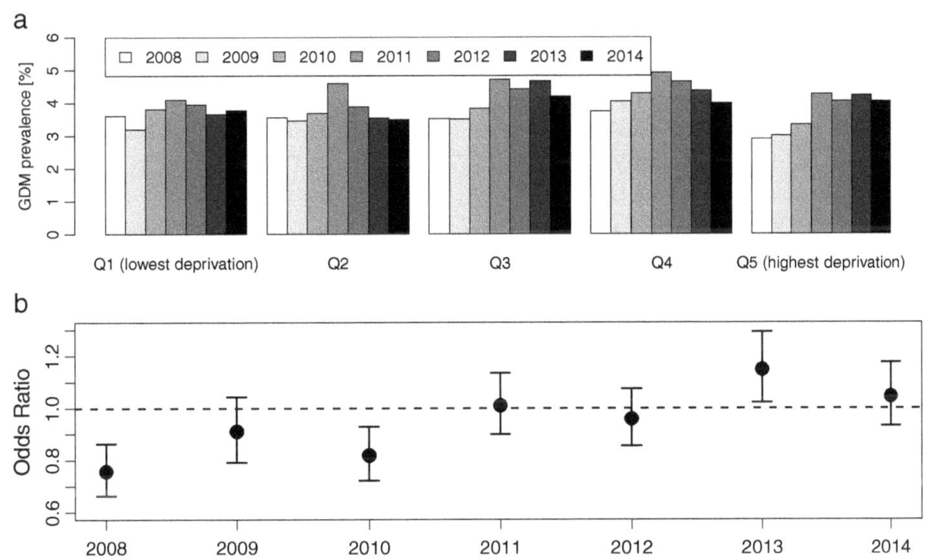

Fig. 1 Yearly rates of gestational diabetes mellitus (GDM) diagnoses from 2008 to 2014 (numbers of pregnancies without pre-gestational diabetes in brackets) in Bavaria, Germany, by deprivation quintiles (Q1-Q5, plot a), and yearly odds ratios with corresponding 95 % confidence intervals for Q5 compared to reference Q1 (plot b, all estimates adjusted for maternal obesity, age, migration background and single mother status). In 2011, the criteria for GDM diagnosis were revised in Germany following WHO recommendations. In 2012, charge-free GDM screening, following a two-step procedure, was established in Germany

Table 2 Odds ratios [95 % confidence intervals] for gestational diabetes mellitus by Bavarian Index of Multiple Deprivation (BIMD) quintile in 2008 and 2014 (based on $n = 81{,}129$ and $n = 92{,}589$ observations, respectively) as categorical variables, and by maternal obesity, age, migration background and single mother status, both crude and mutually adjusted

BIMD	2008, crude	2008, adjusted	2014, crude	2014, adjusted
Quintile 1 (least deprived)	Reference	Reference	Reference	Reference
Quintile 2	0.99 [0.85, 1.15]	0.99 [0.85, 1.15]	0.92 [0.80, 1.06]	0.93 [0.81, 1.08]
Quintile 3	0.97 [0.86, 1.10]	0.92 [0.81, 1.04]	**1.12 [1.001, 1.24]**	1.07 [0.95, 1.20]
Quintile 4	1.04 [0.90, 1.19]	1.01 [0.88, 1.16]	1.06 [0.94, 1.20]	1.09 [0.96, 1.24]
Quintile 5 (most deprived)	**0.79 [0.70, 0.90]**	**0.76 [0.66, 0.86]**	1.07 [0.96, 1.19]	1.05 [0.93, 1.18]
Maternal obesity	**3.07 [2.81, 3.35]**	**3.19 [2.92, 3.49]**	**3.53 [3.28, 3.80]**	**3.71 [3.43, 4.00]**
Maternal age ≥35 years	**1.54 [1.42, 1.67]**	**1.56 [1.44, 1.69]**	**1.64 [1.53, 1.75]**	**1.69 [1.57, 1.82]**
Migration background	**1.44 [1.32, 1.56]**	**1.52 [1.39, 1.67]**	**1.60 [1.49, 1.71]**	**1.68 [1.55, 1.82]**
Single mother status	**1.56 [1.34, 1.81]**	**1.46 [1.25, 1.71]**	**1.31 [1.14, 1.50]**	**1.27 [1.10, 1.46]**

Significant associations ($p < 0.05$) are shown in bold face

Although the screening fees were only about 10–25 €, we assume that this may already have constituted a financial barrier for an unemployed single woman in Germany receiving state benefits of only 364 € ("Hartz IV") monthly in 2011. This would agree well with findings from other studies, indicating that especially people with low SES tended to avoid or delay physician visits after a practice charge for physicians (10 € per calendar quarter) was introduced in Germany in 2004 [24], and that financial barriers may be relevant for participation in colorectal cancer screening [25, 26].

In general, the trends of GDM prevalence in our data appear plausible, although they could only partly be explained by concomitant increases in the prevalence of risk factors such as maternal obesity or increased maternal age. Indeed, we observed an increase in the prevalence of both risk factors in our data, which is in line with long-term temporal trends in Germany [27, 28]. However, we think that it appears likely that the marked increase in GDM prevalence in 2011 in our data was due to the revision of the GDM diagnosis criteria in Germany in the same year, which may have particularly improved the detection of milder GDM cases (as only one instead of two elevated blood glucose values was deemed sufficient for GDM diagnosis). The lower prevalence in the following years may be due to introduction of the glucose-challenge pretest in 2012, which is known to miss about 20 % of all GDM cases [29]. Interestingly, we observed almost no such decrease in prevalence in women from mostly deprived areas, possibly indicating that the introduction of charge-free screening levelled out the numbers missed by pretesting in this subgroup. We are, however, hesitant to overinterpret GDM prevalence rates from 2011 and 2012, as changes introduced in these years may not have been immediately adopted by physicians [30] thus possibly leading to regional differences in this respect. Unfortunately, we are not aware of any other study reporting temporal trends of GDM prevalence in Germany before and after 2011–2012 to support our assumptions.

A major strength of the presented results is seen in the large number of pregnancies available for analysis. However, the data were collected for purposes not related to the study hypothesis. Data quality is high as completeness of the data is monitored annually across obstetric units as an integral part of benchmarking health-care provision: The BAQ, providing the data for our study, is part of an established national program to

Table 3 Odds ratios [95 % confidence intervals] for gestational diabetes mellitus by Bavarian Index of Multiple Deprivation (BIMD) domains in 2008 and 2014 (based on $n = 81{,}129$ and $n = 92{,}589$ observations, respectively), both crude and adjusted for maternal obesity, age, migration background and single mother status

BIMD domain	2008, crude	2008, adjusted	2014, crude	2014, adjusted
Income deprivation	**0.84 [0.80, 0.87]**	**0.84 [0.80, 0.88]**	**0.91 [0.88, 0.95]**	**0.92 [0.89, 0.96]**
Employment deprivation	1.00 [0.96, 1.04]	0.98 [0.94, 1.02]	**1.07 [1.03, 1.10]**	**1.05 [1.02, 1.09]**
Educational deprivation	**0.88 [0.84, 0.91]**	**0.88 [0.84, 0.91]**	0.97 [0.94, 1.003]	0.98 [0.94, 1.01]
Municipal revenue deprivation	**0.92 [0.88, 0.96]**	**0.93 [0.89, 0.97]**	**0.94 [0.91, 0.97]**	**0.96 [0.93, 0.999]**
Social capital deprivation	**0.87 [0.83, 0.90]**	**0.88 [0.84, 0.91]**	**0.97 [0.93, 0.999]**	0.99 [0.95, 1.02]
Environment deprivation	**1.10 [1.06, 1.14]**	**1.08 [1.03, 1.12]**	**1.11 [1.08, 1.15]**	**1.08 [1.04, 1.12]**
Security deprivation	**1.09 [1.05, 1.13]**	**1.08 [1.04, 1.12]**	**1.06 [1.03, 1.10]**	**1.06 [1.02, 1.10]**

Significant associations ($p < 0.05$) are shown in bold face

generate annual statistics depicting an individual obstetric units' deviations from national targets. This program has been run within all federal states over the last three decades. Quality assurance data from the UK and the USA have similarly been analysed in other studies on determinants of pregnancy outcomes [31–35].

Unfortunately, the BAQ data do not contain a valid indicator of the mother's SES so that we were not able to distinguish between the associations of individual and area level deprivation on GDM prevalence. It should further be noted that the BIMD quintiles were calculated based on the number of municipalities, as opposed to the population size of each municipality. Therefore, the proportions of pregnant women were not equally distributed across BIMD quintile. This was similar to previous studies [17, 18], however, and we do not think that this might constitute a potential source of severe bias.

In summary, our findings indicate that women living in highly deprived areas have a higher risk of developing GDM, and that even moderate charges may constitute an obstacle for participation in GDM screening. Thus, access to charge-free GDM screening and to appropriate treatment may be an important step towards more equality in pregnancy-related health care.

Abbreviations

BAQ: Bayerische Arbeitsgemeinschaft für Qualitätssicherung; BIMD: Bavarian index of multiple deprivation; BMI: Body mass index; CI: Confidence interval; GDM: Gestational diabetes mellitus; OR: Odds ratio; SES: Socioeconomic status; WHO: World Health Organization

Funding

The work was supported by grants from the Kompetenznetz Diabetes mellitus (Competence Network for Diabetes mellitus), funding from the German Federal Ministry of Education and Research (BMBF) to the German Center for Diabetes Research (DZD e.V.), and by iMed–the Helmholtz Initiative on Personalized Medicine.
The funders had no impact on design, conduct and reporting of the study; collection, management, analysis, and interpretation of the data; and preparation, review, or approval of the manuscript.

Authors' contributions

The authors' responsibilities were as follows: AB (guarantor) formulated the study hypothesis together with WM, performed the statistical analyses and contributed to the first and final draft of the manuscript. DK, AGZ, NL and WM contributed to interpretation of the study results and to the first and final draft of the manuscript. NL was responsible for provision and interpretation of the data.

Competing interests

Nothing to declare.

Author details

[1]Institute of Diabetes Research, Helmholtz Zentrum München, Neuherberg, Germany. [2]Forschergruppe Diabetes der Technischen Universität München, [3]Munich, Germany. Department of Health Services Management, Munich School of Management, Ludwig-Maximilians-Universität München, Munich, Germany. [4]Forschergruppe Diabetes e.V. am Helmholtz Zentrum München, Munich, Germany. [5]German Center for Diabetes Research (DZD), Partner, Neuherberg, Germany. [6]German Bavarian Quality Assurance Institute for Medical Care, Munich, Germany. [7]Institute of Health Economics and Health Care Management, Helmholtz Zentrum München, Neuherberg, Germany.

References

1. American Diabetes Association. Standards of medical care in diabetes–2011. Diabetes Care. 2011;34 Suppl 1:S11–61.
2. Poston L. Maternal obesity, gestational weight gain and diet as determinants of offspring long term health. Best Pract Res Clin Endocrinol Metab. 2012;26(5): 627–39.
3. Dabelea D, Snell-Bergeon JK, Hartsfield CL, Bischoff KJ, Hamman RF, McDuffie RS, Kaiser Permanente of Colorado GDMSP. Increasing prevalence of gestational diabetes mellitus (GDM) over time and by birth cohort: Kaiser Permanente of Colorado GDM Screening Program. Diabetes Care. 2005; 28(3):579–84.
4. Metzger BE, Gabbe SG, Persson B, Buchanan TA, Catalano PA, Damm P, Dyer AR, Leiva A, Hod M, Kitzmiler JL, et al. International association of diabetes and pregnancy study groups recommendations on the diagnosis and classification of hyperglycemia in pregnancy. Diabetes Care. 2010;33(3):676–82.
5. Farren M, Daly N, O'Higgins AC, McKeating A, Maguire PJ, Turner MJ. The interplay between maternal obesity and gestational diabetes mellitus. J Perinat Med. 2015;43(3):311–7.
6. Cleary-Goldman J, Malone FD, Vidaver J, Ball RH, Nyberg DA, Comstock CH, Saade GR, Eddleman KA, Klugman S, Dugoff L, et al. Impact of maternal age on obstetric outcome. Obstet Gynecol. 2005;105(5 Pt 1):983–90.
7. Savitz DA, Janevic TM, Engel SM, Kaufman JS, Herring AH. Ethnicity and gestational diabetes in New York City, 1995–2003. BJOG. 2008;115(8):969–78.
8. Cypryk K, Szymczak W, Czupryniak L, Sobczak M, Lewinski A. Gestational diabetes mellitus - an analysis of risk factors. Endokrynol Pol. 2008;59(5):393–7.
9. Hedderson MM, Gunderson EP, Ferrara A. Gestational weight gain and risk of gestational diabetes mellitus. Obstet Gynecol. 2010;115(3):597–604.
10. Ruiz-Gracia T, Duran A, Fuentes M, Rubio MA, Runkle I, Carrera EF, Torrejon MJ, Bordiu E, Valle LD, Garcia de la Torre N, et al. Lifestyle patterns in early pregnancy linked to gestational diabetes mellitus diagnoses when using IADPSG criteria. The St Carlos gestational study. Clin Nutr. 2016;35(3):699–705.
11. Kahr MK, Suter MA, Ballas J, Ramin SM, Monga M, Lee W, Hu M, Shope CD, Chesnokova A, Krannich L, et al. Geospatial Analysis of Food Environment Demonstrates Associations with Gestational Diabetes. Am J Obstet Gynecol. 2016;214(1):110.e1–9.
12. Dode MA, dos Santos IS. Non classical risk factors for gestational diabetes mellitus: a systematic review of the literature. Cad Saude Publica. 2009;25 Suppl 3:S341–359.
13. Janghorbani M, Stenhouse EA, Jones RB, Millward BA. Is neighbourhood deprivation a risk factor for gestational diabetes mellitus? Diabet Med. 2006; 23(3):313–7.
14. Sampson L, Dasgupta K, Ross NA. The association between socio-demographic marginalization and plasma glucose levels at diagnosis of gestational diabetes. Diabet Med. 2014;31(12):1563–7.
15. Heslehurst N. Identifying 'at risk' women and the impact of maternal obesity on National Health Service maternity services. Proc Nutr Soc. 2011;70(4):439–49.
16. Maier W, Holle R, Hunger M, Peters A, Meisinger C, Greiser KH, Kluttig A, Volzke H, Schipf S, Moebus S, et al. The impact of regional deprivation and individual socio-economic status on the prevalence of Type 2 diabetes in Germany. A pooled analysis of five population-based studies. Diabet Med. 2013;30(3):e78–86.
17. Grundmann N, Mielck A, Siegel M, Maier W. Area deprivation and the prevalence of type 2 diabetes and obesity: analysis at the municipality level in Germany. BMC Public Health. 2014;14:1264.
18. Maier W, Scheidt-Nave C, Holle R, Kroll LE, Lampert T, Du Y, Heidemann C, Mielck A. Area level deprivation is an independent determinant of prevalent type 2 diabetes and obesity at the national level in Germany. Results from the National Telephone Health Interview Surveys 'German Health Update' GEDA 2009 and 2010. Plos One. 2014;9(2):e89661.
19. Kleinwechter H, Schäfer-Graf U, Bührer C, Hoesli I, Kainer F, Kautzky-Willer A, Pawlowski B, Schunck K, Somville T, Sorger M, et al. Gestational diabetes

mellitus (GDM) diagnosis, therapy and follow-up care: Practice Guideline of the German Diabetes Association (DDG) and the German Association for Gynaecologyand Obstetrics (DGGG). Exp Clin Endocrinol Diabetes. 2014; 122(7):395–405.

20. Beyerlein A, Lack N, von Kries R. Within-population average ranges compared with institute of medicine recommendations for gestational weight gain. Obstet Gynecol. 2010;116(5):1111–8.
21. Beyerlein A, Schiessl B, Lack N, von Kries R. Associations of gestational weight loss with birth-related outcome: a retrospective cohort study. BJOG. 2011;118(1):55–61.
22. Maier W, Fairburn J, Mielck A. Regional deprivation and mortality in Bavaria. Development of a community-based index of multiple deprivation. Gesundheitswesen. 2012;74(7):416–25.
23. Noble M, Wright G, Smith G, Dibben C. Measuring multiple deprivation at the small-area level. Environ Plan A. 2006;38(1):169–85.
24. Rückert IM, Böcken J, Mielck A. Are German patients burdened by the practice charge for physician visits ('Praxisgebuehr')? A cross sectional analysis of socio-economic and health related factors. BMC Health Serv Res. 2008;8:232.
25. Klabunde CN, Vernon SW, Nadel MR, Breen N, Seeff LC, Brown ML. Barriers to colorectal cancer screening: a comparison of reports from primary care physicians and average-risk adults. Med Care. 2005;43(9):939–44.
26. Green AR, Peters-Lewis A, Percac-Lima S, Betancourt JR, Richter JM, Janairo MP, Gamba GB, Atlas SJ. Barriers to screening colonoscopy for low-income Latino and white patients in an urban community health center. J Gen Intern Med. 2008;23(6):834–40.
27. Scholz R, Voigt M, Schneider KT, Rochow N, Hagenah HP, Hesse V, Straube S. Analysis of the German perinatal survey of the years 2007–2011 and comparison with data from 1995–1997: maternal characteristics. Geburtshilfe Frauenheilkd. 2013;73(12):1247–51.
28. Mensink GB, Schienkiewitz A, Haftenberger M, Lampert T, Ziese T, Scheidt-Nave C. Overweight and obesity in Germany: results of the German health interview and examination survey for adults (DEGS1). Bundesgesundheitsblatt Gesundheitsforschung Gesundheitsschutz. 2013;56(5–6):786–94.
29. Naylor CD, Sermer M, Chen E, Farine D. Selective screening for gestational diabetes mellitus. Toronto Trihospital Gestational Diabetes Project Investigators. N Engl J Med. 1997;337(22):1591–6.
30. Görig T, Schneider S, Bock C, Maul H, Kleinwechter H, Diehl K. Screening for gestational diabetes mellitus in Germany: a qualitative study on pregnant womens attitudes, experiences, and suggestions. Midwifery. 2015;31(11):1026–31.
31. Park S, Sappenfield WM, Bish C, Salihu H, Goodman D, Bensyl DM. Assessment of the Institute of Medicine Recommendations for Weight Gain During Pregnancy: Florida, 2004–2007. Maternal Child Health J. 2011;15(3):289–301.
32. Donahue SM, Kleinman KP, Gillman MW, Oken E. Trends in birth weight and gestational length among singleton term births in the United States: 1990–2005. Obstet Gynecol. 2010;115(2 Pt 1):357–64.
33. Khashan AS, Kenny LC. The effects of maternal body mass index on pregnancy outcome. Eur J Epidemiol. 2009;24(11):697–705.
34. Bhattacharya S, Campbell DM, Liston WA. Effect of body mass index on pregnancy outcomes in nulliparous women delivering singleton babies. BMC Public Health. 2007;7:168.
35. Bodnar LM, Siega-Riz AM, Simhan HN, Himes KP, Abrams B. Severe obesity, gestational weight gain, and adverse birth outcomes. Am J Clin Nutr. 2010;91(6):1642–48.

18

Serum level and polymorphisms of retinol-binding protein-4 and risk for gestational diabetes mellitus

Shimin Hu[1], Qian Liu[1,2], Xin Huang[1] and Hongzhuan Tan[1*]

Abstract

Background: Retinol-binding protein-4 (RBP4) has been reported to be potentially involved in the pathogenesis of gestational diabetes mellitus (GDM); however, the findings are inconsistent. Our aims were to review the studies that investigated the association of serum levels and polymorphisms of RBP4 with GDM risk, and to provide recommendations for future research.

Methods: The databases PubMed, EBSCO, ScienceDirect, and Web of Knowledge were searched up to October 2015 to find out studies evaluating the relationship between serum RBP4 level/ RBP4 polymorphisms and GDM risk. In the meta-analysis of serum RBP4 levels the key inclusion was that studies were designed as BMI-matched studies or had observed non-significant differences in BMI between cases and controls.

Results: Fourteen case–control studies (647 cases and 620 controls) reporting the association between serum RBP4 level and GDM risk, and three studies (1012 cases and 1605 controls) investigating the association between *RBP4* polymorphisms and GDM risk were involved. Our results showed that high serum RBP4 levels represent a risk factor for GDM (pooled standardized mean difference =0.758, 95 % confidence interval [0.387, 1.128]). The results of subgroup analyses based on "gestational age at blood sampling" or "diagnostic criteria" are consistent with the overall results. However, the postpartum subgroup and "before 24 weeks" subgroup both only include one article and indicate no association between serum RBP4 level and GDM risk. The meta-analysis on the association between rs3758539 polymorphism and GDM risk shows that *RBP4* rs3758539 polymorphism is not associated with the development of GDM.

Conclusions: The results of this meta-analysis support the hypothesis that RBP4 is a modest independent risk factor for GDM (i.e., nonobese patients with GDM might express RBP4 at abnormal levels). The serum RBP4 level is associated with the risk of GDM. However, the association in the first-trimester and postpartum period should be validated by further research. The association between RBP4 rs3758539 polymorphism and GDM risk was not confirmed.

Keywords: Retinol-binding protein-4, Gestational diabetes mellitus, Meta-analysis

Background

Gestational diabetes mellitus (GDM) is defined as varying degrees of glucose intolerance that is first detected during pregnancy [1]. The prevalence of GDM is increasing in decades and floating from 1.7 to 11.6 % among populations [2]. Although considerable research effort has been focused on GDM, the pathophysiology of the disease remains incompletely understood. During pregnancy, insulin resistance will be enhanced physiologically. Insulin resistance can be further strengthened by some factors such as obesity, leading to high risk of GDM [3–5].

Retinol-Binding Protein-4 (RBP4) is mainly synthesized by hepatocytes and adipose tissues. It was identified in 2005 as an adipocytokine with potential capability in reducing insulin sensitivity and enhancing hepatic gluconeogenesis [6]. A multi-center clinical study [7] revealed that serum RBP4 levels correlated with the magnitude of

* Correspondence: tanhz99@qq.com
[1]Department of Epidemiology and Health Statistics, School of Public Health of Central South University, Changsha, Hunan 410007, PR China

insulin resistance in subjects with obesity, impaired glucose tolerance, or type 2 diabetes and in nonobese, nondiabetic subjects with a strong family history of type 2 diabetes. In nonobese subjects, decreased expression of glucose transporter type 4 (GLUT-4) in adipocytes predicts increased serum RBP4 levels and insulin resistance. Adipose-specific deletion of GLUT-4 was reported to lead to secondary defects in insulin action in muscle and liver. The mechanism by which a decrease in adipocyte GLUT-4 results in an increase in RBP4 expression is unknown, but it might involve sensing of glucose by adipocytes. RBP4 is regulated by GLUT-4. The downstream of RBP4's regulatory mechanism is that an increase in serum RBP4 levels can induce hepatic expression of phosphoenolpyruvate carboxykinase, a gluconeogenic enzyme, to increase gluconeogenesis, and impair insulin signaling in muscles through decreasing the expression of phosphoinositide-3 kinase [8].

In patients with a history of GDM, insulin resistance exists before pregnancy but worsens during gestation. Insulin secretion is insufficient to compensate for the insulin resistance and this leads to hyperglycemia, which can be detected through routine glucose screening during pregnancy. Thus, chronic insulin resistance is a central component of the pathophysiology of GDM [9]. Furthermore, the cellular GLUT-4 content also decreases in patients with GDM [10]. The aforementioned findings have predictably given rise to the hypothesis that RBP4 might contribute to insulin resistance in GDM, much as it does in type 2 diabetes.

To date, several genetic variants that affect *RBP4* expression levels (e.g., rs3758539 and rs12265684) have been investigated for their potential association with the risk of GDM, but the reported findings are inconsistent [11–13]. False-negative results, inadequate statistical power, small sample sizes, and ethnic differences may contribute to the lack of reproducibility in genetic-association studies [14, 15]. Among the *RBP4* genetic variants examined in the studies to date, only the rs3758539 variant was analyzed more than once, in the USA, China, and Mexico, and therefore we only analyzed the association between *RBP4* genetic variants (rs3758539) and GDM in the present study.

The association between serum RBP4 levels and GDM risk has also been investigated, and, the reported results are also inconsistent [12, 13, 16–33]. Statistical association does not necessarily mean causal association. We propose 3 hypotheses regarding the positive statistical association between RBP4 levels and GDM risk: (1) GDM pathophysiology is related to obesity but not RBP4 levels, and serum RBP4 levels are elevated because of the increased size of adipocytes [7]; (2) RBP4 is a pathophysiological link between obesity and insulin resistance; (3) RBP4 is a modest independent risk factor for GDM (i.e., nonobese patients with GDM might express RBP4 at abnormal levels). If we want to prove serum RBP4 level is associated with GDM risk, considerable attention must be paid to body mass index (BMI) matched strategy. The positive results of studies with BMI-matched strategy are more credible to convince us that RBP4 is a modest independent risk factor for GDM. In meta-analysis about serum RBP4 level, we only included those studies in which BMI was matched, or showed a similar distribution in case and control groups, and then analyzed whether RBP4 is an independent risk factor for GDM.

Our aims were to review previous studies that investigated the association of serum RBP4 levels and *RBP4* polymorphisms with GDM risk, and to provide recommendations for future research.

Methods

Literature search

First, the databases PubMed, EBSCO, ScienceDirect, and Web of Knowledge were searched up to October 2015 to find out studies evaluating the relationship between serum RBP4 level and GDM risk. The following keywords were used: ("gestational diabetes mellitus" OR "gestational diabetes" OR GDM) AND ("retinol-binding protein-4" OR "retinol binding protein-4" OR "retinol binding protein 4" OR "retinol-binding protein 4" OR RBP4 OR RBP-4). Next, we systematically searched the same databases for studies that examined RBP4 polymorphisms in patients with GDM. The following keywords were used in this step: ("gestational diabetes mellitus" OR "gestational diabetes" OR "GDM") AND ("polymorphism" OR "variant") AND ("retinol-binding protein-4" OR "retinol binding protein-4" OR "retinol binding protein 4" OR "retinol-binding protein 4" OR "RBP4" OR "RBP-4"); furthermore, the names of specific polymorphisms were combined with "gestational diabetes." All reference lists of the resulting primary research reports and relevant reviews were manually searched to identify additional eligible studies.

Eligible studies and data extraction

Eligible studies included in this meta-analysis: (1) investigated the relationship between serum RBP4 levels and GDM risk, or between GDM and at least 1 genetic variant of *RBP4*; (2) included a case group of patients with GDM and a control group; (3) diagnosed GDM according to the oral glucose-tolerance test (OGTT); (4) provided data with mean and standard deviation (SD) or median and interquartile range (in the case of the meta-analysis of serum RBP4 levels); (5) were not animal studies; (6) were designed as BMI-matched studies or had observed nonsignificant differences in BMI between cases and controls (in the case of the meta-analysis of serum RBP4 levels).

Studies with overlapping data were excluded from our analysis. We identified only one study that required additional information: Ping et al. [12] had not reported the *P* value of the difference in BMI between cases and controls in their analysis of serum RBP4 levels. However, we obtained Ping's PhD dissertation, written in Chinese, and extracted this information from it. Data were extracted independently by two reviewers in consultation with a third, from each study included. The information regarding the first author, year of publication, study population (country and ethnicity), number of patients and controls, and diagnostic criteria were extracted. For genetic-association studies, information was extracted on the frequency of genotypes, the Hardy-Weinberg equilibrium (HWE) status, and the genotyping method used. For studies investigated serum RBP4 levels, information was extracted on serum RBP4 measurements, the mean and SD of serum RBP4 levels, and the gestational age at the time of blood sampling. When the standard error of the mean (SEM) was reported, SD was calculated as $SD = SEM/\sqrt{n}$. If the case or control groups were further divided into subgroups, the data from the subgroups were merged as $n = n_1 + n_2$, $\bar{x} = \frac{n_1\bar{x}_1 + n_2\bar{x}_2}{n_1+n_2}$ and $SD = \sqrt{\frac{(n_1-1)SD_1^2+(n_2-1)SD_2^2+\frac{n_1 n_2}{n_1+n_2}\left(\bar{x}_1^2+\bar{x}_2^2-2\bar{x}_1\bar{x}_2\right)}{n_1+n_2-1}}$ [34]. When a study provided medians and interquartile ranges (instead of means and SDs), without the minimum or maximum values, we treated the medians as means and calculated the SDs, as SD = interquartile range/1.35 [35]. If the study provided the minimum and maximum, we imputed the means and SDs as described by Hozo et al. [36]. When a study had tested the blood sample by two or more different methods, the result of the enzyme immunometric assay was chosen here because it is the most commonly used method in the studies included in our meta-analysis.

Statistical methods

The association between serum RBP4 level and GDM risk was estimated by calculating the pooled standardized mean difference (SMD) and 95 % confidence interval (CI). To analyze the potential influences of gestational age at blood sampling and diagnostic criteria, we performed subgroup analysis. Based on the gestational age at blood sampling, the subjects were divided into 4 subgroups: (1) before 24 weeks, (2) 24–28 weeks, (3) after 28 weeks, and (4) postpartum; For two studies [26, 28], the gestational ages at blood sampling considerably overlapped within 24–28 weeks; thus, these two studies were assigned to the gestational age subgroup of 24–28 weeks. And according to the diagnostic criteria studies were divided into two subgroups: (1) based on the American Diabetes Association (ADA) criteria [37], and (2) based on the more rigorous criteria established by the National Diabetes Data Group (NDDG) [38], the World Health Organization (WHO) [39], and Sun et al. [20]. The association between genetic factors (e.g., genotypes and alleles) and GDM was examined by using the Chi-square test or the Fisher exact test. The association of the *RBP4* rs3758539 polymorphism with GDM risk was assessed, by calculating the pooled odds ratio (OR) and 95 % CI, according to general, dominant, and recessive genetic models, and an allelic model [40, 41]. The significance of the pooled OR and SMD was determined using Z test, and the level was set at $p < 0.05$.

Heterogeneity among studies was assessed using the *Q* test and the I^2 statistic [42, 43]. When significant heterogeneity was observed ($P < 0.1$ in the *Q* test, and $I^2 >$ 50 %), a random effects model was used for pooling data from the primary studies; if the heterogeneity was not significant, a fixed effects model was used. The HWE compliance of the controls in each study was assessed using the Chi-square test. Sensitivity analysis was performed by sequentially excluding individual studies to assess the stability of the results. Funnel-plot asymmetry was assessed using Egger's linear regression test, $P < 0.05$ representing significant publication bias. If asymmetry was observed, contour-enhanced meta-analysis funnel plots were used to distinguish publication bias from other causes of asymmetry [44, 45]. All analyses were performed using STATA 12.0 software (Stata Corporation, College Station, TX), and all *p* values were 2-tailed.

Results

Main characteristics of eligible studies

With respect to the association between serum RBP4 levels and GDM risk, an initial search identified 232 records of potentially relevant studies from the databases included. Of these, 202 records were excluded based on their title and/or abstract: these were repetitive publications, reviews, reports of animal studies, and/or reports of studies that investigated either outcomes irrelevant to this meta-analysis or adipokines other than RBP4. A further 16 full-text articles were excluded because: ① six papers contain data that overlapped with other articles, ② seven papers reported different BMI distributions between the case and control groups ($P < 0.05$), ③ and three papers with the plasma RBP4 concentrations or unavailable data. Final selected 14 case–control studies included 647 cases and 620 controls were included in our meta-analysis (Table 1, Additional file 1: Table S1); the process of study selection is shown in Additional file 2: Figure S1(a).

With respect to the association between *RBP4* rs3758539 polymorphism and GDM risk, the initial database search identified 147 reports of potentially relevant studies. Of these, 143 records were excluded based on their title and/

Table 1 Detailed characteristics of all eligible studies for the association with serum RBP4 levels and GDM

Study	Year	Country	No of case	No of control	Diagnose criteria[b]	Gestational age at blood sampling	Test	BMI[c]	RBP4(μg/ml)[d]		P-value
									Case	Control	
Chan a [16]	2007	China, Han	20	20	NDDG	24–28 weeks	ELISA	Matched	0.0424 ± 0.0138	0.0320 ± 0.0087	0.007
Chan b [16]	2007	China, Han	20	20	NDDG	immediately after delivery	ELISA	Matched	0.0301 ± 0.0110	0.0309 ± 0.0100	0.811
Kim [17]	2008	South Korea	10	9	ADA	24–28 weeks	ELISA	P > 0.05	39.1 ± 6.3	30.0 ± 10.0	0.026
Lewandowski[a] [19]	2008	Austria	15	35	ADA	28 weeks	Unclear	Matched	53.9 ± 18.7	34.4 ± 12.4	<0.001
Sun [20]	2009	China, Han	32	30	OGTT confirmed	24 h before delivery	ELISA	Matched	27.0 ± 1.2	19.4 ± 1.8	<0.001
Klein a [21]	2010	Austria, Caucasian	63	38	ADA	24–28 weeks	ELISA	Matched	18.0 ± 3.7	16.9 ± 5.1	0.213
Klein b [21]	2010	Austria, Caucasian	63	38	ADA	33 weeks	ELISA	Matched	20.3 ± 7.2	17.9 ± 6.1	0.089
Su [23]	2010	China, Han	63	58	ADA	24–28 weeks	ELISA	Matched	41.6 ± 12.2	34.5 ± 9.8	<0.001
Tepper [24]	2010	USA, mixed	12	10	ADA	24–28 weeks	EIA	Matched	25.2 ± 2.1	25.2 ± 2.1	1.000
Kuzmicki a[a] [26]	2011	Poland	68	68	WHO	24–30 weeks	EIA	P > 0.05	58.1 ± 25.3	51.0 ± 18.1	0.062
Kuzmicki b[a] [26]	2011	Poland	20	18	WHO	36–40 weeks	EIA	P > 0.05	62.4 ± 31.0	42.9 ± 19.0	0.027
Chen [25]	2011	China, Han	52	46	NDDG	before delivery	ELISA	Matched	31.93 ± 7.21	26.92 ± 8.5	0.002
Ping [12]	2012	China, Han	74	69	ADA	24–28 weeks	ELISA	P > 0.05	21.53 ± 5.96	20.84 ± 4.31	<0.001
Skvarca[a] [28]	2012	Slovenia	30	44	ADA	26.81 ± 3.46 weeks	ELISA	P > 0.05	15.00 ± 6.11	15.57 ± 8.35	0.750
Liang [31]	2014	China, Han	35	35	NDDG	24–28 weeks	ELISA	P > 0.05	22.90 ± 3.09	17.90 ± 3.91	<0.001
Fruscalzo [32]	2015	Germany, mixed	32	44	ADA	11–13 weeks	ELISA	P > 0.05	24.78 ± 6.51	27.93 ± 7.98	0.071
Du [33]	2015	China	38	38	NDDG	37–42 weeks	ELISA	Matched	39.08 ± 8.29	21.42 ± 3.85	<0.001

[a]Raw data in the article are presented as median (interquartile range)
[b]Diagnostic criteria: *NDDG* National Diabetes Data Group criteria, *ADA*, American Diabetes Association criteria, *WHO* World Health Organization criteria
[c]BMI: matched, the control subjects had been matched with the GDM subjects for BMI; $P > 0.05$, difference of BMI between case and control had no statistical significance
[d]Data are presented as mean ± standard deviation

Table 2 Detailed characteristics of all eligible studies for the association with RBP4 gene polymorphisms and GDM

Gene polymorphisms	Author	Year	Country	Ethnicity	Case include	No of case	No of control	Genotype[a]		P for HWE
								Case	Control	
rs3758539	Hiraoka a[d] [11]	2011	America	Utah Caucasian	GDM	88	315	56/31/1	228/77/10	0.27
	Hiraoka b[d] [11]	2011	America	Hawai'i Filipino	GDM	82	286	63/16/3	226/55/5	0.44
	Hiraoka c[d] [11]	2011	America	Hawai'i Pacific Islander	GDM	19	32	18/1/0	23/9/0	0.35
	Ping[e] [12]	2012	China	Han	GDM + GIGT[c]	723	872	375/75/5	462/143/8	0.41
	Saucedo[d] [13]	2014	Mexico	Unclear	GDM	100	100	93/7	91/9	P > 0.05[b]
rs12265684	Ping[e] [12]	2012	China	Han	GDM + GIGT[c]	723	872	382/106/5	483/168/14	0.89
rs3758538	Ping[d] [12]	2012	China	Han	GDM + GIGT[c]	723	872	414/63/4	562/76/2	0.74
rs10882273	Ping[d] [12]	2012	China	Han	GDM + GIGT[c]	723	872	363/107/8	451/174/13	0.42
rs116736522	Saucedo[d] [13]	2014	Mexico	Unclear	GDM	100	100	97/3	96/4	P > 0.05[b]
rs34571439	Saucedo[d] [13]	2014	Mexico	Unclear	GDM	100	100	91/9	88/12	P > 0.05[b]

[a]Genotype for rs3758539, GG/AG/AA (For Saucedo, GG/GA + AA); rs12265684, CC/CG/GG; rs3758538, AA/AC/CC; rs10882273, TT/TC/CC; rs116736522, GG/GC + CC; rs34571439, AA/AC + CC
[b]No sufficient data to calculate the P for HWE. Authors mentioned "all variants are in the Hardy-Weinberg equilibrium" in the article
[c]*GIGT* gestational impaired glucose tolerance
[d]No significant differences was found in allelic frequencies between case and control groups
[e]Significant differences was found in allelic frequencies between case and control groups

Table 3 Summary of different comparative results of serum RBP4 level with GDM risk

Category		No of study	No of case	No of control	SMD (95 % CI)	Z	*p* value	I^2%	P_{het}
overall		17	647	620	0.816 [0.411–1.122]	3.94	0.000	91.0	0.000
Gestational age at blood sampling	Before 24 weeks	1	32	44	-0.426 [-0.886–0.035]	1.81	0.070	-	-
	24-28 weeks	10	390	386	0.561 [0.252–0.870]	3.56	0.000	74.8	0.000
	After 28 weeks	5	205	170	1.830 [0.580– 3.080]	2.87	0.004	96.0	0.000
	Postpartum	1	20	20	-0.076 [-0.696–0.544]	0.24	0.810	-	-
Diagnostic criteria	ADA criteria	8	347	310	0.205 [-0.063–0.472]	1.50	0.134	61.7	0.011
	Rigorous criteria	9	300	310	1.388 [0.665–2.110]	3.77	0.000	91.0	0.000

P_{het} = *p* value for heterogeneity, *OR* = adds ratio, *CI* = confidence interval, *ADA* = American Diabetes Association criteria, More rigorous criteria contained National Diabetes Data Group criteria, World Health Organization criteria and the criteria of Sun et al

or abstract: these were repetitive publications, reviews, reports of animal studies, and/or reports of studies that investigated either outcomes irrelevant to this meta-analysis or genes other than *RBP4*. In addition, 1 full-text review was excluded because it contained data overlapped with other primary papers. Finally, 3 eligible studies that included 1,012 cases and 1,605 controls were included in the meta-analysis (Table 2); the process of study selection is shown in Additional file 2: Figure S1(b).

Association between serum RBP4 level and GDM Risk

The meta-analysis for serum RBP4 level includes 14 articles (17 results) with a total of 647 cases and 620 controls. The results show that serum RBP4 level and GDM risk are significantly associated (SMD = 0.816, 95 % CI [0.411, 1.122]) (Table 3, Fig. 1). The "24–28 weeks" subgroup, "after 28 weeks" subgroup and the rigorous criteria subgroup indicate that higher serum RBP4 level is related to GDM risk (24–28 weeks subgroup:

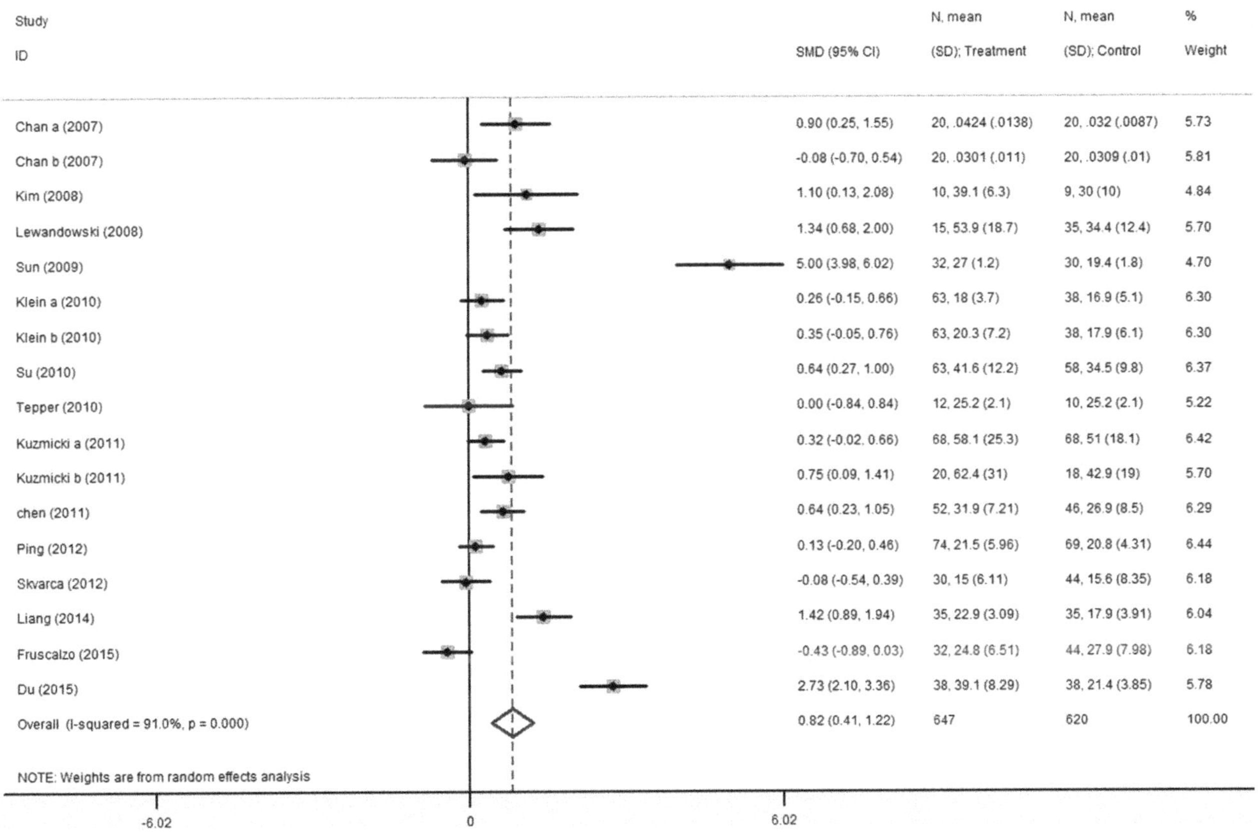

Fig. 1 Meta-analysis for the association of serum RBP4 level with GDM risk using a random-effects model

SMD = 0.561, 95 % CI [0.252, 0.870]; after 28 weeks: SMD = 1.830, 95 % CI [0.580–3.080]; the rigorous criteria subgroup: SMD = 1.388, 95 % CI [0.665, 2.110]). The "before 24 weeks" subgroup and postpartum subgroup both include only 1 study and show non-significant association between serum RBP4 level and GDM risk (before 24 weeks subgroup: SMD = -0.426, 95 % CI [-0.886, 0.870]; postpartum subgroup SMD = -0.076, 95 % CI [-0.696, 0.472]). Non-significant result is also observed in the ADA criteria subgroup (SMD = 0.205, 95 % CI [-0.063, 0.472]) (Table 3, Figs. 2 and 3).

In the sensitivity analysis, 1 eligible study was excluded at a time in order to assess the influence of each dataset on the pooled SMD. We observed no changes in the corresponding pooled SMD or in the significance of the results (Additional file 3: Figure S2), which indicated that our results were significantly robust to the study-selection process.

Publication bias was assessed using Begg's funnel plot and Egger's test. The results of Begg's funnel plot reveal the presence of significant asymmetry. These results are consistent with the modified Egger linear regression test and Begg's test ($t = 2.50$, $p = 0.025$; $Z = 2.27$, $p = 0.023$). In order to analyze the potential causes to the funnel plot asymmetry, we treated the contour-enhanced funnel plots with the trim-and-fill method. This treatment resulted in 4 filled studies, which were all in the region of $p < 0.05$ (Fig. 4). Hence, the cause of the asymmetry may be more likely to be due to factors other than publication bias, such as variable study quality. After the "unpublished" (filled) studies are included, higher serum RBP4 level is still related to GDM risk (SMD = 0.300, 95 % CI [0.189, 0.411])."

Association between rs3758539 Polymorphisms and GDM Risk

The meta-analysis concerning rs3758539 included three studies with a total of 1012 cases and 1605 controls. The dominant genetic model shows non-significant association between GG vs. GA + AA (OR = 1.133, 95 % CI [0.695, 1.846]). The following results were obtained only including two studies [8, 9]: G allele vs. A allele

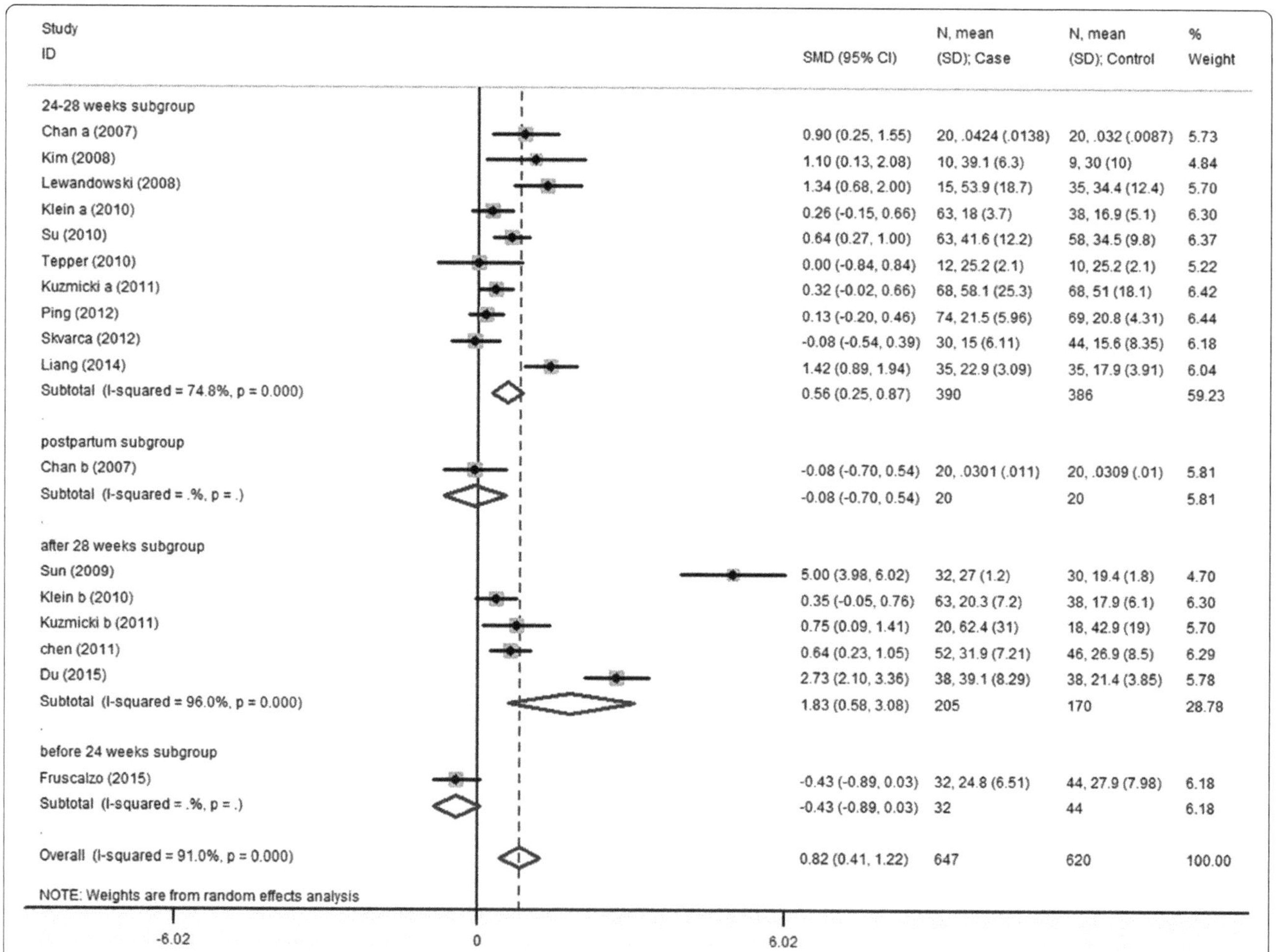

Fig. 2 Gestational age at blood sampling subgroup analysis using a random-effects model

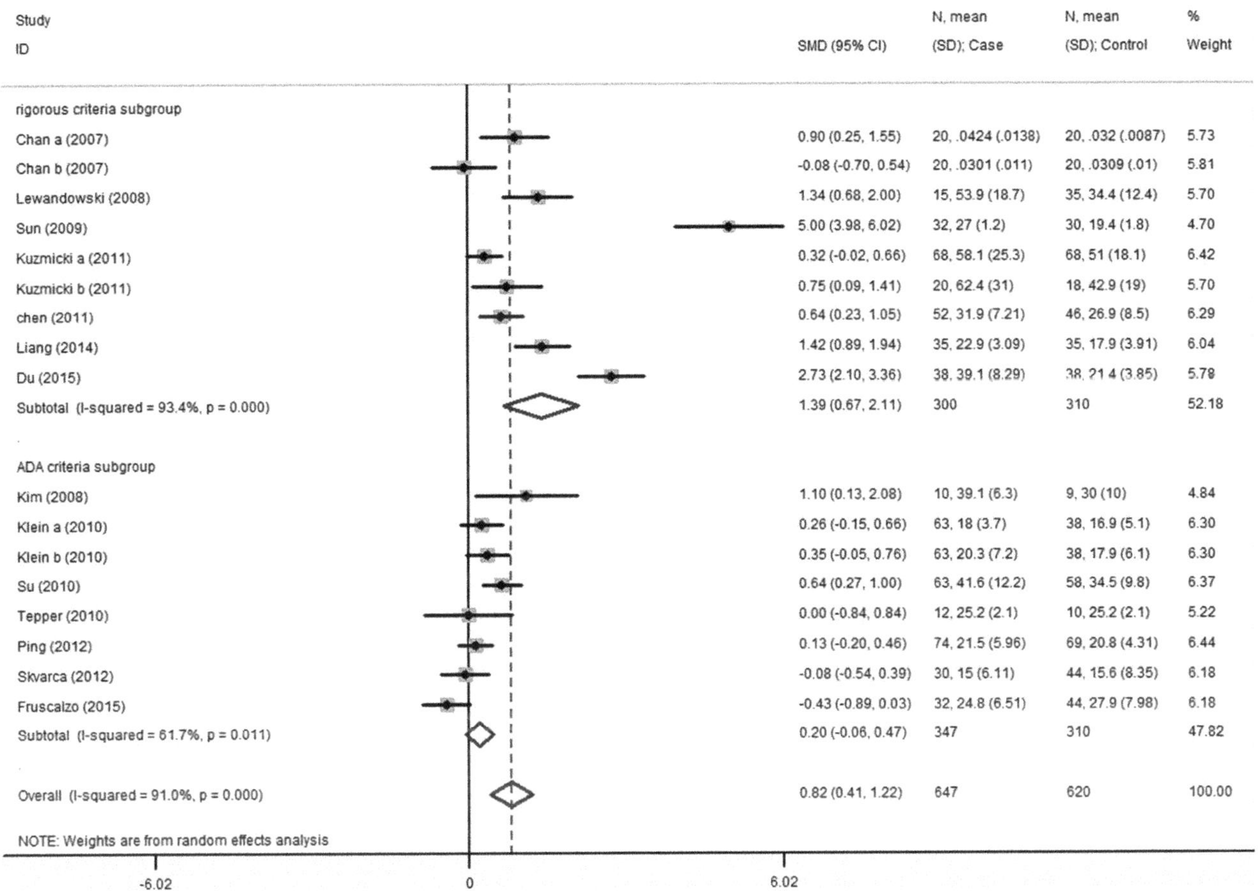

Fig. 3 Diagnostic criteria subgroup analysis using a random-effects model

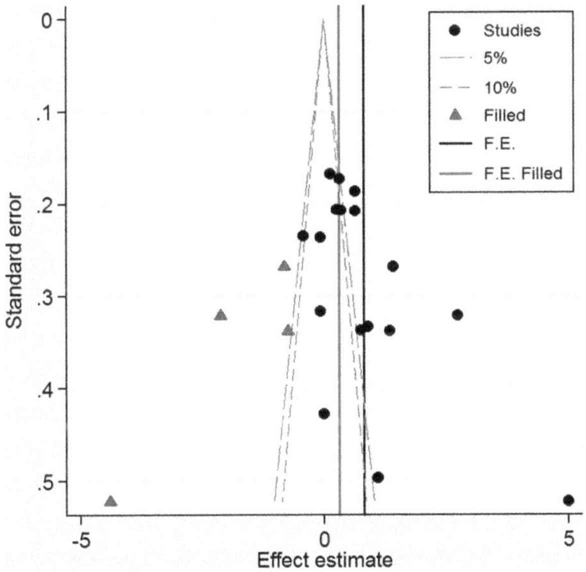

Fig. 4 Contour-enhanced funnel plots for funnel plot asymmetry analysis of serum RBP4 level with GDM risk

(OR = 1.093, 95 % CI [0.687, 1.739]), GG + GA vs. AA (OR = 1.123, 95 % CI [0.508, 2.483]), and GG vs. AA (OR = 1.124, 95 % CI [0.505, 2.502]) (Table 4, Fig. 5). Publication bias was not detected owing to the small number of available studies. During the sensitivity analysis, one eligible study was excluded each time to investigate the influence of the individual dataset on the pooled OR. The results show that the corresponding pooled OR and significant results did not change materially (Additional file 4: Figure S3), indicating that our results were significantly robust.

Discussion

Main findings

Our meta-analysis shows that higher prenatal serum RBP4 level is related to GDM risk, but this association cannot be shown in the first-trimester and postpartum periods. The GDM diagnostic criteria affected the strength of association between RBP4 level and GDM risk. Adopting a higher threshold of OGTT would result in a larger difference of serum RBP4 level between GDM

Table 4 Summary of different comparative results of rs3758539 polymorphism

Genetic model		No of case	No of control	OR (95 % CI)	Z	*p* value	I^2%	P_{het}	Effect model
Dominant	GG versus GA + AA	1012	1605	1.133 [0.695–1.846]	0.50	0.617	65.2	0.022	R
Recessive	GG + GA versus AA	893	1473	1.123 [0.508–2.483]	0.29	0.775	8.3	0.336	F
Additive	GG versus AA	893	1473	1.124 [0.505–2.502]	0.29	0.775	0.9	0.365	F
Allele	G versus A	912	1505	1.093 [0.687–1.739]	0.37	0.709	68.3	0.024	R

P_{het} = *p* value for heterogeneity, *OR* = adds ratio, *CI* = confidence interval, *F* = fixed-effect model, *R* = random-effect model

women and controls. *RBP4* rs3758539 polymorphisms may not be associated with GDM risk.

Interpretation

We pooled 17 studies (647 cases and 620 controls) in which the BMI-matched strategy was used, and then analyzed the relationship between serum RBP4 levels and GDM risk. Our results indicated that high serum RBP4 levels were related to GDM risk. We performed subgroup analyses of the effects of gestational age at blood sampling and diagnostic criteria. The studies included in the meta-analysis covered all periods during the pregnancy and only one study concerned the postpartum situation. The pooled results of second- and third-trimester subgroups were consistent with the overall result, GDM gravidas have higher serum RBP4 level than the controls. No statistically significant association was found between serum RBP4 levels and GDM risk in the postpartum subgroup and first-trimester subgroup. In the postpartum study blood samples were collected immediately after delivery. High exertion at delivery, which requires high output of energy, might temporarily enhance insulin sensitivity [16], and specific metabolic state at delivery might produce a difference between postpartum and prenatal results. The negative result of first-trimester subgroup reveals that with the insulin resistance level increasing during pregnancy, the magnitude of the effect of RBP4 may change. However, the inclusion of only a single study in postpartum subgroup and "before 24 weeks" subgroup could potentially make the stratified analysis unreliable. Therefore, the results must be interpreted with caution, and need to be validated using additional studies that include a large number of samples covering various periods during pregnancy and after delivery. In the subgroup analyses based on diagnostic criteria, both of the two subgroups show results consistent with the overall meta-analysis. And the pooled SMD of rigorous criteria subgroup is

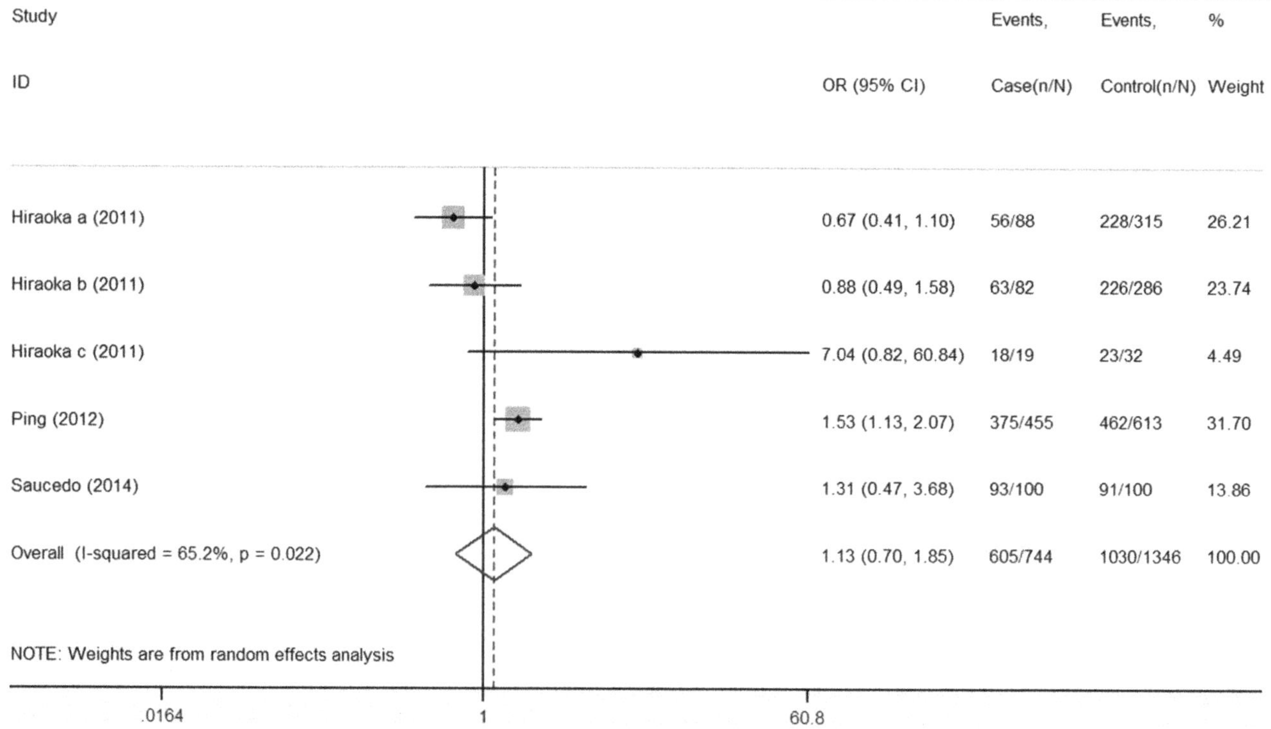

Fig. 5 Meta-analysis for the association of rs3758539 polymorphism with GDM risk (GG vs. (GA + AA))

higher than the pooled SMD of ADA criteria subgroup. Although the result of ADA criteria subgroup had no statistical significance, we still can get further hints: higher blood glucose level at fasting and OGTT is associated with higher serum RBP4 levels. This finding was consistent with several published articles [17, 18, 21, 23, 31], which revealed that blood glucose and serum RBP4 levels presents a modest dose–response relationship. Thus, the results of subgroup analysis based on diagnostic criteria confirmed our hypothesis that RBP4 is related to glycometabolism in GDM.

Two articles reported the odds ratio about serum RBP4 level between women with and without GDM estimated from logistic regression models. The study by Abetew et al. [29] revealed that women in the highest quartile for serum RBP4 had a 1.89-fold higher risk of GDM compared with women in the lowest quartile (95 % CI: 1.05–3.43). However, this relationship did not reach statistical significance after adjustment for maternal race/ethnicity, family history of diabetes, and pre-pregnancy overweight status (adjusted OR: 1.54; 95 % CI: 0.82–2.90). In the study by Fruscalzo et al. [32], serum RBP4 level was not involved in the final multivariate logistic regression model after adjustment for maternal age, pre-pregnancy BMI, tobacco smoke, macro-region of origin, familial history of diabetes and so on.

The coding region of *RBP4* is located at chromosome 10q23–24 in humans, contains 5 exons and 6 introns, and has been linked to increased risk for type 2 diabetes in various populations [46, 47]. Numerous single nucleotide polymorphisms (SNPs), including +5,398 C > T, +8,201 T > A, +8,204 T > A, rs17484721, rs36035572, rs3758539, rs3758539, rs10882273, rs36014035, and rs34571439, have been identified as genetic markers for type 2 diabetes or insulin resistance [48–56]. Some of these SNPs are associated with circulating RBP4 level or RBP4 expression in visceral adipose tissues [48, 55, 57]. In this study, we investigated the relationship between the *RBP4* rs3758539 polymorphism and susceptibility to GDM, but did not find any significant association. Among the five races included in the meta-analysis, significant results were only observed in Han Chinese. However, given the low frequency of the minor allele of rs3758539 in these ethnic groups [11, 13] and the small OR [12], non-significant results could be attributed to the small sample size. Therefore, additional studies of a comparatively larger scale are required to further validate this result.

To the best of our knowledge, this is the first meta-analysis that has evaluated the relationship between genetic variants of *RBP4* and the risk of GDM. However, the study has certain limitations. First, the subgroup analysis performed based on gestational age at blood sampling included only one postpartum study, which makes the stratified analysis unreliable. Moreover, the meta-analysis of RBP4 polymorphisms involved a small number of samples and studies. Therefore, the results must be interpreted with caution. Second, funnel-plot asymmetry can confound the interpretation of meta-analyses. Here, the observed funnel-plot asymmetry might have resulted from poor methodological quality related to the small size and heterogeneity of the studies, in addition to publication bias [35, 44, 45]. Third, the sample size of each individual study of RBP4 levels and GDM is relatively small and all these studies are case–control studies. These factors affect the quality of individual studies included in the meta-analysis. Last, our study only included articles that featured English-language abstracts, and the main text written in English or Chinese, and this might have resulted in a language bias.

Conclusions

The results of this meta-analysis support the hypothesis that RBP4 is a modest independent risk factor for GDM (i.e., nonobese patients with GDM might express RBP4 at abnormal levels). The serum RBP4 level is associated with the risk of GDM. However, the association in the first-trimester and postpartum period should be validated by further research. The association between *RBP4* rs3758539 polymorphism and GDM risk was not confirmed.

Additional files

Additional file 1: Table S1. Adjusted covariates of all eligible studies for the association with serum RBP4 levels and GDM.

Additional file 2: Figure S1. PRISMA flow diagram of study selection process (a) genetic variants and (b) serum concentration. (TIFF 4988 kb)

Additional file 3: Figure S2. The results of sensitivity analysis of serum RBP4 level with GDM risk.

Additional file 4: Figure S3. The results of sensitivity analysis of rs3758539 (GG vs. GA + AA) with GDM risk.

Abbreviations

ADA: American Diabetes Association; BMI: body mass index; CI: confidence interval; GDM: gestational diabetes mellitus; HWE: Hardy–Weinberg equilibrium; NDDG: National Diabetes Data Group; OGTT: oral glucose tolerance test; OR: odds ratio; PEPCK: phosphoenolpyruvate carboxykinase; RBP4: retinol-binding protein-4; SD: standard deviation; SEM: standard error of mean; SMD: standardized mean difference; SNPs: single nucleotide polymorphisms; WHO: World Health Organization.

Competing interests

The authors declare that they have no competing interests.

Authors' contributions

SH and QL has searched the databases and extracted the information. XH, as the third reviewer, reviewed the processes of literature search and data extraction. SH did statistical analysis. SH and HT drafted the manuscript. All authors read and approved the final manuscript.

Author details
[1]Department of Epidemiology and Health Statistics, School of Public Health of Central South University, Changsha, Hunan 410007, PR China. [2]Criminal Investigation Division, Changsha Public Security Bureau, Hunan 410004, China.

References

1. Buchanan TA, Xiang AH. Gestational diabetes mellitus. J Clin Invest. 2005; 115(3):485–91.
2. Schneider S, Bock C, Wetzel M, Maul H, Loerbroks A. The prevalence of gestational diabetes in advanced economies. J Perinat Med. 2012;40(5):511–20.
3. Stupin JH, Arabin B. Overweight and obesity before, during and after pregnancy: Part 1: pathophysiology, molecular biology and epigenetic consequences. Geburtshilfe Frauenheilkd. 2014;74(7):639–45.
4. Athukorala C, Rumbold AR, Willson KJ, Crowther CA. The risk of adverse pregnancy outcomes in women who are overweight or obese. BMC Pregnancy Childbirth. 2010;10:56.
5. Ovesen P, Rasmussen S, Kesmodel U. Effect of prepregnancy maternal overweight and obesity on pregnancy outcome. Obstet Gynecol. 2011; 118(2 Pt 1):305–12.
6. Yang Q, Graham TE, Mody N, Preitner F, Peroni OD, Zabolotny JM, Kotani K, Quadro L, Kahn BB. Serum retinol binding protein 4 contributes to insulin resistance in obesity and type 2 diabetes. Nature. 2005;436(7049):356–62.
7. Graham TE, Yang Q, Bluher M, Hammarstedt A, Ciaraldi TP, Henry RR, Wason CJ, Oberbach A, Jansson PA, Smith U, et al. Retinol-binding protein 4 and insulin resistance in lean, obese, and diabetic subjects. N Engl J Med. 2006; 354(24):2552–63.
8. Tamori Y, Sakaue H, Kasuga M. RBP4, an unexpected adipokine. Nat Med. 2006;12(1):30–1.
9. Barbour LA, McCurdy CE, Hernandez TL, Kirwan JP, Catalano PM, Friedman JE. Cellular mechanisms for insulin resistance in normal pregnancy and gestational diabetes. Diabetes Care. 2007;30 Suppl 2:S112–9.
10. Garvey WT, Maianu L, Zhu JH, Hancock JA, Golichowski AM. Multiple defects in the adipocyte glucose transport system cause cellular insulin resistance in gestational diabetes. Heterogeneity in the number and a novel abnormality in subcellular localization of GLUT4 glucose transporters. Diabetes. 1993; 42(12):1773–85.
11. Hiraoka M, Urschitz J, Sultan O, Ward K. A polymorphism in the retinol binding protein 4 gene is not associated with gestational diabetes mellitus in several different ethnic groups. Hawaii Med J. 2011;70(8):164–7.
12. Ping F, Xiang HD, Li M, Li W, Liu JT, Nie M, Hui YC. Effects of variation in retinol binding protein 4 gene and adipose specific expression of gestational diabetes in Beijing, China. Diabetes Res Clin Pract. 2012; 97(2):283–9.
13. Saucedo R, Zarate A, Basurto L, Hernandez M, Puello E, Mendoza-Lorenzo P, Ostrosky-Wegman P. RBP4 gene variants are associated with insulin resistance in women with previous gestational diabetes. Dis Markers. 2014; 2014:269208.
14. Hirschhorn JN, Lohmueller K, Byrne E, Hirschhorn K. A comprehensive review of genetic association studies. Genet Med. 2002;4(2):45–61.
15. Cardon LR, Bell JI. Association study designs for complex diseases. Nat Rev Genet. 2001;2(2):91–9.
16. Chan TF, Chen HS, Chen YC, Lee CH, Chou FH, Chen IJ, Chen SY, Jong SB, Tsai EM. Increased serum retinol-binding protein 4 concentrations in women with gestational diabetes mellitus. Reprod Sci. 2007;14(2):169–74.
17. Kim SH, Choi HJ, Im JA. Retinol-binding protein 4 responses during an oral glucose tolerance testing in women with gestational diabetes mellitus. Clin Chim Acta. 2008;391(1-2):123–5.
18. Krzyzanowska K, Zemany L, Krugluger W, Schernthaner GH, Mittermayer F, Schnack C, Rahman R, Brix J, Kahn BB, Schernthaner G. Serum concentrations of retinol-binding protein 4 in women with and without gestational diabetes. Diabetologia. 2008;51(7):1115–22.
19. Lewandowski KC, Stojanovic N, Bienkiewicz M, Tan BK, Prelevic GM, Press M, Tuck S, O'Hare PJ, Randeva HS. Elevated concentrations of retinol-binding protein-4 (RBP-4) in gestational diabetes mellitus: Negative correlation with soluble vascular cell adhesion molecule-1 (sVCAM-1). Gynecol Endocrinol. 2008;24(6):300–5.
20. Sun L-F, Chen W-P, Li J, Ye Y-H. Correlation of retinol binding protein 4 expression in maternal serum and subcutaneous adipose tissue with insulin resistance in gestational diabetes mellitus. Zhonghua Fu Chan Ke Za Zhi. 2009;44(12):915–9.
21. Klein K, Bancher-Todesca D, Leipold H, Knofler M, Haslinger P, Handisurya A, Kautzky-Willer A, Worda C Retinol-binding protein 4 in patients with gestational diabetes mellitus. J Womens Health (Larchmt. 2010;19(3):517–21.
22. Maghbooli Z, Hossein-nezhad A, Mirzaei K, Karimi F, Besharati A, Omidfar K, Larijani B. Association between retinol-binding protein 4 concentrations and gestational diabetes mellitus and risk of developing metabolic syndrome after pregnancy. Reprod Sci. 2010;17(2):196–201.
23. Su YX, Hong J, Yan Q, Xu C, Gu WQ, Zhang YF, Shen CF, Chi ZN, Dai M, Xu M, et al. Increased serum retinol-binding protein-4 levels in pregnant women with and without gestational diabetes mellitus. Diabetes Metab. 2010;36(6 Pt 1):470–5.
24. Tepper BJ, Kim YK, Shete V, Shabrova E, Quadro L. Serum retinol-binding protein 4 (RBP4) and retinol in a cohort of borderline obese women with and without gestational diabetes. Clin Biochem. 2010;43(3):320–3.
25. Chen Z-y, Du J. Change of serum retinol-binding protein-4 level in pregnancy obese subjects and GDM and related factors. J China Med Univ. 2011;40(5):465–8.
26. Kuzmicki M, Telejko B, Wawrusiewicz-kurylonek N, Nikolajuk A, Zwierz-gugala D, Jelski W, Kolodziejczak M, Zonenberg A, Wilczynski J, Kretowski A, et al. Retinol-binding protein 4 in adipose and placental tissue of women with gestational diabetes. Gynecol Endocrinol. 2011;27(12):1065–9.
27. Khovidhunkit W, Pruksakorn P, Plengpanich W, Tharavanij T. Retinol-binding protein 4 is not associated with insulin resistance in pregnancy. Metab Clin Exp. 2012;61(1):65–9.
28. Skvarca A, Tomazic M, Krhin B, Blagus R, Janez A. Adipocytokines and insulin resistance across various degrees of glucose tolerance in pregnancy. J Int Med Res. 2012;40(2):583–9.
29. Abetew DF, Qiu C, Fida NG, Dishi M, Hevner K, Williams MA, Enquobahrie DA. Association of retinol binding protein 4 with risk of gestational diabetes. Diabetes Res Clin Pract. 2013;99(1):48–53.
30. Nanda S, Nikoletakis G, Markova D, Poon LCY, Nicolaides KH. Maternal serum retinol-binding protein-4 at 11-13 weeks' gestation in normal and pathological pregnancies. Metabolism. 2013;62(6):814–9.
31. Liang Z, Du M, Fang Q, Chen D. Significance of RBP4 in patients with gestational diabetes mellitus: a case-control study of Han Chinese women. Gynecol Endocrinol. 2014;30(2):161–4.
32. Fruscalzo A, Londero AP, Driul L, Henze A, Tonutti L, Ceraudo M, Zanotti G, Berni R, Schweigert FJ, Raila J. First trimester concentrations of the TTR-RBP4-retinol complex components as early markers of insulin-treated gestational diabetes mellitus. Clin Chem Lab Med. 2015;53(10):1643–51.
33. Du M, Wang B, Liang Z, Dong M, Chen D. The Relationship between Retinol-Binding Protein 4 Concentrations and Gestational Diabetes Mellitus in Chinese Women. Gynecol Obstet Invest. 2015. doi: 10.1159/000398794.
34. Zhang T, Zhong W (editors). Applied methodology for evidence-based medicine. Changsha, China: Central South University Press; 2011.
35. Higgins JPT, Green S (editors). Cochrane Handbook for Systematic Reviews of Interventions Version 5.1.0 [updated March 2011]. The Cochrane Collaboration, 2011. Available from http://handbook.cochrane.org/.
36. Hozo SP, Djulbegovic B, Hozo I. Estimating the mean and variance from the median, range, and the size of a sample. BMC Med Res Methodol. 2005;5:13.
37. The Expert Committee on the Diagnosis Of Diabetes Mellitus. Report of the expert committee on the diagnosis and classification of diabetes mellitus. Diabetes Care. 2003;26 Suppl 1:S5–20.
38. National Diabetes Data Group. Classification and diagnosis of diabetes mellitus and other categories of glucose intolerance. Diabetes. 1979;28(12):1039–57.
39. Department of Noncommunicable Disease Surveillance. Definition, diagnosis, and classi-fication of diabetes mellitus and its complications. Report of a WHO Consultation. Part 1: Diagnosis and classification of diabetes mellitus. WHO/NCD/NCS/99.2. Geneva: WHO; 1999.
40. Clarke GM, Anderson CA, Pettersson FH, Cardon LR, Morris AP, Zondervan KT. Basic statistical analysis in genetic case-control studies. Nat Protoc. 2011; 6(2):121–33.
41. Li X, Shen L, Tan HZ. Polymorphisms and plasma level of transforming growth factor-beta 1 and risk for preeclampsia: a systematic review. Plos One. 2014;9(5):e97230.
42. Whitehead A, Whitehead J. A general parametric approach to the meta-analysis of randomized clinical trials. Stat Med. 1991;10(11):1665–77.
43. Higgins JP, Thompson SG. Quantifying heterogeneity in a meta-analysis. Stat Med. 2002;21(11):1539–58.
44. Palmer TM, Peters JL, Sutton AJ, Moreno SG. Contour-enhanced funnel plots for meta-analysis. Stata J. 2008;8(2):242–54.

45. Peters JL, Sutton AJ, Jones DR, Abrams KR, Rushton L. Contour-enhanced meta-analysis funnel plots help distinguish publication bias from other causes of asymmetry. J Clin Epidemiol. 2008;61(10):991–6.
46. Meigs JB, Panhuysen CI, Myers RH, Wilson PW, Cupples LA. A genome-wide scan for loci linked to plasma levels of glucose and HbA(1c) in a community-based sample of Caucasian pedigrees: The Framingham Offspring Study. Diabetes. 2002;51(3):833–40.
47. Shepherd PR, Kahn BB. Glucose transporters and insulin action–implications for insulin resistance and diabetes mellitus. N Engl J Med. 1999;341(4):248–57.
48. Hu C, Jia W, Zhang R, Wang C, Lu J, Wu H, Fang Q, Ma X, Xiang K. Effect of RBP4 gene variants on circulating RBP4 concentration and type 2 diabetes in a Chinese population. Diabet Med. 2008;25(1):11–8.
49. Hung YP, Lee NY, Lin SH, Chang HC, Wu CJ, Chang CM, Chen PL, Lin HJ, Wu YH, Tsai PJ, et al. Effects of PPARgamma and RBP4 gene variants on metabolic syndrome in HIV-infected patients with anti-retroviral therapy. PLoS One. 2012;7(11):e49102.
50. Liu J, Gao JY, Zhang JP, Li PQ, Liu JX, Liu J, Xie XD. Evaluation of the association between retinal binding protein 4 polymorphisms and type 2 diabetes in Chinese by DHPLC. Endocrine. 2008;34(1-3):23–8.
51. Wu Y, Li H, Loos RJ, Qi Q, Hu FB, Liu Y, Lin X. RBP4 variants are significantly associated with plasma RBP4 levels and hypertriglyceridemia risk in Chinese Hans. J Lipid Res. 2009;50(7):1479–86.
52. Nair AK, Sugunan D, Kumar H, Anilkumar G. Case-control analysis of SNPs in GLUT4, RBP4 and STRA6: association of SNPs in STRA6 with type 2 diabetes in a South Indian population. PLoS One. 2010;5(7):e11444.
53. Munkhtulga L, Nakayama K, Utsumi N, Yanagisawa Y, Gotoh T, Omi T, Kumada M, Erdenebulgan B, Zolzaya K, Lkhagvasuren T, et al. Identification of a regulatory SNP in the retinol binding protein 4 gene associated with type 2 diabetes in Mongolia. Hum Genet. 2007;120(6):879–88.
54. Craig RL, Chu WS, Elbein SC. Retinol binding protein 4 as a candidate gene for type 2 diabetes and prediabetic intermediate traits. Mol Genet Metab. 2007;90(3):338–44.
55. Kovacs P, Geyer M, Berndt J, Kloting N, Graham TE, Bottcher Y, Enigk B, Tonjes A, Schleinitz D, Schon MR, et al. Effects of genetic variation in the human retinol binding protein-4 gene (RBP4) on insulin resistance and fat depot-specific mRNA expression. Diabetes. 2007;56(12):3095–100.
56. van Hoek M, Dehghan A, Zillikens MC, Hofman A, Witteman JC, Sijbrands EJ. An RBP4 promoter polymorphism increases risk of type 2 diabetes. Diabetologia. 2008;51(8):1423–8.
57. Munkhtulga L, Nagashima S, Nakayama K, Utsumi N, Yanagisawa Y, Gotoh T, Omi T, Kumada M, Zolzaya K, Lkhagvasuren T, et al. Regulatory SNP in the RBP4 gene modified the expression in adipocytes and associated with BMI. Obesity (Silver Spring). 2010;18(5):1006–14.

19

Assessing use of a printed lifestyle intervention tool by women with borderline gestational diabetes and their achievement of diet and exercise goals

Shanshan Han[1*], Philippa F. Middleton[1,2], Thach S. Tran[3] and Caroline A. Crowther[1,4]

Abstract

Background: The purpose of this study is to assess use of a booklet by pregnant women to record and assist dietary and lifestyle changes; to describe diet and exercise goals set during the initial lifestyle discussions; and to assess achievement of goals.

Methods: Participants were women with borderline gestational diabetes who received a printed pregnancy record booklet, as part of a randomised trial, to record and set monthly goals for diet and exercise. Outcomes included women's use of the booklets and their achievement of dietary and exercise goals after 1 month.

Results: Fifty-six women returned their used pregnancy record booklets and were included in this study. These women set a total of 197 dietary goals and 65 exercise goals. In the first month, over 80 % of dietary goals that targeted grains, dairy and overall diet were achieved, but only 20–30 % of goals about vegetables, and foods high in fat, sugar and/or salt were achieved. After 1 month, women had achieved 86.4 % of their exercise goals to maintain their current level of activity, but only 25.0 % exercise goals to increase walking during pregnancy.

Conclusions: Women who used pregnancy record booklets reported good achievement rates for goals related to grains, fruits, dairy and overall diet, but they were less likely to be successful in achieving goals to increase intake of vegetables, and limit foods that high in fat, sugar and/or salt. Maintaining an active lifestyle during pregnancy was feasible for women although increases in physical activity were less often achieved.
Using a pregnancy record booklet may be helpful in assisting and encouraging behavioural changes, although further investigations of long-term effects and in different populations are warranted.

Keywords: Borderline gestational diabetes mellitus, Pregnant women, Diet, Exercise, Printed lifestyle intervention tool, Descriptive study

* Correspondence: shan.han@adelaide.edu.au
[1]Australian Research Centre for Health of Women and Babies (ARCH), Robinson Research Institute, School of Medicine, Discipline of Obstetrics and Gynaecology, The University of Adelaide, 72 King William Road, North Adelaide 5006, South Australia, Australia
Full list of author information is available at the end of the article

Background

Gestational diabetes mellitus (GDM) is defined as hyperglycaemia first recognised during pregnancy [1, 2]. Due to the increasing rates of maternal obesity and type two diabetes mellitus and the trend towards older maternal age, the prevalence of GDM is increasing worldwide [3–6].

GDM is associated with a range of adverse health outcomes for both the mothers and their babies [7–10]. Behavioural management, involving dietary and exercise interventions, has been found to be beneficial for women with pregnancy hyperglycaemia [11–15]. Medical nutrition therapy (MNT) has been recommended as the primary therapeutic strategy for managing pregnancy hyperglycaemia [16–19].

Printed lifestyle intervention tools have been frequently used for providing interventions and facilitating behavioural modifications in women with GDM [20–22]. However, there are few reports about the usefulness of these strategies for women with pregnancy hyperglycaemia.

This descriptive study was nested within a multicentre, randomised controlled trial that commenced in 2008, investigating the effect of dietary and lifestyle advice for women with borderline gestational diabetes [defined as a positive 50 g oral glucose challenge test (OGCT) (1 h venous plasma glucose ≥7.8 mmol/L) followed by a normal 75 g oral glucose tolerance test (OGTT) (fasting venous plasma glucose <5.5 mmol/L and a 2 h glucose <7.8 mmol/L)] (the IDEAL Study) [23]. As outlined in the published study protocol, women between 24^0 and 34^6 weeks' gestation with a singleton pregnancy, classified as having borderline GDM were eligible for the IDEAL Study [23]. Women were randomised into either the 'Intervention Group' or the 'Routine Care Group' [23]. Those in the Intervention Group had a lifestyle discussion with a dietitian as soon as they enrolled in the study and were given the pregnancy record booklets as part of the study intervention [23]. Women in the Routine Care Group received standard antenatal care with no lifestyle discussion or pregnancy record booklet provided [23].

The present study aimed to assess women's use of pregnancy record booklets provided to assist their dietary and lifestyle changes; to describe the woman's diet and exercise goals set during the initial lifestyle discussion; and to describe goals achieved after 1 month.

Methods

Participants and procedure

Women in the IDEAL study Intervention Group who received pregnancy record booklets during their initial lifestyle discussions with a dietitian, were invited to return their pregnancy record booklet after their babies were born. To facilitate booklet return via post, a reply paid envelope was attached to the pregnancy record booklet and women were made aware of it at the initial lifestyle discussion. Women were advised to bring their pregnancy record booklet when attending antenatal appointments and when admitted for childbirth. Women who returned and used their booklets at least once were included in this study.

The pregnancy record booklet

The pregnancy record booklet was designed for women to record their existing diet and exercise patterns and to set diet and exercise goals for the coming month (see Additional file 1 for sample pages), based on published recommendations and the best available evidence at that time [24, 25]. During the initial lifestyle discussion, the woman's diet and exercise were reviewed and diet and exercise goals aiming for adequate nutrient intake and optimal glycaemic control were set for the next month. Factors including the woman's age, pre-pregnancy weight, activity level, current dietary intake and weight gain for the current and any previous pregnancies were considered when advising women about their diet and exercise goals [23].

Individualised dietary and lifestyle goals focused on the quantity and quality of food consumption. Diet quantity was prespecified in the pregnancy record booklet as daily intakes of food from the categories of bread/cereal (grains), vegetable, fruit, dairy, meat and protein-rich food and foods high in fat, sugar and/or salt. Diet quality included choosing low glycaemic index foods, low fat dairy, higher fibre food varieties, lean meat, and using unsaturated oils and limiting fats and oils. Women's exercise goals focused on the type, duration, frequency and intensity of the physical activity, which were tabulated in the pregnancy record booklet.

One month after the initial lifestyle discussion, by using the pregnancy record booklet, women reviewed their dietary and exercise habits, set and documented new goals for the next month. Women were requested to review and reset their diet and exercise goals each month during pregnancy. If women had any concerns and/or questions around their diet and exercise after the initial lifestyle discussion, they were encouraged to talk with their attending midwives or obstetricians.

Analysis

Information recorded in the woman's pregnancy booklet was entered into the study database. Dietary data about quantity and quality of food consumed were transcribed, coded and categorized into seven categories as prespecified in the pregnancy record booklet including bread/cereal (grains), vegetable, fruit, dairy, meat and protein rich food, foods high in fat, sugar and/or salt and overall dietary goal. Exercise data were transcribed and coded, and analysed thematically by systematic comparisons based on grounded theory methods [26]. Women's use of pregnancy record booklet during pregnancy was analysed using SAS software version 9.3 (SAS Institute Inc., Cary, NC, USA).

Results

Participants and booklet use

A total of 56 women, who completed their initial lifestyle discussion at a mean (standard deviation) gestation of 31.6 (1.7) weeks, used booklets at least once by the end of pregnancy and were included in the study.

Women who used the booklet compared with all women who received a booklet from the randomised trial, were more likely to be primiparous (66.1 % versus 50.6 %), of Asian ethnicity (21.4 % versus 16.2 %), have a family history of diabetes (51.8 % versus 37.5 %) or hypertension (51.8 % versus 36.8 %); but were less likely to be obese (9.4 % versus 19.9 %), smoke (9.1 % versus 16.9 %) or be socially disadvantaged (12.5 % versus 21.8 %) (Table 1).

Table 1 Baseline characteristics: women who used pregnancy record booklet versus all women who received booklet

Characteristics	Women who returned booklets and used at least once (*n* = 56)	Women who received booklets (*n* = 358)
Maternal age (years)[a]	31.3 (4.5)	30.6 (5.1)
Primiparity	37 (66.1)	181 (50.6)
BMI Category		
-Underweight (<18.5 kg/m^2)	3 (5.7)	8 (2.3)
-Normal (18.5–24.9 kg/m^2)	30 (56.6)	182 (52.6)
-Overweight (25–29.9 kg/m^2)	15 (28.3)	87 (25.1)
-Obese (≥30 kg/m^2)	5 (9.4)	69 (19.9)
Race		
-White	43 (76.8)	265 (74.0)
-Asian	12 (21.4)	58 (16.2)
-Other	1 (1.8)	35 (9.8)
Smoker	5 (9.1)	59 (16.9)
Family history of diabetes	29 (51.8)	133 (37.5)
Family history of hypertension	29 (51.8)	130 (36.8)
Socioeconomic status[b]		
-Most disadvantaged	7 (12.5)	78 (21.8)
-Disadvantaged	10 (17.9)	56 (15.6)
-Average	15 (26.8)	72 (20.1)
-Advantaged	14 (25.0)	83 (23.2)
-Most advantaged	10 (17.9)	69 (19.3)

Figures are number and percentage
BMI body mass index
[a]Mean and standard deviation
[b]As measured by the Australian Bureau of Statistics Socio-Economic Indexes for Areas [29]

Use of the booklet by women included review of their current diet, dietary goal setting, their exercise pattern and exercise goal setting. Of the 56 women, all used the booklet at least once for reviewing their diet and 52 (92.9 %) used the booklet for setting their dietary goals for the next month; 53 (94.6 %) women used their booklets at least once for reviewing their exist pattern of exercise and 44 (78.6 %) used the booklet for setting exercise goals for the next month.

Dietary goal setting and achievement

Dietary goals were set from seven different food categories as prespecified in the pregnancy record booklet, including bread/cereal (grains); vegetable; fruit; dairy; meat and protein rich food; foods high in sugar, fat and/or salt, or not belonging to the categories above; and overall dietary goals which focused on the overall quantity or quality of the diet (Table 2). The most frequently targeted dietary goal was to reduce foods high in sugar, fat and/or salt, followed by overall dietary goals of maintaining good dietary patterns and/or habits.

Bread/ cereal (grains) group

The grains group was targeted by the fewest women (*n* = 20, 38.5 %) among the seven goal categories. Of the 22 goals, 11 were set to improve diet quality by choosing low glycaemic index food (GI) such as brown rice and pasta or higher fibre food varieties such as wholemeal bread (Table 2). The remaining goals were set to increase daily intake of food from this group. Of these, only two goals (20.0 %) were set to meet recommendations (Table 3).

After 1 month, the majority of women (*n* = 17, 85.0 %) achieved their goals, which included choosing low GI food or higher fibre food varieties (10 goals) and increasing daily serves according to the dietary recommendation (seven goals). Two (10.0 %) women who set two goals to increase their daily intake of bread and/or cereal (grains), improved their bread and/or cereal (grains) intake after 1 month, but did not reach their goals.

Vegetable group

Twenty-two (42.3 %) women set a total of 22 dietary goals relating to vegetables during the initial visit (Table 2). Almost all goals (*n* = 21, 95.5 %) aimed to increase daily vegetable intake (Table 2). Of these, 11 (52.4 %) met dietary recommendations and seven (33.3 %) partially met the recommendation (Table 3).

After 1 month, only seven (31.8 %) women achieved their goals, which included increasing vegetable intake (six goals) and reducing starchy vegetables (one goal). One (4.5 %) woman, who set a goal to increase her vegetable intake, reported decreased vegetable intake after 1 month (Table 2).

Table 2 Dietary goals women set and whether achieved after 1 month by category

Women's goal setting and achievement	Set goals	Achieved goals	Improved but did not achieve	Did not change	Worsened	Unknown
Dietary goals	*N*[a] (%)	*N* (%[b])	*N* (%)	*N* (%)	*N* (%)	*N* (%)
Bread, cereal (grains) group						
22 goals set by 20 women	20 (38.5)	17 (85.0)	2 (10.0)	2 (10.0)	-	-
–Increase overall daily intake –Choose low GI food varieties –Choose wholemeal/wholegrain bread –Choose wholemeal flour –Choose wholemeal pasta –Reduce gluten free bread						
Vegetable						
22 goals set by 22 women	22 (42.3)	7 (31.8)	4 (18.2)	6 (27.3)	1 (4.5)	4 (18.2)
–Increase daily vegetable intake –Less potato and sweet potato						
Fruit						
26 goals set by 25 women	25 (48.1)	18 (72.0)	3 (12.0)	2 (8.0)	-	3 (12.0)
-Increase overall daily fruit intake -Reduce overall daily fruit intake -Reduce daily fruit juice intake -Limit tropical fruit						
Dairy						
27 goals set by 25 women	25 (48.1)	20 (80.0)	1 (4.0)	2 (8.0)	-	2 (8.0)
-Choose low fat dairy -Increase dairy intake -Reduce dairy intake						
Meat and protein rich food						
26 goals set by 25 women	25 (48.1)	15 (60.0)	1 (4.0)	5 (20.0)	2 (8.0)	3 (12.0)
-Reduce overall meat intake -Increase overall meat intake -Choose lean meat -Increase red meat intake						
Extra food[c]						
40 goals set by 35 women	35 (67.3)	8 (22.9)	2 (5.7)	4 (11.4)	-	23 (65.7)
-Limit food high in fat, sugar and/or salt -Limit fat and oil-Change the type of fat used in cooking -Replace buttered toast with cereal and milk -Reduce coffee						
Overall dietary goal						
34 goals set by 23 women	23 (44.2)	22 (95.7)	-	-	-	2 (8.7)
-Maintain current dietary intake (quantity) -Maintain current good dietary habits (quality) -Reduce the overall food serving sizes						

GI Glycaemic Index
[a]Table subtotals do not add to 100 % because women may have set multiple goals for one goal category
[b]percentage of women who set goals
[c]includes food high in fat, sugar and/or salt, and those do not belong to any of the five main food groups

Fruit group

During the initial lifestyle discussion, 25 (48.1 %) women set 26 goals relating to fruit (Table 2). Most goals ($n = 19$, 73.1 %) were to adjust the serves of daily fruit intake according to the dietary recommendations, including 16 goals to increase fruit intake and three goals to reduce daily fruit intake (Table 2). For optimal glycaemic control, other goals included limiting high GI fruit such as tropical fruits (five goals) and limiting fruit juice intake (two goals) (Table 2). Of the 19 goals to adjust daily serves, about half ($n = 10$, 52.6 %) met the dietary recommendations, three (15.8 %) were more than the recommendations and another three (15.8 %) were less than the dietary recommendations (Table 3).

Table 3 Dietary goals women set in relation to dietary recommendations[a]

Food groups	Met dietary recommendation	More than dietary recommendation	Less than dietary recommendation	Unknown	Total
Bread, cereal	2 (20.0)	0 (0.0)	6 (60.0)	2 (20.0)	10
Vegetable	11 (52.4)	0 (0.0)	7 (33.3)	3 (14.3)	21
Fruit	10 (52.6)	3 (15.8)	3 (15.8)	3 (15.8)	19
Dairy	12 (85.7)	1 (7.1)	0 (0.0)	1 (7.1)	14
Meat	4 (21.1)	10 (52.6)	3 (15.8)	2 (10.5)	19

Figures are number and percentage
1. Bread/cereal group: 4–6 serves/ day
2. Vegetable: 5–6 serves/ day
3. Fruit: 2–4 serves/ day
4. Dairy: 2–3 serves/ day
5. Meat/ other protein: 1.5 serves/ day

[a]According to Australian Guide to Healthy Eating (1998) [24]

After 1 month, most ($n = 18$, 72.0 %) women achieved their dietary goals of increased fruit intake (9 goals), reduced tropical fruit (5 goals) and reduced fruit intake (4 goals). Three (12.0 %) women who set three goals of increased fruit intake reported increased intake but did not achieve their goals after 1 month (Table 2).

Dairy group

During the initial lifestyle discussion, 25 (48.1 %) women set 27 goals relating to dairy (Table 2). Of the goals set, 13 goals focused on improving diet quality by choosing low fat dairy products (Table 2). The remaining 14 goals were to adjust number of serves per day according to the dietary recommendations, including 13 goals to increase dairy intake and one goal to reduce dairy intake. Of these, the majority were set to meet the dietary recommendations (12, 85.7 %) and one (7.1 %) was more than the recommendation (Table 3).

After 1 month, the majority of women ($n = 20$, 80 %) successfully achieved 22 goals they set, which included increasing dairy intake (10 goals) and choosing low fat dairy food (12 goals). One (4.0 %) woman, who set one goal to reduce her daily dairy intake, reported reduced daily dairy intake but did not achieve her goal.

Meat and other protein-rich food group

During the initial lifestyle discussion, 25 (48.1 %) women set 26 goals relating to meat and other protein rich food (Table 2). Of the goals set, seven goals aimed to improve diet quality by choosing lean meat (6 goals) and including more red meat in diet (1 goal). The remaining 19 goals were to adjust the daily serves of protein food intake, including 14 goals aimed to reduce and five goals to increase meat intake. Of these, only four (21.1 %) met the recommendations, 10 (52.6 %) were more than the recommended daily serves, and three (15.8 %) were less than the recommendations.

After 1 month, most women ($n = 15$, 60.0 %) achieved their goals including reducing meat intake (six goals), increasing meat intake (five goals) and choosing lean meat (four goals). One (4.0 %) woman who set a goal to reduce her daily meat intake reported decreased meat intake after 1 month but did not completely achieve her goal. Two (8.0 %) women, who planned to reduce their daily meat intake, reported an increased intake after 1 month (Table 2).

Extra food group including foods high in sugar, fat and/or salt and those do not belong to any of the above mentioned five main food groups

This food group was the most frequently targeted by the women among the seven dietary goal categories. Thirty-five (67.3 %) women set a total of 40 goals during the initial lifestyle discussion (Table 2). The most frequently proposed goal was to limit food high in sugar, fat and/or salt (27 goals) followed by limiting fats and oil intake (eight goals) (Table 2). After 1 month, eight (22.9 %) women achieved eight goals they set included reducing fat, oil and/or sweets intake; two (5.7 %) women who set two goals reported they reduced their intake of soft drink and chocolate but had not fully achieved their goals; four (11.4 %) women who set four goals did not achieve their goals of decreasing chips, biscuits, ice-cream and cakes after 1 month (Table 2). For 23 (65.7 %) women who set a total of 26 goals, whether they achieved their goals is not known as there was insufficient information recorded in the booklets returned (Table 2).

Overall goals

Twenty-three (44.2 %) women set a total of 34 overall goals. Of these goals set, 20 aimed for maintaining their existing dietary intake, 13 were set to maintain their existing good dietary habits and one goal was set to reduce overall serve sizes across the five main food groups as the woman had a relatively balanced, but oversized, diet (Table 2).

After 1 month, 22 (95.7 %) women achieved 32 goals they set to either maintain their existing dietary intake or existing good dietary habits.

Exercise goal and achievement

During the initial lifestyle discussion, 53 women proposed a total of 65 exercise goals from six different categories including to increase walking, maintain existing active lifestyle, increase recreational exercise, increase incidental exercise, adjust exercise intensity and improve overall fitness (Table 4).

The most frequently proposed exercise goal by women was to increase walking (28 women, 28 goals). After 1 month, seven (25.0 %) women had achieved their goals, six (21.4 %) women had improved their walking exercise but had not achieved their goals, eight (28.6 %) women did not change their walking exercise, two (7.1 %) women reported a poorer exercise pattern where their walking exercise was decreased and for five (17.9 %) women it is not known if they had achieved their goals (Table 4).

A total of 22 (50.0 %) women set a goal of maintaining their existing active exercise pattern (Table 4). The majority of women (19 women, 86.4 %) achieved their goals successfully after 1 month but three (13.6 %) women reported a poorer exercise pattern during the review after 1 month where their physical activity levels were decreased.

During the initial lifestyle discussion, eight (18.2 %) women set a total of eight goals to increase their recreational exercise that included hydrotherapy, swimming, yoga, Pilates and pelvic floor exercises (Table 4). After 1 month, four (50.0 %) women achieved their goals; one (12.5 %) woman increased her recreational exercise but did not achieve the goal she set; one (12.5 %) woman did not change her recreational exercise pattern and for two women it is unknown if they achieved their recreational exercise goals (Table 4).

During the initial lifestyle discussion, four (9.1 %) women set four goals for increasing incidental exercise that included gardening and housework. After 1 month, two women (50 %) achieved their goals and the remaining two women (50 %) did not change their incidental exercise pattern (Table 4).

Two (4.5 %) women set two goals to adjust their exercise intensity during pregnancy, which included increased walking intensity and decreased gym exercise intensity. After 1 month, one (50 %) woman achieved her goal and the other 50 % woman did not report if she achieved her goal (Table 4).

Discussion

We found that, after a month, women were likely to achieve goals for grains, fruits, dairy foods and overall diet, but less likely to meet goals targeting vegetables and limiting extra foods (including foods high in fat, sugar and/or salt and those not belonging to any of the five main food groups).

In our study, a high proportion of women reported their dietary intakes were lower than the recommendations for categories of grains, vegetables, fruits and dairy, therefore most goals were to increase daily intakes of food from these categories. While women's daily intakes for meat and alternatives, and food from the extra food group category were more likely to be more than the recommendation, with most goals set to reduce daily intakes. Our findings were consist with the results from large observational studies, where Australian pregnant women reported lower consumption of all food groups, except for meat (and alternatives) and discretionary foods [27, 28]. Only a small proportion of women in our study seemed able to set and achieve a goal to meet the dietary recommendations by increasing their grain intakes or decreasing meat intakes.

For exercise goals, women who were already active and aimed to maintain their existing exercise pattern were more likely to be successful. Other exercise goals proposed by women, including increasing walking, increasing recreational exercise, adjusting exercise intensity and improving level of fitness all had a relatively low achievement rate after 1 month.

Few studies have reported on the use of a printed lifestyle tool to assist women with pregnancy hyperglycaemia in making changes to their dietary and exercise habits. Our findings help to provide in-depth understanding of the use by women of a printed lifestyle tool, their ability to assess their current diet and exercise patterns and their willingness to set lifestyle goals. This

Table 4 Exercise goals women set and whether achieved after 1 month

Exercise goal categories	Set goals N (%)	Achieved goals N (%)	Improved but did not achieved N (%)	Did not change N (%)	Worsened N (%)	Unknown N (%)
Increase walking	28 (63.6)	7 (25.0)	6 (21.4)	8 (28.6)	2 (7.1)	5 (17.9)
Maintain exercise pattern	22 (50.0)	19 (86.4)	-	-	3 (13.6)	-
Increase recreational exercise	8 (18.2)	4 (50.0)	1 (12.5)	2 (25.0)	-	1 (12.5)
Increase incidental exercise	4 (9.1)	2 (50.0)	-	2 (50.0)	-	-
Adjust exercise intensity	2 (4.5)	1 (50.0)	-	-	-	1 (50.0)
Improve overall fitness	1 (2.3)	-	-	-	-	1 (100.0)

information may help to design behavioural intervention tools in the future and providing tailored care for women needing such advice.

A limitation of this study is that women were invited, but not required, to return booklets, and only a minority of women did so; in addition, the majority of women (94.6 %) who returned their booklets were from two geographical areas (Adelaide, South Australia and Melbourne, Victoria, Australia), which may limit generalisability of the study findings. In our study, information from the pregnancy record booklet about women's diet and exercise changes was self-reported, so there may be differences between what women reported and what their diet and exercise patterns actually were. We were unable to assess whether goals achieved within the first month were sustained beyond this time. Longer term follow-up to assess the goals women set and whether able to be achieved over a longer period will be worth considering in any future studies.

Conclusions

This descriptive study suggests that most dietary and exercise goals are achieved by women with borderline GDM who used a printed pregnancy record booklet. Women's dietary goals targeting grains, fruits, dairy foods and overall dietary pattern are more likely to be achieved while dietary goals for improving vegetable and foods high in fat, sugar and/or salt and those do not belong to any of the five main food groups were less often achieved. Maintaining women's existing active lifestyle is feasible during pregnancy although goals to increase physical activities are not as likely to be reached.

Providing a printed pregnancy record booklet may be beneficial in encouraging and assisting behavioural changes during pregnancy, although further assessment in different populations with longer term follow-up is warranted.

Ethics approval and consent to participate

Human research ethics approval was obtained from the Children, Youth and Women's Health Service (CYWHS) Human Research Ethics Committee (REC 1860/8/12) for the IDEAL Study [23]. Written consent from participants was obtained. The lead investigator for the IDEAL Study, C A Crowther, provided permission for use of the IDEAL Study data for this manuscript.

Consent for publication

Not applicable.

Abbreviations

ARCH: Australian Research Centre for Health of Women and Babies; BMI: Body mass index; GDM: Gestational diabetes mellitus; GI: Glycaemic index; IDEAL Study: Investigation of dietary advice and lifestyle for women with borderline gestational diabetes; MNT: Medical nutrition therapy; OGCT: Oral glucose challenge test; OGTT: Oral glucose tolerance test.

Competing interests

None of the authors have any financial or non-financial competing interests associated with the publication of this manuscript.

Authors' contributions

SH contributed to the conception and design of the study, transcribed and coded diet and exercise data, performed data analysis, drafted the manuscript and revised according to other author's comments and contributions. PFM contributed to the conception and design of the study, provided advice on data analysis, commented on and edited all drafts of the manuscript. TST performed and provided advice on data analysis, commented on all drafts of the manuscript. CAC contributed to the conception and design of the study, commented on and edited all drafts of the manuscript. All authors read and approved the final manuscript.

Acknowledgements

All the women who participated in the study; Mr Vincent Ball and Mr Sasha Zhang for preparing and managing the study database; Ms Elen Shute and Ms Claire Binnion for assisting booklet data entry; Dr Joanna Tieu for assisting in the initial booklet design.

Author details

[1]Australian Research Centre for Health of Women and Babies (ARCH), Robinson Research Institute, School of Medicine, Discipline of Obstetrics and Gynaecology, The University of Adelaide, 72 King William Road, North Adelaide 5006, South Australia, Australia. [2]Women's and Children's Health Research Institute, 72 King William Road, North Adelaide 5006, South Australia, Australia. [3]Garvan Institute of Medical Research, 384 Victoria Street, Darlinghurst 2010, NSW, Australia. [4]Liggins Institute, The University of Auckland, Private Bag 92019 Victoria Street West, West Auckland 1142, Auckland, New Zealand.

References

1. Metzger BE, Coustan DR. Summary and recommendations of the fourth international workshop-conference on gestational diabetes mellitus. The organizing committee. Diabetes Care. 1998;21(2):B161–167.
2. Alberti KG, Zimmet PZ. Definition, diagnosis and classification of diabetes mellitus and its complications. Part 1: diagnosis and classification of diabetes mellitus provisional report of a WHO consultation. Diabet Med. 1998;15:539–53.
3. Bottalico JN. Recurrent gestational diabetes: risk factors, diagnosis, management, and implications. Semin Perinatol. 2007;31:176–84.
4. Debelea D, Snell-Bergeon JK, Hartsfield CL, Bischoff KJ, Hamman RF, McDuffie RS, et al. Increasing prevalence of gestational diabetes mellitus (GDM) over time and by birth cohort: Kaiser Permanente of Colorado GDM screening program. Diabetes Care. 2005;28:579–84.
5. Mulla W, Henry T, Homko C. Gestational diabetes screening after HAPO: has anything changed? Curr Diab Rep. 2010;10:224–8.
6. Ferrara A. Increasing prevalence of gestational diabetes mellitus: a public health perspective. Diabetes Care. 2007;30 Suppl 2:S141–146.
7. International association of diabetes and pregnancy study groups (IADPSG). International association of diabetes and pregnancy study groups recommendations on the diagnosis and classification of hyperglycemia in pregnancy. Diabetes Care. 2010;33:676–82.
8. Ju H, Rumbold AR, Willson KJ, Crowther CA. Borderline gestational diabetes mellitus and pregnancy outcomes. BMC Pregnancy Childbirth. 2008;8:31.
9. The HAPO Study Cooperative Research Group. Hyperglycemia and adverse pregnancy outcome (HAPO) study: associations with neonatal anthropometrics. Diabetes. 2009;58:453–9.
10. Reece EA, Leguizamón G, Wiznitzer A. Gestational diabetes: the need for a common ground. Lancet. 2009;373:1789–97.

11. Bonomo M, Corica D, Mion E, Gonçalves D, Motta G, Merati R, et al. Evaluating the therapeutic approach in pregnancies complicated by borderline glucose intolerance: a randomized clinical trial. Diabet Med. 2005;22:1536–41.
12. Crowther CA, Hiller JE, Moss JR, McPhee AJ, Jeffries WS, Robinson JS, et al. Effect of treatment of gestational diabetes mellitus on pregnancy outcomes. N Engl J Med. 2005;352:2477–86.
13. Landon MB, Spong CY, Thom E, Carpenter MW, Ramin SM, Casey B, et al. A multicenter, randomized trial of treatment for mild gestational diabetes. N Engl J Med. 2009;361:1339–48.
14. Alwan N, Tuffnell DJ, West J. Treatments for gestational diabetes. *Cochrane Database Syst Rev.* 2009; doi: 10.1002/14651858.CD003395.pub2
15. Han S, Crowther CA, Middleton P, Heatley E. Different types of dietary advice for women with gestational diabetes mellitus. Cochrane Database Syst Rev. 2013; doi: 10.1002/14651858.CD009275.pub2
16. American College of Obstetricians and Gynecologists (ACOG). ACOG practice bulletin. Clinical management guidelines for obstetrician-gynecologists. Number 30, september 2001 (replaces technical bulletin number 200, December 1994). gestational diabetes. Obstet Gynecol. 2001;98:525–38.
17. Hoffman L, Nolan C, Wilson JD, Oats JJ, Simmons D. Gestational diabetes mellitus-management guidelines. The Australasian diabetes in pregnancy society. Med J Aus. 1998;169:93–7.
18. National Institute for Health and Care Excellence (NICE). Diabetes in pregnancy: management of diabetes and its complications from preconception to the postnatal period. 2015. https://www.nice.org.uk/guidance/ng3. Accessed March 23, 2015.
19. American Diabetes Association. Standards of medical care in diabetes-2015. Diabetes Care. 2015;38:S1–S93.
20. Grant SM, Wolever TM, O'Connor DL, Nisenbaum R, Josse RG. Effect of a low glycaemic index diet on blood glucose in women with gestational hyperglycaemia. Diabetes Res Clin Pract. 2011;91:15–22.
21. Louie JC, Markovic TP, Perera N, Foote D, Petocz P, Ross GP, et al. A randomized controlled trial investigating the effects of a low-glycemic index diet on pregnancy outcomes in gestational diabetes mellitus. Diabetes Care. 2011;34:2341–6.
22. Moses RG, Barker M, Winter M, Petocz P, Brand-Miller JC. Can a low-glycemic index diet reduce the need for insulin in gestational diabetes mellitus? A randomized trial. Diabetes Care. 2009;32:996–1000.
23. Crowther CA, Hague WM, Middleton PF, Baghurst PA, McPhee AJ, Tran TS, et al. The IDEAL study: investigation of dietary advice and lifestyle for women with borderline gestational diabetes: a randomised controlled trial - study protocol. BMC Pregnancy Childbirth. 2012;12:106.
24. Smith A, Kellett E, Schmerlaib Y. Australian guide to healthy eating. Department of Health and Ageing: Canberra; 1998. http://nht.org.au/wp-content/uploads/2014/03/AustralianGuidetoHealthyEating.pdf. Accessed November 20, 2014.
25. Han S, Crowther CA, Middleton P. Interventions for pregnant women with hyperglycaemia not meeting gestational diabetes and type 2 diabetes diagnostic criteria. Cochrane Database Syst Rev. 2012; doi: 10.1002/14651858.CD009037.pub2
26. Glaser B, Strauss A. The discovery of grounded theory: strategies for qualitative research. Chicago: Aldine; 1967.
27. Mishra G, Schoenaker D, Mihrshahi S, Dobson A. How do women's diets compare with the new Australian dietary guidelines? Public Health Nutr. 2014;18(2):218–25.
28. Malek L, Umberger W, Makrides M, Zhou J. Adherence to the Australian dietary guidelines during pregnancy: evidence from a national study. Public Health Nutr. 2015;31:1–9.
29. Australian Bureau of Statistics (ABS). Census of population and housing: socio-economic indexes for areas (SEIFA), Australia- data only 2006 (cat. no. 2033.0.55.001). 2008.

Differences in pregnancy outcomes and characteristics between insulin- and diet-treated women with gestational diabetes

Katrien Benhalima[1*], Karolien Robyns[1], Paul Van Crombrugge[2], Natascha Deprez[2], Bruno Seynhave[3], Roland Devlieger[4], Johan Verhaeghe[4], Chantal Mathieu[1] and Frank Nobels[2]

Abstract

Background: Our aim was to evaluate the difference in pregnancy outcomes and characteristics between insulin- and diet-treated women with gestational diabetes (GDM).

Methods: Retrospective analysis of the medical files from 2010–2013 of women with GDM diagnosed with the Carpenter & Coustan criteria attending two clinics, one in a university and another in a non-university hospital. Characteristics associated with insulin use were analyzed. Multivariable logistic regression was used to adjust for confounders. For women attending the university hospital, indices of insulin sensitivity such as the reciprocal of the homeostasis model assessment of insulin resistance (1/HOMA-IR) and an index of beta-cell function, the Insulin Secretion-Sensitivity Index-2 (ISSI-2) were calculated.

Results: Over a 4 year period, 601 women were identified with GDM of whom 22.9 % were obese at first prenatal visit. 24.2 % needed insulin. Insulin did not prevent adverse outcomes, as women on insulin had higher rates of large-for-gestational age infants (LGA) (28.5 % vs. 13.1 %, $p < 0.0001$) and more cesarean sections (44.1 % vs. 27.0 %, $p = 0.001$), remaining significant after adjustment for confounders. Compared to diet-treated women, women on insulin more often had an ethnic minority background (33.3 % vs. 21.6 %, $p = 0.004$), more often had a history of GDM (21.5 % vs. 10.4 %, $p = 0.002$), were more often multiparous (59.3 % vs. 47.6 %, $p = 0.044$) and were diagnosed with GDM earlier in pregnancy (weeks 25.3 ± 4.9 vs. 27.1 ± 3.7, $p < 0.0001$). When undergoing an oral glucose tolerance test, women treated with insulin had a higher fasting glycaemia (97.6 ± 18.8 vs.87.7 ± 10.3, $p < 0.0001$), a higher 1-hour glycaemia (197.7 ± 30.1 vs.184.5 ± 25.8, $p < 0.0001$), a higher 2-hour glycaemia (185.2 ± 28.5 vs. 175.0 ± 22.8, $p < 0.0001$), more often 3 and 4 abnormal values (58.1 % vs. 37.8 %, $p < 0.0001$ and 24.8 % vs. 7.7 %, $p < 0.0001$) and higher HbA1c levels (5.5 ± 0.6 vs 5.2 ± 0.5, $p < 0.0001$). ISSI-2 (1.3 ± 0.5 vs. 1.7 ± 0.5, $p < 0.0001$) and 1/HOMA-IR [0.01 (0.001–0.002) vs. 0.02 (0.01–0.03), $p = 0.027$] were lower in women on insulin. Women on insulin more often received corticoids in preparation of preterm delivery (11.0 % vs. 2.4 %, $p < 0.0001$).

Conclusion: Compared to diet-treated women with GDM, women treated with insulin have a higher risk profile, impaired beta-cell function and lower insulin sensitivity. Rates of LGA and cesarean sections were higher in insulin-treated women.

Keywords: Gestational diabetes, Treatment, Insulin, Diet

* Correspondence: katrien.benhalima@uzleuven.be
[1]Department of Endocrinology, UZ Gasthuisberg, KU Leuven, Herestraat 49, 3000 Leuven, Belgium
Full list of author information is available at the end of the article

Background

Gestational diabetes (GDM) is a frequent medical condition during pregnancy and was historically defined as 'any degree of glucose intolerance with onset or first recognition during pregnancy' [1]. GDM has long been known to raise the risk of a large-for-gestational age infant (LGA) and macrosomia resulting in increased rates of shoulder dystocia and caesarian deliveries [2, 3]. Shortly after the delivery the glucose values are generally restored to normal, but women with GDM have a sevenfold increased risk of developing type 2 diabetes (T2DM) [4]. Two large randomized intervention trials have demonstrated improvement in perinatal outcomes in the group of women who received treatment of mild GDM, especially in the frequency of LGA and preeclampsia [5, 6]. Initial treatment of GDM involves diet modification, glucose monitoring and moderate exercise [7]. If lifestyle is insufficient to maintain the glycemic targets, pharmacological therapy becomes necessary. Insulin has been the treatment of choice when lifestyle measures do not maintain glycemic control during pregnancy. Recent studies have suggested that metformin and glibenclamide (glyburide) may be safe and acceptable alternatives but there is a paucity of long-term follow up data on children exposed to oral agents in utero [8, 9]. Recent data also point towards the fact that sulfonylurea do cross the placenta when used in high doses [10]. The American Diabetes Association (ADA) therefore only recommends insulin as pharmacotherapy for GDM [7]. The difference in pregnancy outcomes between insulin- and diet-treated women with GDM and the profile of women where insulin-therapy is warranted, remain unclear. The aim of our study was therefore to evaluate the pregnancy outcomes and characteristics in insulin- versus diet-treated women with GDM in Belgian patients.

Methods

Retrospective analysis of the electronic medical files of all women with GDM diagnosed with the Carpenter & Coustan criteria attending two large obstetrical centers in Belgium (the University Hospital UZ Leuven and the non-university hospital OLV Aalst-Asse-Ninove) from 01–01–2010 till 31–12–2013. The study was approved by the Institutional Review Board of UZ Leuven (ML 10085) and by the Institutional Review Board of the hospital OLV Aalst-Asse-Ninove (B126201422577). Due to the retrospective nature of the study there was no need for informed consent from the participants as in compliance with the Belgian Law of December 8,1992 on the protection of privacy and the Belgian Law of August 22, 2002 on the rights of the patient.

Approximately 2400 women are delivered annually at UZ Leuven and about 1700 women at the hospital OLV Aalst-Asse-Ninove. The background prevalence of T2DM in the adult Belgian population is 6.5 % [11]. In the general adult population 28 % of women are overweight and 13 % are obese [12]. Accurate data on the prevalence of GDM are lacking in Belgium and the current practice for screening for GDM varies across different centers [13]. In both centers, women were not yet universally screened for overt diabetes early in pregnancy. All pregnant women were screened and diagnosed for GDM according to the Fifth International Workshop Conference criteria [14]. Women received a 50 g glucose challenge test (GCT) between 24–28 weeks and those testing positive [threshold after 1-h ≥ 140 mg/dl (7.8 mmol/l)] had a 3-hour 100 g oral glucose tolerance test (OGTT) within two weeks after the GCT using the Carpenter & Coustan criteria for GDM [fasting plasma glucose (FPG) ≥ 95 mg/dl (5.3 mmol/l), 1-hour glycaemia ≥ 180 mg/dl (10.0 mmol/l), 2-hour glycaemia ≥ 155 mg/dl (8.6 mmol/l) and 3-hour glycaemia ≥ 140 mg/dl (7.8 mmol/l), diagnosis of GDM if ≥ 2 values are abnormal]. Although there are no specific recommendations in both centers on which women should receive screening for GDM before 24 weeks of pregnancy, screening for GDM with a 50 g GCT is sometimes performed before 24 weeks of pregnancy in high risk women such as women with a history of GDM. Women with GDM were treated with insulin when despite lifestyle measures the FPG was ≥ 95 mg/dl (5.3 mmol/l) and/or 2-hour postprandial glycaemia ≥120 mg/dl (6.7 mmol/l). To uniform the initiation for insulin therapy as much as possible, the 'Weekly Average Glycaemia' (WAG) is calculated based on the self-monitoring values of the blood glucose (fasting and postprandial) during the first weeks after the diagnosis. Therapy with insulin is initiated when the fasting WAG and/or the postprandial WAG is above target during two weeks in a row. The treatment and follow up policies were identical in both centers. In both centers oral anti-diabetes drugs such as metformin and glibenclamide (glyburide) are not routinely used during pregnancy.

Outcomes were obtained from review of the electronic database. Maternal characteristics recorded were age, ethnicity, weight, body mass index (BMI) at first prenatal visit and at delivery, overweight (BMI ≥25 Kg/m^2), obesity (BMI ≥ 30 Kg/m^2), weight gain (difference in weight between first prenatal visit and the delivery), parity, a history of a first degree or second degree relative with diabetes and history of GDM. Excessive weight gain was defined according to the most recent Institute of Medicine (IOM) guidelines [15]. Other data that were recorded are: the glucose values and the insulin values (only for UZ Leuven) based on the 100 g OGTT during pregnancy (0 min-60 min-120 min-180 min), gestational age at delivery, the timing and result of the GCT, the gestational age at the diagnosis of GDM, HbA1c at the time of the 100 g OGTT during pregnancy, whether women received treatment with corticoids during pregnancy, need of insulin, type of insulin and number of injections and the gestational age at the start of insulin.

The following maternal pregnancy outcomes were recorded: gestational hypertension (blood pressure ≥ 140/90 mmHg), preeclampsia [hypertension with proteinuria or in combination with reduced fetal growth or the 'Hemolysis Elevated Liver enzymes and Low Platelets' (HELPP)-syndrome], preterm delivery (<37 weeks of gestation) and cesarean section (planned + emergency sections combined). The following neonatal outcomes were recorded: birth weight, macrosomia (birth weight > 4 kg), large-for-gestational age infants (LGA, birth weight >90 percentile adjusted for sex and parity), small-for-gestational age infants (SGA, birth weight <10 percentile adjusted for sex and parity), shoulder dystocia, Apgar score (at five minutes) and admission at the neonatal intensive care unit (NICU).

Since insulin levels were not available from women from the OLV Aalst-Asse-Ninove hospital, indices of insulin sensitivity and an index of beta-cell function were only analyzed from women attending the university hospital UZ Leuven. Insulin sensitivity was measured using the insulin sensitivity index of Matsuda, a well-established measure of whole-body insulin sensitivity [16]. The insulin sensitivity index of Matsuda is defined as 10 000/√ [(FPG x fasting plasma insulin) X (mean glucose during OGTT x mean insulin during OGTT)] [16]. As a secondary measure of insulin sensitivity (largely hepatic), we also calculated the reciprocal of the homeostasis model assessment of insulin resistance (1/HOMA-IR) [17]. HOMA-IR is calculated as the product of FPG and fasting plasma insulin divided by 22.5 [17]. Beta-cell function was assessed by the insulin secretion sensitivity index (ISSI-2), an OGTT-derived measure that is analogous to the disposition index obtained from the frequently sampled intravenous glucose tolerance test [18, 19]. Glycaemia was assessed by the area under the glucose curve (AUC glucose) during the OGTT, calculated using the trapezoidal rule [18, 19]. ISSI-2 is defined as the product of 1) insulin secretion measured by the ratio of the AUC insulin to the AUC glucose and 2) insulin sensitivity measured by the insulin sensitivity index of Matsuda [18, 19]. All these measures have been validated for use in pregnancy.

In UZ Leuven, HbA_{1c} was measured by reversed-phase cation-exchange chromatography (ADAMS HA-8160, Menarini Diagnostics Benelux, Zaventem, Belgium) and in OLV Aalst-Asse-Ninove hospital with a capillary zone electrophoresis on a Capillarys 2 Flex Piercing (Sebia). Hba1c is reported in compliance with the National Glycohemoglobin Standardization Program (NGSP). In Both centers plasma glucose was measured by an automated colorimetric-enzymatic method (hexokinase-glucose-6-phosphate-dehydrogenase, application 668) on a Hitachi/Roche-Modular P analyzer. Insulin was measured by the immunometric ECLIA (Roche Modular E170, Basel, Switserland).

Statistical analyses

Statistical analyses were performed using SPSS 22.0. Continuous variables were presented as mean and standard deviation if normally distributed and as median otherwise.

Categorical variables were presented as percentage. To compare variables between two groups independent samples *t*-tests were used for normally distributed continuous variables, Mann–Whitney's *U*-test for non-normally distributed continuous variables and chi-squared tests for categorical variables. A univariable analysis was done initially, and then clinical variables that were identified as most significantly associated with the need for insulin use were included in a multivariable logistic regression. Treatment with corticoids was a significant variable in the univariable analysis but this was not included in multivariable logistic regression since it could not be excluded that treatment with corticoids preceded the use of insulin in some patients. Multivariable logistic regression was also used to analyse the impact of possible confounders such as age, BMI, ethnicity, multi-parity, excessive weight gain and center on pregnancy outcomes and on the indices of insulin sensitivity and beta-cell function. Although the treatment protocol for GDM was similar in both centers, a center was also used as a variable to adjust for differences in population characteristics and potential differences in obstetrical management between both centers. A *p*-value of <0.05 (two-tailed) was considered significant.

Results

Over a 4 year period, 644 women were identified with GDM. After evaluation of the medical files, 43 files were not included in the analysis due to insufficient data (29) or because women took part in a study using the 'International Association of Diabetes and Pregnancy Study groups' (IADPSG) criteria for GDM (14), leaving a cohort of 601 women with GDM for analysis. Of the whole cohort 269 women (44.8 %) attended the university hospital and 332 women (55.2 %) attended the non-university hospital. The prevalence of GDM at the time of the study was 3.3 % in the university center and 5.1 % in the non-university center. Of the whole cohort, 29.7 % had an abnormal fasting glycaemia on the OGTT,

64.1 % had an abnormal 1-hour value, 90.5 % had an abnormal 2-hour value and 68.7 % had an abnormal 3-hour value. In 47.4 % of women the 3-hour value on the OGTT contributed to the diagnosis of GDM. Table 1 gives an overview of the general characteristics of the cohort. Of all women with GDM 24.5 % were from an ethnic minority background (EMB): South Asian (25.3 %), Northern-African (19.8 %), Black African (18.4 %) and Middle-East (13.0 %). 24.1 % (145) of women needed insulin during pregnancy. Of all women on insulin, 69.1 % (92) received only short acting insulin, 2.3 % (3) received only long-acting insulin and 28.6 % (38) received both short -and long acting insulin. Of all women on short acting insulin, 57.1 % (76) received short acting insulin at each meal. The most commonly used short acting insulins were the insulin analogues aspart or lispo (92.9 %) and the most commonly used long acting insulin was NPH insulin (90.2 %). The insulin was stopped after the delivery except in two women. The general characteristics were pretty similar between both centers. In particular, rates of insulin use were not significantly different between the university and non-university center (27.2 % vs. 21.8 %, $p = 0.291$). Table 1 gives an overview of the similarities and differences between both centers.

Table 2 gives an overview of the differences in pregnancy outcomes of the whole cohort between the insulin- and diet-treated women GDM. Insulin did not prevent adverse outcomes, as women on insulin had higher rates of LGA (28.5 % vs. 13.1 %, $p < 0.0001$) and more cesarean sections (44.1 % vs. 27.0 %, $p = 0.001$), remaining significant after adjustment for age, BMI, excessive weight gain, ethnicity, multi-parity and center.

Table 3 gives an overview of the differences in characteristics of the whole cohort between the insulin- and diet-treated women with GDM. Compared to diet-treated women, women on insulin were more often from an EMB (33.3 % vs. 21.6 %, $p = 0.004$), more often had a history of GDM (21.5 % vs. 10.4 %, $p = 0.002$), were more often multiparous (59.3 % vs. 47.6 %, $p = 0.044$) and were diagnosed with GDM earlier in pregnancy. Women on insulin also had higher glycaemic values on the OGTT and more often 3 and 4 abnormal values with higher HbA1c levels at the time of the OGTT (Table 3). In the multivariable regression analysis fasting glycaemia at the time of the OGTT remained the only independent predictor for antenatal insulin requirement ($p < 0.0001$) (Table 3). Based on a receiver operating characteristics (ROC) curve for FPG with an AUC of 0.676, a FPG cut-of ≥ 88.5 mg/dl (4.9 mmol/l) had the best sensitivity and specificity combined of resp. 62.6 % and 60.6 % to predict insulin requirements. 62.8 % of women who had a FPG ≥ 88.5 mg/dl (4.9 mmol/l) on the OGTT required insulin treatment but with a low positive predictive value of 52.3 %.

Table 4 gives an overview of the differences in insulin sensitivity and beta-cell function between the insulin- and diet-treated women with GDM attending the

Table 1 The general characteristics and the differences between both centers of the cohort of women with GDM

	General cohort N = −601	University hospital N = 269 (44.8 %)	Non-University hospital N = 332 (55.2 %)	*p*-value
Mean age (years)	31.9 ± 4.8	32.0 ± 4.8	31.5 ± 4.8	**0.028**
% first degree relative with diabetes	18.3 % (109)	14.9 % (40)	21.1 % (69)	**<0.0001**
% second degree relative with diabetes	21.8 % (130)	8.2 % (22)	33.0 % (108)	**<0.0001**
% with a history of GDM	13.1 % (78)	12.3 % (33)	13.8 % (45)	**0.023**
% overweight	32.2 % (158)	34.2 % (89)	30.0 % (69)	0.317
% obese	22.9 % (112)	22.3 % (58)	23.5 % (54)	0.758
% excessive weight gain	19.7 % (103)	22.0 % (55)	17.5 % (48)	0.197
% EMB	24.5 % (146)	37.2 % (100)	14.1 % (46)	**<0.0001**
Fasting glycaemia at OGTT in mg/dl (mmol/l)	90.0 ± 13.4 (5.0 ± 0.7)	93.6 ± 15.6 (5.5 ± 0.9)	87.3 ± 10.8 (4.8 ± 0.6)	**<0.0001**
HbA1c, mean in % (mmol/mol)	5.3 ± 0.5 (34 ± 6)	5.4 ± 0.5 (36 ± 6)	5.1 ± 0.4 (32 ± 5)	**<0.0001**
% Insulin use	24.1 % (145)	27.2 % (73)	21.8 % (72)	0.291
% macrosomia	8.7 % (52)	7.5 % (20)	9.7 % (32)	0.329
% LGA	16.9 % (101)	16.8 % (45)	17.1 % (56)	0.927
% Preterm delivery	13.0 % (187)	18.3 % (49)	8.8 % (29)	**<0.0001**
% cesarean section	31.2 % (187)	36.6 %(98)	26.96 % (89)	**0.011**
% shoulder dystocia	1.2 % (7)	2.2 % (6)	0.3 % (1)	**0.029**
% admission NICU	9.6 % (57)	16.4 % (44)	4.0 % (13)	**<0.0001**

GDM gestational diabetes, *EMB* ethnic minority background, *OGTT* oral glucose tolerance test, *LGA* large-for-gestational age infants, *NICU* neonatal intensive care unit, P-values in bold are significant values

Table 2 The differences in pregnancy outcomes between the insulin- and diet-treated women with GDM

	Diet $N = 456$ (75.9 %)	Insulin $N = 145$ (24.1 %)	*p*-value	Adjusted *p*-value
% Gestational hypertension	7.7 % (35)	4.2 % (6)	0.140	
% preeclampsia	4.0 % (18)	7.6 % (11)	0.076	
% Preterm delivery	12.8 % (58)	13.9 % (20)	0.743	
% cesarean section	27.0 % (122)	44.1 % (64)	**<0.0001**	**0.001**
Birth weight (g)	3208.2 ± 600.9	3321.4 ± 589.2	**0.049**	0.144
% macrosomia	7.3 % (33)	12.6 % (18)	**0.049**	0.226
% LGA	13.1 % (59)	28.5 % (41)	**<0.0001**	**<0.0001**
% SGA	11.3 % (51)	8.3 % (12)	0.309	
% shoulder dystocia	1.1 % (5)	1.4 % (2)	0.788	
% low Apgar score	2.2 % (10)	2.8 % (4)	0.702	
% admission NICU	8.7 % (39)	12.5 % (18)	0.174	

g grams, *LGA* large-for-gestational age infants, *SGA* small-for-gestational age infants; low Apgar score: <7 at 5 min; *NICU* neonatal intensive care unit; The *p*-values are adjusted for age, BMI, excessive weight gain, ethnicity, multi-parity and center, P-values in bold are significant values

Table 3 The differences in characteristics between the insulin- and diet-treated women with GDM

	Diet $N = 456$ (75.9 %)	Insulin $N = 145$ (24.1 %)	*p*-value	*Adjusted *p*-value
Age, mean (y)	31.8 ± 4.8	32.5 ± 4.7	0.109	
Gestational age, mean (y)	39.3 ± 16.8	38.0 ± 1.6	0.352	
Mean BMI (Kg/m^2) at first prenatal visit	26.8 ± 12.9	29.1 ± 20.2	0.149	
% overweight	32.4 % (121)	31.6 % (36)	0.877	
% obese	21.4 % (80)	27.2 % (31)	0.196	
% exessive weight gain	18.5 % (73)	22.7 % (29)	0.306	
% EMB	21.6 % (97)	33.3 % (48)	**0.004**	0.939
% first degree relative with diabetes	16.7 % (75)	22.9 % (33)	0.107	
% second degree relative with diabetes	23.1 % (104)	17.4 % (25)	0.107	
% history of GDM	10.4 % (47)	21.5 % (31)	**0.002**	0.142
% multiparous	47.6 % (216)	59.3 % (86)	**0.044**	0.998
% primigravida	36.0 % (163)	23.4 % (34)	**0.020**	0.260
Week of GCT, mean	25.4 ± 3.3	23.6 ± 4.9	**<0.0001**	0.203
Value of GCT, mean in mg/dl (mmol/l)	166.7 ± 19.6 (9.3 ± 1.1)	179.0 ± 40.0 (9.9 ± 2.2)	**<0.0001**	0.304
Week of GDM diagnosis mean	27.1 ± 3.7	25.3 ± 4.9	**<0.0001**	0.278
Fasting glycaemia at OGTT in mg/dl (mmol/l)	87.7 ± 10.3 (4.9 ± 0.6)	97.6 ± 18.8 (5.4 ± 1.0)	**<0.0001**	**<0.0001**
1-hour glycaemia at OGTT in mg/dl (mmol/l)	184.5 ± 25.8 (10.2 ± 1.4)	194.7 ± 30.1 (10.8 ± 1.7)	**<0.0001**	0.417
2-hour glycaemia at OGTT in mg/dl (mmol/l)	175.0 ± 22.8 (9.7 ± 1.3)	185.2 ± 28.5 (10.3 ± 1.6)	**<0.0001**	0.342
3-hour glycaemia at OGTT in mg/dl (mmol/l)	145.4 ± 27.6 (8.1 ± 1.5)	152.7 ± 33.4 (8.5 ± 1.8)	**0.013**	0.238
% ≥3 abnormal values on the OGTT	37.8 % (161)	58.1 % (75)	**<0.0001**	0.915
% ≥4 abnormal values at OGTT	7.7 % (33)	24.8 % (32)	**<0.0001**	0.756
HbA1c, mean in % (mmol/mol)	5.2 ± 0.5 (33 ± 6)	5.5 ± 0.6 (37 ± 6)	**<0.0001**	0.496
% treatment with corticoïds	2.4 % (11)	11.0 % (16)	**<0.0001**	

Y years, *BMI* body mass index, *EMB* ethnic minority background, *GCT* glucose challenge test, *OGTT* oral glucose tolerance test, *GDM* gestational diabetes *Adjusted *p*-value: Clinical variables that were identified as most significantly associated with the need for insulin use were included in the multivariable logistic regression, P-values in bold are significant values

Table 4 The differences in insulin sensitivity and beta-cell function between the insulin- and diet-treated women with GDM from the university hospital

	Diet $N = 196$(73.0 %)	Insulin $N = 73$(27.0 %)	P value	Adjusted p value
ISSI-2 index mean	1.7 ± 0.5	1.3 ± 0.5	**<0.0001**	**<0.0001**
Matsuda index median	2.9 (1.9–3.7)	2.3 (1.4–3.3)	**0.019**	0.206
1/HOMA-IR median	0.02 (0.01–0.03)	0.01 (0.01–0.02)	**<0.0001**	**0.027**

GDM: gestational diabetes; ISSI-2: insulin secretion sensitivity index during pregnancy; Matsuda: insulin sensitivity index of Matsuda during pregnancy; 1/HOMA-IR: the reciprocal of the homeostasis model assessment of insulin resistance during pregnancy. The p-values are adjusted for age, BMI, excessive weight gain, ethnicity and multi-parity, P-values in bold are significant values

university hospital. In women attending the university hospital, ISSI-2 (1.3 ± 0.5 vs. 1.7 ± 0.5, $p < 0.0001$) and 1/HOMA-IR [0.01 (0.001–0.002) vs. 0.02 (0.01–0.03), $p = 0.027$] were significantly lower in women on insulin, remaining significant after adjustment for age, BMI, excessive weight gain, ethnicity and multi-parity.

Discussion

The insulin requirement for the treatment of GDM varies according to the population studied and which screening strategy and diagnostic criteria are used for GDM. Most studies show insulin use in GDM between 10–30 %, in line with the insulin need in our study of 24.1 % [20–22]. Insulin did not prevent adverse outcomes in our study, as women on insulin had higher rates of LGA (28.5 %) and more cesarean sections (44.1 %) compared to diet-treated women (resp. 13.1 %, $p < 0.0001$ and 27.0 %, $p = 0.001$), remaining significant after adjustment for BMI, excessive weight gain, ethnicity, age, multi-parity and center. These data show that especially in women on insulin, rates of LGA and cesarean sections remain much higher compared to the LGA and cesarean rates in pregnant women without GDM of resp. 9.0 % and 23.3 % in our population, as was shown previously by our research group [23]. Controlling hyperglycaemia in pregnancy is certainly not the only essential factor to decrease the problem of LGA newborns. The HAPO study has shown that both maternal GDM and obesity are independently associated with adverse pregnancy outcomes and that the combination of obesity and GDM shows a greater risk of these adverse pregnancy outcomes than either obesity or GDM alone [24]. Gestational weight gain is also a known independent risk factor for accelerated fetal growth [25]. BMI and excessive weight gain were however not different between the two groups in our study but of all women with GDM 32.2 % were overweight and 22.9 % were obese at the first prenatal visit. There is clearly a need for better preconception assessment and counseling for overweight and obese women with the aim to lose weight before pregnancy and also to limit weight gain in pregnancy. In our study oral anti-diabetes drugs were not used during pregnancy. Insulin has been the treatment of choice when lifestyle measures do not maintain glycemic control during pregnancy. The long acting insulins NPH and detemir and the short acting insulins human regular and the insulin analogues lispro and aspart have all been proven to be safe for use during pregnancy [7]. However, insulin is associated with an increased risk for hypoglycaemia and weight gain, which might be a hurdle to reach an optimal glycaemic control and contribute to the increased rates of adverse pregnancy outcomes seen in women with GDM on insulin. Some studies have suggested that metformin may be a safe and acceptable alternative for the treatment of GDM with less maternal weight gain compared to insulin and with no increase in congenital anomalies, despite it crossing the placenta [8, 26, 27]. However there is a paucity of long-term follow up data on children exposed to oral agents in utero. More research is therefore necessary to evaluate whether the addition of metformin to insulin can improve pregnancy outcomes in women with GDM and whether this is also safe on the long term.

Our study also shows that women with GDM on insulin had a more adverse metabolic risk profile compared to diet-treated women with GDM with an earlier diagnosis of GDM, higher glucose values on the OGTT and more often >2 abnormal values on the OGTT. Women on insulin were also more often from an EMB, more often multiparous and more often had a history of GDM. However only the fasting glycaemia at the time of the OGTT was an independent predictor for antenatal insulin requirement in the regression analysis in our population. Other studies have shown independent predictors for antenatal insulin requirement to be a positive family history of diabetes, multiple abnormal values on the OGTT, the BMI, the time of diagnosis, the fasting glucose on the OGTT and HbA1c at the diagnosis of GDM [20–22]. The large variation seen in predictors between the different studies is probably related to the differences in the ethnic origin of the populations studied, the differences in sample size and the different screening strategies used for GDM. Several studies have indicated fasting glucose during the OGTT as a potent predictor of antenatal insulin treatment in GDM, in accordance with our finding [22, 28, 29]. However, depending on the methodology of the study, on the target of glucose levels used or ethnic differences, different cut-off values of fasting glucose varying from 87 mg/dl (4.8 mmol/l) to 105 mg/dl (5.8 mmol/l) have been demonstrated to predict the need for insulin [22, 28, 29]. In our population a FPG cut-off level ≥88.5 mg/dl (4.9 mmol/l) had the best sensitivity and specificity rates but with a low positive predictive value. This FPG cut-off is lower than the general recommended FPG target for the treatment of GDM of < 95 mg/dl (5.3 mmol/l) and is also closer to the FPG cut-off proposed by the IADPSG for the diagnosis of GDM compared to the Carpenter & Coustan criteria we used. This might suggest that a lower FPG target for the treatment of GDM might be indicated but there is a need for large randomized intervention trials evaluating the benefit of lower glycaemic targets for the treatment of GDM on pregnancy outcomes.

Our data also show a reduced insulin sensitivity and impaired beta-cell function in women on insulin, which remained significant after adjustment for confounders such as BMI, age, ethnicity, and excessive weight gain. It has long been thought that the insulin resistance provided a short-term challenge to the beta-cells, with GDM arising in those women whose beta-cells were unable to meet this challenge. Several studies have shown that the defect in beta-cell compensation that characterizes GDM is chronic and probably not just acquired during pregnancy. Shortly after delivery the insulin resistance is generally restored to the pre-pregnancy level but often the chronic beta-cell dysfunction persists [30, 31]. We have previously shown in our population that 39.1 % of women with a recent history of GDM, had glucose intolerance based on the OGTT three months postpartum and that these women also had a persistent impaired beta-cell function and lower insulin sensitivity postpartum [32].

In our cohort, less than one third of women had an abnormal fasting glycaemia on the OGTT while the 2-hour and 3-hour glycaemia values were most frequently abnormal. However, in contrast to the FPG, the 2-and 3-hour glycaemia were not anymore significantly associated with the use of insulin in the multivariable logistic regression. The use of a 2-hour 75 g OGTT with the Carpenter & Coustan criteria for the diagnosis of GDM was accepted as an alternative by the previous ADA recommendations, but this is clearly less validated than the use of the 3-hour 100 g OGTT [1]. If a 2-hour 75 g OGTT would be used in our population with the Carpenter & Coustan criteria for GDM, the prevalence of GDM would decrease importantly since the 3-hour value contributed to the diagnosis of GDM in nearly half of all women with GDM.

Strengths of the study are the detailed characterization of a large cohort of women with GDM using a good database. Variables that were identified as most significantly associated with the need for insulin use were included in a multivariable logistic regression. Pregnancy outcomes and measures of insulin sensitivity and beta-cell function were adjusted for multiple confounders. A limit of the study is the retrospective nature of the analysis and the fact that insulin values were only available from women attending the university hospital.

Conclusions

Compared to diet-treated women with GDM, women treated with insulin have a higher metabolic risk profile, impaired beta-cell function and lower insulin sensitivity. Moreover, insulin did not prevent adverse outcomes, as rates of LGA and cesarean sections were still higher in insulin-treated women. Women with GDM needing insulin remain a high risk population and more research is necessary to improve outcomes in this group.

Competing interests

The authors declare that they have no competing interests.

Authors' contributions

KB, KR, FN, ND, PVC and CM have made substantial contributions to the conception of the study and have been involved in drafting the manuscript. KB and KR have collected the data. KB, KR, FN, ND, PVC, JV, RD and CM have been involved in revising it critically for important intellectual content. All authors have given final approval of the version to be published.

Acknowledgements

KB is the recipient of a Clinical Doctoral Scholarship of 'FWO Vlaanderen' and RD is the recipient of a 'Fundamenteel Klinisch Navorserschap FWO Vlaanderen'.

Author details

[1]Department of Endocrinology, UZ Gasthuisberg, KU Leuven, Herestraat 49, 3000 Leuven, Belgium. [2]Department of Endocrinology, OLV ziekenhuis Aalst-Asse-Ninove, Moorselbaan 164, 9300 Aalst, Belgium. [3]Department of Obstetrics and Gynecology, OLV ziekenhuis Aalst-Asse-Ninove, Moorselbaan 164, 9300 Aalst, Belgium. [4]Department of Obstetrics and Gynecology, UZ Gasthuisberg, KU Leuven, Herestraat 49, 3000 Leuven, Belgium.

References

1. American Diabetes Association. Diagnosis and classification of diabetes mellitus. Diabetes Care. 2009;32:S62–7.
2. Study HAPO, Cooperative Research Group, Metzger BE, Lowe LP, Dyer AR, Trimble ER, et al. Hyperglycemia and adverse pregnancy outcomes. N Engl J Med. 2008;358:1991–2002.
3. Gilmartin AB, Ural SH, Repke JT. Gestational diabetes mellitus. Rev Obstet Gynecol. 2008;1:129–34.
4. Bellamy L, Casas JP, Hingorani AD, Williams D. Type 2 diabetes mellitus after gestational diabetes: a systematic review and meta-analysis. Lancet. 2009;373:1773–9.
5. Crowther CA, Hiller JE, Moss JR, McPhee AJ, Jeffries W, Robinson JS. Australian Carbohydrate Intolerance study in Pregnancy Women (ACHOIS) Trial Group. Effect of treatment of gestational diabetes mellitus on pregnancy outcomes. N Engl J Med. 2005;352:2477–86.
6. Landon MB, Spong CY, Thom E, Carpenter M, Ramin SM, Casey B, et al. A multicenter, randomized trial of treatment for mild gestational diabetes. N Engl J Med. 2009;361:1339–48.
7. American Diabetes Association. Standards of Medical Care in diabetes-2014. Diabetes Care. 2014;37:S14–80.
8. Rowan JA, Hague WM, Gao W, Battin MR, Moore MP, MiG Trial Investigators. Metformin versus insulin for the treatment of gestational diabetes. N Engl J Med. 2008;358:2003–15.

9. Zeng YC, Li MJ, Chen Y, Jiang L, Wang SM, Mo XL, et al. The use of glyburide in the management of gestational diabetes mellitus: a meta-analysis. Adv Med Sci. 2014;59:95–101.
10. Myngheer N, Allegaert K, Hattersley A, McDonald T, Kramer H, Ashcroft FM, et al. Fetal macrosomia with transplacental transfer of sulfonylurea in a mother with KCNJ11-related neonatal diabetes. Diabetes Care. 2014;37:3333–5.
11. International Diabetes Federation, Diabetes e-Atlas, 6th edn, Brussels. http://www.idf.org/sites/default/files/EN_6E_Atlas_Full_0.pdf (2013). Accessed 13 March 2015.
12. Http://statbel.fgov.be/nl/statistieken/cijfers/bevolking/structuur. Accessed 20 December 2012
13. Benhalima K, Van Crombrugge P, Devlieger R, Verhaeghe J, Verhaegen A, De Catte L, et al. Screening for pregestational and gestational diabetes in pregnancy: a survey of obstetrical centers in the northern part of Belgium. Diabetology and Metabolic Syndrome. 2013;5:66. doi:10.1186/1758-5996-5-66.
14. Metzger BE, Buchanan TA, Coustan DR, de Leiva A, Dunger DB, Hadden DR, et al. Summary and recommendations of the Fifth International Workshop-Conference on Gestational Diabetes Mellitus. Diabetes Care. 2007;30 suppl 2:S251–60.
15. Institute of Medicine (US) and National Research Council (US) Committee to Reexamine IOM Pregnancy Weight Guidelines. Weight Gain During Pregnancy: Reexamining the Guidelines. In: Rasmussen KM, Yaktine AL, editors. National Academies Press (US). Washington: The National Academies Collection: Reports funded by National Institutes of Health; 2009.
16. Matsuda M, Defronzo RA. Insulin sensitivity indices obtained from oral glucose tolerance testing. Comparison with the euglycemic insulin clamp. Diabetes Care. 1999;22:1462–70.
17. Matthews DR, Hosker JP, Rudenski AS, Naylor BA, Treacher DF, Turner RC. Homeostasis model assessment: insulin resistance and beta-cell function from fasting plasma glucose and insulin concentrations in man. Diabetologia. 1985;28:412–9.
18. Kirwan JP, Huston-Presley L, Kalhan SC, Catalano PM. Clinically useful estimates of insulin sensitivity during pregnancy: validation studies in women with normal glucose tolerance and gestational diabetes. Diabetes Care. 2001;24:1602–7.
19. Retnakaran R, Qi Y, Goran MI, Hamilton JK. Evaluation of proposed oral disposition index measures in relation to the actual disposition index. Diabet Med. 2009;26:1198–203.
20. Mitra S, Nayak PK, Sahoo J, Mathew A, Padma A, Kamalanathan S, et al. Predictors for antenatal insulin requirements in gestational diabetes. Gynecol Endocrinol. 2014;30:565–8.
21. Wong VW, Jalaludin B. Gestational diabetes mellitus: who requires insulin therapy? Aust NZ J Obstet Gynaecol. 2011;51:432–6.
22. Bakiner O, Bozkirli E, Ozsahin K, Sariturk C, Ertorer E. Risk factors that can predict antenatal insulin need in gestational diabetes. J Clin Med Res. 2013;5:381–8.
23. Benhalima K, Hanssens M, Devlieger R, Verhaeghe J, Mathieu C. Analysis of pregnancy outcomes using the new IADPSG recommendation compared with the Carpenter and Coustan criteria in an area with a low prevalence of gestational diabetes. Int J Endocrinology. 2013. doi:10.1155/2013/248.121.
24. Catalano PM, McIntyre HD, Cruickshank JK, McCance DR, Dyer AR, Metzger BE, et al. The Hyperglycemia and adverse pregnancy outcome study. Associations of GDM and obesity with pregnancy outcomes. Diabetes Care. 2012;35:780–6.
25. Ludwig DS, Currie J. The association between pregnancy weight gain and birthweight: a within-family comparison. Lancet. 2010;376:984–90.
26. Gui J, Liu Q, Feng L. Metformin vs insulin in the management of gestational diabetes: a meta-analysis. Plos One. 2013;8:e64585–5.
27. Balsells M, Garcia-Patterson A, Sola I, Roque M, Gich I, Corcoy R. Glibenclamide, metformin, and insulin for the treatment of gestational diabetes: a systematic review and meta-analysis. BMJ. 2015. doi:10.1136/nmj.h102.
28. Juutinen J, Hartikainen AL, Bloigu R, Tapanainen JS. A retrospective study on 435 women with gestational diabetes: fasting plasma glucose is not sensitive enough for screening but predicts a need for insulin treatment. Diabetes Care. 2000;23:1858–9.
29. Akinci B, Caltik A, Yener S, Yesil S. Is fasting glucose level during oral glucose tolerance test an indicator of the insulin need in gestational diabetes ? Diabetes Res Clin Pract. 2008;82:219–25.
30. Buchanan A, Xiang AH. Gestational diabetes mellitus. J Clin Invest. 2005;115:485–91.
31. Buchanan TA. Pancreatic B-Cell Defects in Gestational Diabetes: Implications for the Pathogenesis and Prevention of Type 2 Diabetes. J Clin Endocrinol Metab. 2001;86:989–93.
32. Benhalima K, Leuridan L, Calewaert P, Devlieger R, Verhaeghe J, Mathieu C. Glucose intolerance after a recent history of gestational diabetes. Int J Endocrinology. 2014. doi:10.1155/2014/727652.

21

Development and initial testing of a GDM information website for multi-ethnic women with GDM

Mary Carolan-Olah[1*], Cheryl Steele[2] and Gillian Krenzin[2]

Abstract

Background: Gestational diabetes mellitus (GDM) affects approximately 5–15 % of pregnant women in Australia. Highest rates are seen among women who are obese, from specific ethnic backgrounds and low socio-economic circumstance. These features also impact on uptake of self-management recommendations. GDM that is not well managed can give rise to serious pregnancy complications. The aim of this project was to develop and test an intervention to improve knowledge of GDM and GDM self-management principles.

Methods: A web-based intervention, consisting of resources aimed at a low level of literacy, was developed and tested among multi-ethnic women at a metropolitan hospital in Melbourne Australia. A basic one-group pre-test/post-test design was used to explore the impact of the intervention on knowledge, in 3 domains: (1) Knowledge of GDM; (2) food values, and;(3) GDM self-management principles. Questionnaire data was analysed using Statistical Package for the Social Sciences (SPSS), version 21.0. Fisher's exact test was used to test for an improvement in each knowledge scale.

Results: Twenty-one women with GDM, from multi-ethnic backgrounds, participated in the testing of the intervention. Results indicated that the intervention was effective at improving knowledge scores and this effect was greatest in the first domain, knowledge of GDM. Although some improvement of knowledge scores occurred in the other two domains, food values and self-management principles, these improvements were less than expected. This finding may relate to a number of misunderstandings in the interpretation of the web resource and survey questions. These issues will need to be resolved prior to proceeding to a clinical trial.

Conclusion: Initial results from this study look promising and suggest that with some improvements, the intervention could prove a useful adjunct support for women with GDM from multi-ethnic and low socio-economic backgrounds. Conducting a randomised controlled trial is feasible in the future and will provide a useful means of examining efficacy of the intervention.

Keywords: Gestational diabetes, Self-management, Knowledge, Intervention, Internet

Background

In Australia, Gestational Diabetes Mellitus (GDM) affects approximately 5 % of pregnant women overall [1] and figures are considerably higher among women from specific ethnic backgrounds, such as Asian and South Asian. In such groups, GDM rates may be 2–3 times higher than national rates [2, 3]. These high rates are a concern as GDM is linked to a number of adverse outcomes for mothers and infants. Mothers are more likely to experience: induction of labour; pre-term birth, caesarean section, hypertension and extended hospital stay [1]. Infants of mothers with GDM are predisposed to hypoglycaemia [4], higher rates of stillbirth, macrosomia and birth injury [5], low apgar scores, admission to special care nursery, and longer hospital stays [1, 4]. Careful management of GDM reduces these risks [4, 6].

Self-care is the most usual approach to GDM management and women are taught to: monitor their blood glucose levels; adjust their dietary intake to GDM recommendations, and; increase physical activity, in a bid to maintain

* Correspondence: Mary.carolan@vu.edu.au
[1]Nursing and Midwifery, College of Health and Biomedicine, Victoria University, St Alban's Campus, PO Box 14228, Melbourne 8001, Australia

blood glucose levels within normal limits. These changes can be very difficult and, for some women quite extensive, due to previous dietary and exercise habits. For these reasons, many women struggle to adhere to GDM recommendations [7–10], particularly as changes must be adopted immediately [8, 11]. Additionally, in order to successfully self-manage the condition, women need to understand GDM, the importance of self-management [4], what constitutes a healthy diet, the impact of different foods on blood glucose levels, and the amount and type of exercise to undertake [8]. Emotional support is critical to motivation and a number of studies indicate that such support contributes positively to GDM skills development [7, 10]. Conversely, a number of factors are identified as likely to impact negatively on the adoption of health recommendations. These factors include: low educational attainment [12], limited health literacy [13], and low levels of English language proficiency [14]. Each of these features increase the likelihood that women will experience significant difficulty self-managing their GDM.

Overall, there is a need for GDM interventions that target low income, ethnically diverse and low literacy groups, as these groups are at high risk of developing GDM. However, despite this clear need, such programs are rare, and only two published studies were identified that reported on interventions to improve levels of knowledge and GDM outcomes among low socio-economic and minority groups [15, 16]. In the first instance, Hoppichler and Lechleitner [16] tested an intervention, which involved repeated intensive dietary counselling, among locally born women with GDM, compared to low literate migrant Turkish women, also with GDM, in Austria. Secondly, Mendelson et al., [15] used a similar approach for low income Mexican-American women with GDM, in California, USA. Both studies considered their interventions successful and also emphasised the importance of ensuring acceptability of educational resources [15, 16]. Furthermore, the literature suggests that in order for GDM interventions to be effective in low income groups, resources need to be pitched at a low level of health literacy [17] and experts in the field recommend using strategies such as pictorial representation of important information and repetition of simple instructions [18]. The provision of culturally sensitive resources is also recognised as important and as likely to improve acceptability and uptake of the intervention [15, 19].

With this information in mind, the website intervention, reported in this paper, aimed to address such issues as cultural sensitivity, low health literacy and low levels of English proficiency, in the belief that women with GDM need resources that they understand and that are culturally relevant to them. The intervention was developed for use in a low socio-economic area of Melbourne [20], where women incur a higher GDM incidence than that recorded nationally [21]. In this area, there are high levels of obesity [22], and as many as one third of the population speak a language other than English at home [23]. In this paper, development and initial testing of the intervention, is discussed. The intervention was planned to serve as an adjunct to routine educational sessions by the dietician and diabetes educator. The team also aimed to test ease of use, relevance and acceptability of the website for the target group of women, and to consider the feasibility of proceeding to a clinical trial.

Theoretical model

The philosophy of the intervention was based on empowerment of pregnant women [24, 25] and the website was developed along the principles of adult learning theory, that is, the understanding that adults will dedicate effort to learning when the aims and objectives are realistic and important to them [26]. Moreover, within adult learning theory there is an assumption that adults draw on personal experience to make sense of and to integrate new information [27]. Thus, the intervention has incorporated a series of steps anchored to the women's previous knowledge of food values and dietary concerns, and includes small incremental changes that are likely to be adopted. This approach acknowledges that pregnant women come from diverse backgrounds with different experiences, motivation and understanding. Another psychological theory that has informed the work, is Leventhal et al.'s common sense theory [28, 29]. Leventhal et al.'s [28] common sense theory suggests that individuals create a mental image of their illness, in this case GDM, based on various forms of information at their disposal. Such information commonly includes lay information, from friends and family, more formal information such as from the doctor or midwife, and the individual's own sense making of their experiences with the illness [29]. We therefore incorporated a number of images to assist with comprehension of GDM, such as the following image, which diagrammatically represents the basis of the disorder:

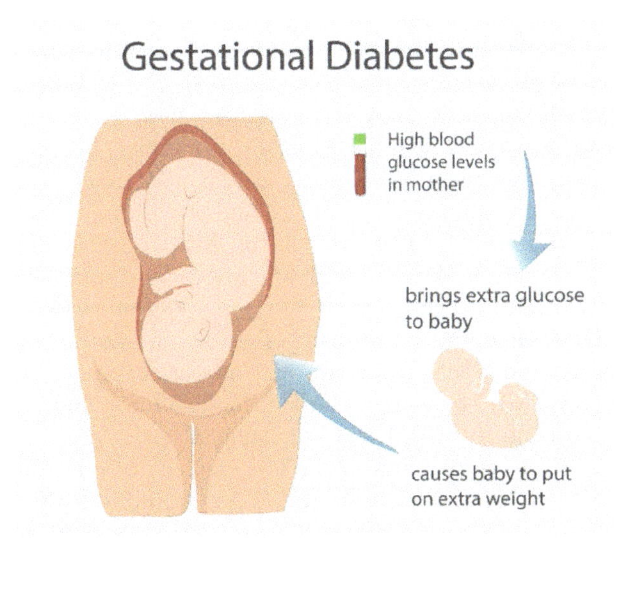

One of the difficulties with GDM is a tendency for women to underestimate the seriousness of the condition, based on it's transient quality and we aimed to address this difficulty by re-iteration of the impact, for the baby, of unmanaged GDM. We choose this approach, as in our earlier study, we found that 'thinking about the baby' was a powerful motivator for women to manage their GDM [10].

The overall challenge was to convey the urgency of behavioural change without unnecessarily alarming the women.

Methods

A basic pre-test/post-test survey questionnaire design was used to measure differences, if any, in knowledge of GDM, food values and GDM self-management principles before and after the intervention. This particular approach was chosen as it is considered suitable for measuring changes in behaviours or attitudes [30] and it has been successfully used in a number of nursing and health related studies [31, 32]. Additionally, we intended this testing of the intervention as a means of identifying any weaknesses in the design, and any deficits in general user-friendliness and acceptability for the target group of women. For these reasons, we included three additional questions in the post-test questionnaire, where participants were asked to give feedback on the intervention, in terms of (1) ease of use; (2) value of the information on the website; and (3) any changes or inclusions they would recommend.

Data collection

Instruments

The instrument used was the Knowledge of GDM questionnaire [33] which is based on an earlier validated questionnaire, the Diabetes Knowledge Scale, developed to measure knowledge and understanding of diabetes types 1 and 2, food values, and maintenance of blood glucose levels [34]. A number of modifications were made to the earlier questionnaire in a bid to make it more relevant to GDM and changes were informed by an expert panel, as reported elsewhere [33]. The Knowledge of GDM questionnaire, has now been used successfully among women with GDM from a number of ethnic groups, including Vietnamese, Indian and locally born Australian women [33], and White American, African American and Asian women in America [35]. The questionnaire is composed of twenty-four questions, which fall into three main domains: (1) Knowledge of GDM, including the impact of GDM on mother and baby, and recognising normal glycemic levels; (2) Knowledge of food, including food values; and, (3) Knowledge of GDM self-management principles (see Fig. 1 for sample questions). The majority of questions had one correct answer and were scored simply as correct/ incorrect. Four questions had more than one correct answer, and were scored as correct (all correct answers identified) or incorrect (did not identify all correct answers). The additional 3 questions which sought the women's views of the website, as above, completed the post-test questionnaire.

Description of intervention

In earlier studies, we found that most pregnant women in the area, despite their low income status, had access to smart phones and/or computer and that this was their preferred medium for learning about GDM [33]. For these reasons, we developed a web-based intervention, for use on home computers, tablets and smart phones. Women accessing the intervention progress through a series of information sheets, which address topics such as *'what is GDM'* and *'what is healthy eating'*. The intervention also offers practical advice and instruction such as *what to do if you are hungry between meals*. Instructions are phrased simply as short sentences, with a green tick, for acceptable foods, and a red x for poor choices. There are a large number of pictures and minimal amounts of text, and these are recognized as useful approaches for addressing low levels of literacy [36, 37]. An explanation of the amount of exercise that is required, and the type of exercise that is safe in pregnancy, is also included. Representation of ethnic specific food (Western, Vietnamese, Indian, Chinese) and portions appropriate for pregnant women, is placed alongside an explanation of the amount of exercise that is required to burn up the calories contained in the food, as below:

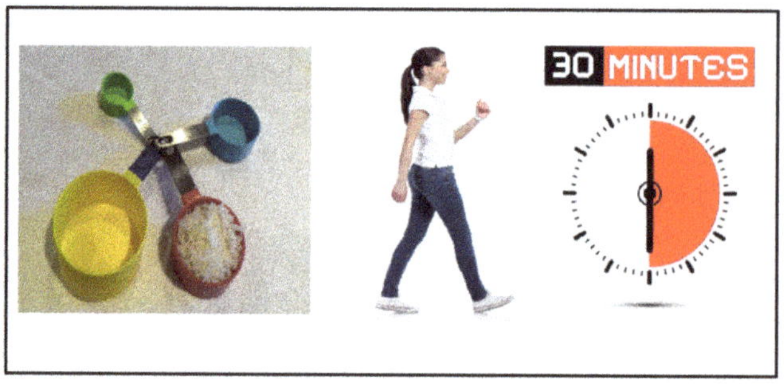

1/2 cup cooked rice = 122 calories = Walking x 30 minutes

Recruitment and data collection

A convenience sample of 21 women from the hospital diabetes clinic tested the first version of the intervention. We used the following inclusion criteria:

- Pregnant
- Diagnosis of GDM
- More than 18 years of age
- Singleton pregnancy

Domain	Question
Domain 1: Knowledge of GDM	Because I have gestational diabetes, my baby may be: **a. larger than usual** b. smaller than usual **c. born early** **d. admitted to special care** e. I don't know
Domain 1: Knowledge of GDM	In uncontrolled diabetes the blood glucose is: a. normal **b. increased** c. decreased d. I don't know
Domain 1: Knowledge of GDM	The normal range for blood glucose is: **a. 3.5-7 mmol/L** b. 7-15 mmol/L c. 2-10 mmol/L d. I don't know
Domain 2: Knowledge of food	Rice is mainly: a. protein **b. carbohydrate** c. fat d. mineral and vitamin e. I don't know
Domain 3: Knowledge of self-management principles	Which of the following snacks are suitable for the woman with gestational diabetes: a. An apple b. Small handful nuts c. Low fat yoghurt d. Cracker and low fat cheese **e. Any of the above**
Domain 3: Knowledge of self-management principles	One serve of carbohydrate might be: a. 1 slice multigrain bread b. I medium potato c. 1 roti/chapati d. 1/3 cup cooked rice **e. Any of the above**

Fig. 1 Sample questions

- Conversational English, as this initial website is in English

Ethics approval was granted by the Western Health (Sunshine Hospital) low risk ethics panel (HREC/11/WH/81). Women were given a verbal description of the intervention and advised that participation was voluntary. Interested women were invited to go through the website using the touchscreen or computer in the clinic waiting room. Those who agreed to participate, provided written consent. Participants filled in a pre-test questionnaire (approximately 5 min), perused the website while waiting for their clinic appointments, and filled in the post-test questionnaire (approximately 5 min) at their next appointment one week later. A research assistant was available to assist the women to navigate the website and to read out the questionnaire and record the participant's responses, if the participant wished. Five participants requested this level of assistance.

Data analysis

A cross table was created comparing the improvement in each of the three scores (GDM, Food, Self-management) against the participant's level of education (Table 2). Fisher's Exact test was used to test for an association between each scale's improvement and the education variable as this test is suitable for small data sets [38]. The *P*-values for these tests are provided below each sub-table.

Results

Demographic characteristics

Twenty one women were included in the pre-test/ post-test evaluation. Participants were predominantly from Vietnamese, Australian, Indian and Chinese backgrounds, which is reflective of the population presenting for gestational diabetes services in our region. Age distribution is also typical, with most women aged < 35 years. Completed years of schooling varied from less than 6 years to more than 12 years, with most participants having attended some high school (Table 1).

Table 1 Demographic detail

Country of birth	n
Vietnam	6
Australia	5
India	5
China	3
Philippines	1
Sudan	1
Total	21
Age	n
21-25 years	4
26-30 years	6
31-35 years	6
36-40 years	3
41-45 years	1
Not declared	1
Total	21
Years of education	n
<6 (did not complete primary school)	1
11 years or fewer – did not completed high school	10
12 years or more –completed high school	9
Not declared	1
Total	21

A small number of questions were left unanswered, and overall, there were 17 complete sets of GDM and Food improvement scores and 19 complete sets of Self-management improvement scores. Although data analysis suggests insufficient evidence to support an association between education level and improvement of any of the three scales, patterns in the results may suggest otherwise. For example, there were more women who improved in the *11 years or fewer* education group compared to *More than 12 years* (Table 2).

It was also possible consider the sample as a whole. The percentage of those who improved (or stayed at 100 % correct) post-intervention is given in Table 3, along with its 95 % confidence interval. The 95 % confidence intervals in Table 3 are wide, showing the imprecision of the percentage estimate, in this small sample. Nonetheless, it is clear that the intervention had the greatest impact on the first domain: Knowledge of GDM with 70 % of women improving their knowledge or staying at 100 % post-intervention. The smallest change was in the area of self-management and little more than one third of women improved or stayed at 100 %.

The initial testing identified a number of questions that participants particularly misunderstood (Fig. 2) and which were answered incorrectly more often in the post-test than in the pre-test. A number of factors contributed to this situation. For example, question 1 (Fig. 2) had more than one correct answer and participants were likely to identify being overweight and specific ethnicity as predictors of GDM, but did not recognise maternal age and parity >3, as predictors. For question 2, many women were unable to recognise the food value of butter and very often choose (a.) *protein* or (e.) *I don't know.* In question 3, participants choose (b.) *should exercise more than women who do not have gestational diabetes* more often than (a.) *should take moderate exercise such as walking* and in question 4, many women identified one or two snacks as suitable for women with GDM, but not all.

In the final group of questions, results indicated that the majority of participants found the intervention acceptable and pertinent to their information needs around GDM (Table 4). Almost all (20/21) found the intervention easy/fairly easy to use and useful/fairly useful. Comments in the final free text question provide some additional insights and participants indicated a number of improvements that they would like, including larger pictures (10 out of the sample of 21 women (10/21), more ethnic specific foods (11/21), less ethnic specific foods (7/21), less text (3/21), more information (6/21), including specifically recipes suitable for GDM. Areas the women identified as particularly useful were the 'healthy shopping list' and information about 'what to do if I am still hungry?

Discussion

This paper reports on the development and initial testing of a new intervention, which aims to support women, from multi-ethnic and low health literacy backgrounds, to self-manage their GDM. This intervention has been developed in English initially and there are plans to later amend the program for the Vietnamese community, who have low levels of English language fluency. The aim of this stage of the project was to test the acceptability, ease of use, and usefulness of the intervention for the target population. We also aimed to identify any issues with the website and content and to ascertain both the improvements necessary and the feasibility of proceeding to a clinical trial. Overall, the findings suggest that women found the intervention useful and easy to use. The testing also revealed a number of areas that were effective at promoting greater knowledge scores and a further number of areas that required some improvement. Both of these findings are discussed below.

In the first instance, the intervention proved effective at increasing women's knowledge scores. The largest improvement occurred in domain 1: Knowledge of GDM and over 70 % of women improved their knowledge scores or stayed at 100 % post-intervention. This is an important effect as knowledge acquisition is established as a necessary first step in understanding and motivation

Table 2 Knowledge scores by education level

		Education				Total
		11 years or fewer - Not completed high school		More than 12 years - Completed high school		
GDM score change from pre to post*	Improved or stayed at 100 %		7		5	12
		87.5 %		55.6 %		70.6 %
	Stayed the same if below 100 %, or worsened		1		4	5
		12.5 %		44.4 %		29.4 %
	Total		8		9	17
		100.0 %		100.0 %		100.0 %
Food score change from pre to post**	Improved or stayed at 100 %		6		3	9
		66.7 %		33.3 %		50.0 %
	Stayed the same if below 100 %, or worsened		3		6	9
		33.3 %		66.7 %		50.0 %
	Total		9		9	18
		100.0 %		100.0 %		100.0 %
Self-management score change from pre to post***	Improved or stayed at 100 %		5		2	7
		55.6 %		20.0 %		36.8 %
	Stayed the same if below 100 %, or worsened		4		8	12
		44.4 %		80.0 %		63.2 %
	Total		9		10	19
		100.0 %		100.0 %		100.0 %

*Fisher's Exact test *P*-value for an association between GDM score improvement and Education = 0.294
**Fisher's Exact test *P*-value for an association between Food score improvement and Education = 0.347
***Fisher's Exact test *P*-value for an association between Self-management score improvement and Education = 0.170

for behavioural change [39]. Moreover, a number of prior studies indicate that women with GDM often complain that the information they receive is insufficient, incomplete or does not meet their needs [11, 33, 40]. Participants in these studies indicate that their efforts to self-manage their GDM are often frustrated by a lack of such knowledge [10, 11]. Feedback in this study suggests that our intervention assists by providing material that participants consider useful and accessible.

In the second domain, knowledge of food, there was a modest improvement in knowledge scores, although the improvement was less than anticipated. This finding may in part be explained by two factors. Firstly, a number of women answered question 2 (Fig. 2, food value of butter) incorrectly, and the percentage getting the question wrong increased considerably in the post-test, which had a negative impact on overall improvement scores. This finding may relate to the fact that many women in the area do not use butter for cooking or food preparation, and therefore may be unfamiliar with this food. However, this explanation does not explain why scores disimproved so markedly from pre-test to post-test. For the future, we plan to simplify and change this question to butter/oil/ghee, which is more in line with local cooking practices. Secondly, a further explanation of repeated incorrect answers about food values may reflect entrenched cultural beliefs about food, and this is something that requires further exploration. In particular, a qualitative exploration of food beliefs and taboos is planned among pregnant women, from specific ethnicities, in our area.

The smallest improvement was recorded in the third domain, knowledge of self-management, where little more than one third of women improved their knowledge scores or remained at 100 %. This finding is in part

Table 3 Knowledge scores composite

	Percentage of sample who improved or stayed at 100 % correct post-intervention	95 % Confidence interval
GDM	70.6 %	(44.0 %, 89.7 %)
Food	50.0 %	(26.0 %, 74.0 %)
Self-management	36.8 %	(16.3 %, 61.6 %)

1. Women are more likely to develop gestational diabetes if they: **a. are overweight** **b. have had more than 3 children** **c. are over 30 years** **d. are from India, Asia or the Middle east** e. I don't know
2. Butter is mainly: a. protein b. carbohydrate **c. fat** d. mineral and vitamin e. I don't know
3. Women with gestational diabetes should: **a. take moderate exercise such as walking** b. exercise more than women who do not have gestational diabetes c. rest more than women who do not have gestational diabetes d. I don't know
4. Which of the following snacks are suitable for the woman with gestational diabetes: a. An apple b. Small handful nuts c. Low fat yoghurt d. Cracker and low fat cheese **e. Any of the above**

Fig. 2 Questions commonly misunderstood

explained by the misinterpretation of question 3 (Fig. 2), where many women got the answer correct in the first instance and then incorrect in the post-test. Based on this feedback, we plan to amend the text about exercise both in the intervention and in the questionnaire. Participants also got some questions, with more than one correct answer, partially correct, by identifying one variable rather than all correct variables. As these questions required identification of all correct variables to score, this partial knowledge was not recorded. Question 4 (Fig. 2) provides a good example and many women identified one or two healthy snacks but not all four. Nonetheless, these questions provide valuable feedback and allow identification of areas where the required knowledge uptake is insufficient. For example, for question 4, most participants recognise an apple and yoghurt as appropriate snacks, while many do not recognise nuts or crackers and cheese as appropriate. To address this deficit, we may need to further clarify the section, in the intervention, outlining snacks and perhaps add some additional ethnic specific snacks to the questionnaire.

Table 4 Ease of use

Easy to use		n	Percent %
	Very easy	18	85.7
	Fairly easy	2	9.5
	Quite difficult	1	4.7
	Total	21	100 %
Useful		n	Percent %
	Very useful	18	85.7
	Fairly useful	2	9.5
	Not very useful	1	4.7
	Total	21	100 %

Greater improvement of scores were seen among women with lower rather than higher educational levels. It is not immediately clear what this finding means, however, one possible explanation is that women of lower educational levels may be the most likely to benefit from this intervention, as they are the most likely to have low levels of health literacy [41]. They may also have limited access or ability to decipher health information [42]. Thus, the intervention may offer more support for learning for women with lower educational levels compared to higher levels.

In the literature, fostering knowledge and beliefs, is seen as a necessary first step to health related behavioural change [39] and self-management skill development [43]. This approach is also considered to be in line with adult learning theory [39], where the individual is empowered and motivated by understanding the importance of change [26]. Similarly, a number of studies have found that women are highly motivated to adopt healthy behaviours, in pregnancy to protect the unborn baby [44]. This effect may be even stronger during GDM self-management, if women fully understand the implications of GDM for the child's future health [8, 45]. Additionally, knowledge of food values, and the basic constituents of a healthy diet, have been positively associated with good nutritional practices, such as eating sufficient fruit and vegetables [46, 47]. Worsley suggests that education may play a part in effecting such behavioural change by encouraging a different set of beliefs about food ([46], p. 583).

However, caution is also advised and a number of studies suggest that knowledge of prudent health behaviours alone, is not sufficient to bring about behavioural change [9, 46, 48]. These studies recognise that dietary changes are difficult and impacted by many factors such as food preferences, cravings and social eating [9] and socio-economic circumstance, food habits and food availability [48].

Strengths and limitations

The aim of this basic one-group pre-test/post-test study was to explore the impact of the newly developed intervention on knowledge scores in three domains: Knowledge of GDM; food values, and GDM self-management principles. The study has been successful in that it has provided useful feedback that will enable the researchers to improve the intervention. In particular, we plan to clarify the content, amend inconsistencies and ambiguities and add additional information where indicated. These efforts will lead to an improvement of the intervention and a tailoring of the intervention to the needs of the target population. Nonetheless, although the study has achieved the stated aims, some limitations are also present and the small sample size has limited the value of statistical evaluation. For example, p values are very large and although differences in knowledge scores are evident, a larger sample size is required in order to be confident that the associations observed are not just chance. Similarly, there were more women who improved in the *11 years or fewer* education group compared to *more than 12 years* and the meaning of this finding might also be clearer in a larger sample. Finally, only women who spoke conversational English were eligible to participate in this initial testing of the intervention, and this is a limitation that we aim to address in the next phase of the project.

Implications for practice

The development and testing of the intervention described here has a number of important implications for practice. In the first instance, the demographic profile of GDM, with increased risk factors for multi-ethnic, low socio-economic and poorly educated women, highlights the need for culturally acceptable educational resources pitched at a low level of literacy. Addressing this need is very important as rates of GDM are continuing to increase dramatically in these groups with potentially devastating consequences for mothers and infants and multi-generational effects for families.

Conclusion

In conclusion, the intervention was effective at improving knowledge scores for women with GDM in the three tested domains: Knowledge of GDM; knowledge of food; and, knowledge of GDM self-management principles, and also that the intervention is a useful adjunct to the routine education sessions women with GDM attend, in our area. Testing has revealed a number of issues, such as ambiguity of information around physical exercise in GDM and some foods. These issues require attention prior to proceeding to a trial.

Competing interests

The authors declare that they have no competing interests.

Authors' contributions

MCO conceived of the study, and participated in its design and coordination and drafted the manuscript. CS contributed to the day to day management of the project and contributed intellectually to the manuscript development. HM and GK advised and assisted with development of the project, data collection and analysis and contributed intellectually to the manuscript. All authors read and approved the final manuscript.

Acknowledgements

Many thanks to dietetics team at Western Health, Sunshine Hospital for their assistance, recommendations and advice during the development of dietary resources. Thanks also to the participants who were involved in testing the intervention. This study was made possible through funding from the Ian Potter Foundation, Melbourne, grant reference 201200017.

Author details

[1]Nursing and Midwifery, College of Health and Biomedicine, Victoria University, St Alban's Campus, PO Box 14228, Melbourne 8001, Australia. [2]Western Health, Diabetes Education Service, Western Hospital, Gordon St., Footscray, VIC 3011, Australia.

References

1. Australian Institute of Health and Welfare (AIHW). Diabetes in pregnancy: its impact on Australian women and their babies. Canberra: AIHW; 2010.
2. Carolan M. Gestational diabetes mellitus among women born in South East Asia: A review of the evidence. Midwifery. 2013;29(9):1019–26.
3. Carolan M, Davey MA, Biro MA, Kealy M. Maternal age, ethnicity and gestational diabetes mellitus. Midwifery. 2012;28(6):778–83.
4. Cheung NW. The management of gestational diabetes. Vasc Health Risk Manag. 2009;5:153–64.
5. Yogev Y, Visser GHA. Obesity, gestational diabetes and pregnancy outcome. Semin Fetal Neonatal Med. 2009;14(2):77–84.
6. Glastras S, Fulcher G. Guidelines for the management of gestational diabetes in pregnancy. Clin Pract. 2012;9(2):161–70.
7. Persson M, Winkvist A, Mogren I. 'From stun to gradual balance'- women's experiences of living with gestational diabetes mellitus. Scand J Caring Sci. 2010;24(3):454–62.
8. Carolan M. Women's experiences of gestational diabetes self-management: A qualitative study. Midwifery. 2013;29(6):637–45.
9. Hui AL, Sevenhuysen G, Harvey D, Salamon E. Food choice decision-making by women with gestational diabetes. Can J Diabetes. 2014;38(1):26–31.
10. Carolan M, Gill GK, Steele C. Women's experiences of factors that facilitate or inhibit gestational diabetes self-management. BMC Pregnancy Childbirth. 2012;12:99.
11. Evans MK, O'Brien B. Gestational diabetes: the meaning of an at-risk pregnancy. Qual Health Res. 2005;15(1):66–81.
12. Chung JH, Voss KJ, Caughey AB, Wing DA, Henderson EJ, Major CA. Role of patient education level in predicting macrosomia among women with gestational diabetes mellitus. J Perinatol. 2006;26(6):328–32.
13. Zanchetta MS, Poureslami IM. Health literacy within the reality of immigrants' culture and language. Can J Public Health. 2006;97 Suppl 2:S26–30.
14. Pope C. Addressing limited English proficiency and disparities for hispanic postpartum women. J Obstet Gynecol Neonatal Nurs. 2005;34(4):512–20.
15. Mendelson S, McNeese-Smith D, Koniak-Griffin D, Nyamathi A, Lu MC. A community-based parish nurse intervention program for Mexican American women with gestational diabetes. JOGNN/NAACOG. 2008;37(4):415–25.
16. Hoppichler F, Lechleitner M. Counseling programs and the outcome of gestational diabetes in Austrian and Mediterranean Turkish women. Patient Educ Couns. 2001;45(4):271–4.
17. Rosal MC, Goins KV, Carbone ET, Cortes DE. Views and preferences of low-literate hispanics regarding diabetes education: Results of formative research. Health Educ Behav. 2004;31(3):388–405.
18. Negarandeh R, Mahmoodi H, Noktehdan H, Heshmat R, Shakibazadeh E. Teach back and pictorial image educational strategies on knowledge about diabetes and medication/dietary adherence among low health literate patients with type 2 diabetes. Prim Care Diabetes. 2013;7(2):111–8.
19. Rosal MC, Ockene IS, Restrepo A, White MJ, Borg A, Olendzki B, et al. Randomized trial of a literacy-sensitive, culturally tailored diabetes self-management intervention for low-income Latinos: Latinos en control. Diabetes Care. 2011;34(4):838–44.
20. ABS: Australian Bureau of Statistics. 2033.0.55.001 - Census of Population and Housing: Socio-Economic Indexes for Areas (SEIFA). Canberra: Australian Bureau of Statistics; 2006.
21. Department of Human Services. Well being and lifestyle - the evidence 2006, North West Region. Melbourne, Victoria: Department of Human Services; 2008.
22. INWMML. Inner North West Melbourne Medicare Local. Inner North West Melbourne Medicare Local Whole of Region Needs Assessment. 2012.
23. Department of Human Services. Western Metropolitan Region Health and Social Wellbeing Profile. Public Health and Strategic Melbourne 2002 [cited 2013 25 February 2013]; Available from: http://www.health.vic.gov.au/archive/archive2014/nphp/publications/phpractice/phpractice_project/findingsandrecs.pdf.

24. Homko CJ, Sivan E, Reece EA. The impact of self-monitoring of blood glucose on self-efficacy and pregnancy outcomes in women with diet-controlled gestational diabetes. Diabetes Educat. 2002;28(3):435–43.
25. Murphy A, Guilar A, Donat D. Nutrition education for women with newly diagnosed gestational diabetes mellitus: small-group vs. individual counselling. Can J Diabetes. 2004;28(2):147–51.
26. Speck M. Best practice in professional development for sustained educational change. Spring: ERS Spectrum; 1996. p. 33–41.
27. Knowles MS. Andragogy, not pedagogy. Adult Leader. 1968;16(10):350–2. 10.
28. Leventhal H, Meyer D, Nerenz D. The common-sense representation of illness danger. Contributions to medical psychology. 2nd ed. New York: Pergamon; 1980.
29. Hagger MS, Orbell S. A meta-analytic review of the common-sense model of illness representations. Psychol Health. 2003;18(2):141–84.
30. Polit DF, Beck CT. Nursing Research: **Generating and Assessing Evidence for Nursing Practice**. 9th ed. Philadelphia: Wolters Kluwer/ Lippincott; 2012.
31. Wallström A, Frisman GH. Facilitating early recovery of bowel motility after colorectal surgery: A systematic review. J Clin Nurs. 2014;23(1–2):24–44.
32. Wilkinson A, Whitehead L, Ritchie L. Factors influencing the ability to self-manage diabetes for adults living with type 1 or 2 diabetes. Int J Nurs Stud. 2014;51(1):111–22.
33. Carolan M, Steele C, Margetts H. Knowledge of gestational diabetes among a multi-ethnic cohort in Australia. Midwifery. 2010;26(6):579–88.
34. Dunn SM, Bryson JM, Hoskins PL, Alford JB, Handelsman DJ, Turtle JR. Development of the diabetes knowledge (DKN) scales: forms DKNA, DKNB, and DKNC. Diabetes Care. 1984;7(1):36–41.
35. Gastrich MD, Peck S, Janevic T, Bachmann G, Lotwala N, Siyam A. Gestational diabetes mellitus: An educational opportunity. J Diabetes Nurs. 2013;17(6):220–4.
36. Nicolas-Rocca TS, Schooley B, Joo SJ. Design and development of a patient-centered e-health system to improve patient understanding at discharge. Comm Assoc Inform Syst. 2014;34(1):453–76.
37. Yin HS, Gupta RS, Tomopoulos S, Wolf MS, Mendelsohn AL, Antler L. Readability, suitability, and characteristics of asthma action plans: Examination of factors that may impair understanding. Pediatrics. 2013;131(1):e116–26.
38. Preacher KJ, Briggs, NE. Calculation for Fisher's Exact Test: An interactive calculation tool for Fisher's exact probability test for 2 × 2 tables. Available from: http://www.quantpsy.org/fisher/fisher.htm. 2001.
39. Porcheret M, Main C, Croft P, McKinley R, Hassell A, Dziedzic K. Development of a behaviour change intervention: A case study on the practical application of theory. Implement Sci. 2014;9(1):42.
40. Heuberger R. Increasing empathy, knowledge, and skills regarding gestational diabetes. Top Clin Nutr. 2010;25(3):250–5.
41. Nutbeam D. Health literacy as a public health goal: a challenge for contemporary health education and communication strategies into the 21st century. Health Promot Int. 2000;15(3):259–67.
42. Morahan-Martin JM. How internet users find, evaluate, and Use online health information: a cross-cultural review. CyberPsychology and Behavior. 2004;7(5):497–510.
43. Ryan P. Integrated theory of health behavior change: background and intervention development. Clinical nurse specialist CNS. 2009;23(3):161–70. quiz 71–72.
44. Bassett-Gunter RL, Levy-Milne R, Naylor PJ, Symons Downs D, Benoit C, Warburton DER. Oh baby! Motivation for healthy eating during parenthood transitions: A longitudinal examination with a theory of planned behavior perspective. Int J Behav Nutr Phys Act. 2013;10:88.
45. Nielsen KK, Kapur A, Damm P, de Courten M, Bygbjerg IC. From screening to postpartum follow-up - the determinants and barriers for gestational diabetes mellitus (GDM) services, a systematic review. BMC Pregnancy and Childbirth. 2014;14(1).
46. Worsley A. Nutrition knowledge and food consumption: can nutrition knowledge change food behaviour? Asia Pac J Clin Nutr. 2002;11 Suppl 3:S579–85.
47. Wardle J, Parmenter K, Waller J. Nutrition knowledge and food intake. Appetite. 2002;34:269–75.
48. Rutherford L, Reid S. Knowledge, attitudes and motivations to health: A module of the Scottish Health Survey 2008–2011. Edinburgh: NHS Health Scotland; 2013.

Permissions

All chapters in this book were first published in P&C, by BioMed Central; hereby published with permission under the Creative Commons Attribution License or equivalent. Every chapter published in this book has been scrutinized by our experts. Their significance has been extensively debated. The topics covered herein carry significant findings which will fuel the growth of the discipline. They may even be implemented as practical applications or may be referred to as a beginning point for another development.

The contributors of this book come from diverse backgrounds, making this book a truly international effort. This book will bring forth new frontiers with its revolutionizing research information and detailed analysis of the nascent developments around the world.

We would like to thank all the contributing authors for lending their expertise to make the book truly unique. They have played a crucial role in the development of this book. Without their invaluable contributions this book wouldn't have been possible. They have made vital efforts to compile up to date information on the varied aspects of this subject to make this book a valuable addition to the collection of many professionals and students.

This book was conceptualized with the vision of imparting up-to-date information and advanced data in this field. To ensure the same, a matchless editorial board was set up. Every individual on the board went through rigorous rounds of assessment to prove their worth. After which they invested a large part of their time researching and compiling the most relevant data for our readers.

The editorial board has been involved in producing this book since its inception. They have spent rigorous hours researching and exploring the diverse topics which have resulted in the successful publishing of this book. They have passed on their knowledge of decades through this book. To expedite this challenging task, the publisher supported the team at every step. A small team of assistant editors was also appointed to further simplify the editing procedure and attain best results for the readers.

Apart from the editorial board, the designing team has also invested a significant amount of their time in understanding the subject and creating the most relevant covers. They scrutinized every image to scout for the most suitable representation of the subject and create an appropriate cover for the book.

The publishing team has been an ardent support to the editorial, designing and production team. Their endless efforts to recruit the best for this project, has resulted in the accomplishment of this book. They are a veteran in the field of academics and their pool of knowledge is as vast as their experience in printing. Their expertise and guidance has proved useful at every step. Their uncompromising quality standards have made this book an exceptional effort. Their encouragement from time to time has been an inspiration for everyone.

The publisher and the editorial board hope that this book will prove to be a valuable piece of knowledge for researchers, students, practitioners and scholars across the globe.

List of Contributors

Margareta Persson
School of Health and Social Studies, Dalarna University, Falun, Sweden
Department of Nursing, Umeå University, SE - 901 87 Umeå, Sweden

Anna Winkvist
Department of Internal Medicine and Clinical Nutrition, Sahlgrenska Academy, University of Gothenburg, Gothenburg, Sweden

Ingrid Mogren
Department of Clinical Sciences, Obstetrics and Gynecology, Umeå University, Umeå, Sweden

Helena H. Hauta-alus, Elisa M. Holmlund-Suila, Maria Enlund-Cerullo, Jenni Rosendahl, Saara M. Valkama, Otto M. Helve, Timo K. Hytinantti and Sture Andersson
Children's Hospital, University of Helsinki and Helsinki University Hospital, Biomedicum 2 C, 00020 HUS Helsinki, Finland

Heli T. Viljakainen
Children's Hospital, University of Helsinki and Helsinki University Hospital, Biomedicum 2 C, 00020 HUS Helsinki, Finland
Folkhälsan Research Center, Haartmaninkatu 8, 00014 Helsinki, Finland

Outi M. Mäkitie
Children's Hospital, University of Helsinki and Helsinki University Hospital, Biomedicum 2 C, 00020 HUS Helsinki, Finland
Folkhälsan Research Center, Haartmaninkatu 8, 00014 Helsinki, Finland
Center for Molecular Medicine, Karolinska Institute and Clinical Genetics, Karolinska University Hospital, 171 76 Solna, Stockholm, Sweden

Michela Meregaglia and Helen Banks
CERGAS (Centre for Research on Health and Social Care Management), Bocconi University, Via Roentgen 1, 20136 Milan, Italy

Livia Dainelli and Patrick Detzel
Nestlé Research Center, Nestec SA, Route du Jorat 57, 1000 Lausanne, Switzerland

Chiara Benedetto
Department of Gynecology & Obstetrics, S. Anna Hospital, University of Turin, Via Ventimiglia 3, 10126 Turin, Italy

Giovanni Fattore
CERGAS (Centre for Research on Health and Social Care Management), Bocconi University, Via Roentgen 1, 20136 Milan, Italy
Department of Policy Analysis and Public Management, Bocconi University, Via Roentgen 1, 20136 Milan, Italy

Claudia Chi and Cherie Choong
Department of Obstetrics & Gynaecology, National University Hospital, Singapore 119074, Singapore

See Ling Loy and Jerry Kok Yen Chan
Department of Reproductive Medicine, KK Women's and Children's Hospital, Singapore 229899, Singapore
Duke-NUS Medical School, Singapore 169857, Singapore

Kok Hian Tan
Department of Maternal Fetal Medicine, KK Women's and Children's Hospital, Singapore 229899, Singapore

Shiao-Yng Chan and Yap-Seng Chong
Department of Obstetrics & Gynaecology, National University Hospital, Singapore 119074, Singapore
Singapore Institute for Clinical Sciences, Agency for Science, Technology and Research (A*STAR), Singapore 117609, Singapore
Department of Obstetrics & Gynaecology, Yong Loo Lin School of Medicine, National University of Singapore, National University Health System, Singapore 119228, Singapore

Shirong Cai
Department of Obstetrics & Gynaecology, Yong Loo Lin School of Medicine, National University of Singapore, National University Health System, Singapore 119228, Singapore

Shu E. Soh
Singapore Institute for Clinical Sciences, Agency for Science, Technology and Research (A*STAR), Singapore 117609, Singapore
Department of Paediatrics, Yong Loo Lin School of Medicine, National University of Singapore, Singapore 119228, Singapore

Fabian Yap
Duke-NUS Medical School, Singapore 169857, Singapore
Department of Paediatrics, KK Women's and Children's Hospital, Singapore 229899, Singapore
Lee Kong Chian School of Medicine, Nanyang Technological University, Singapore 636921, Singapore

Peter D. Gluckman
Singapore Institute for Clinical Sciences, Agency for Science, Technology and Research (A*STAR), Singapore 117609, Singapore
Liggins Institute, University of Auckland, Auckland 1142, New Zealand

Keith M. Godfrey
Medical Research Council Lifecourse Epidemiology Unit, University of Southampton, Southampton SO16 6YD, UK
National Institute for Health Research Southampton Biomedical Research Centre, University of Southampton and University Hospital Southampton National Health Service Foundation Trust, Southampton SO16 6YD, UK

Lynette Pei-Chi Shek
Department of Paediatrics, Yong Loo Lin School of Medicine, National University of Singapore, Singapore 119228, Singapore
Khoo Teck Puat-National University Children's Medical Institute, National University Hospital, National University Health System, Singapore 119074, Singapore

Michael S. Kramer
Department of Obstetrics & Gynaecology, Yong Loo Lin School of Medicine, National University of Singapore, National University Health System, Singapore 119228, Singapore
Department of Pediatrics, McGill University Faculty of Medicine, 845 Rue Sherbrooke Ouest, Montreal, QC H3A 0G4, Canada
Department of Epidemiology, Biostatistics and Occupational Health, McGill University Faculty of Medicine, 845 Rue Sherbrooke Ouest, Montreal, QC H3A 0G4, Canada

Ruth Martis, Julie Brown and Caroline A. Crowther
Liggins Institute, The University of Auckland, Auckland 1142, New Zealand

Judith McAra-Couper
Faculty of Health & Environmental Sciences, AUT, Auckland University of Technology, Private Bag 92006, Auckland 1142, New Zealand

Abdulrahman Al-Ajlan
Department of Clinical Lab Sciences, College of Applied Medical Sciences, King Saud University, Riyadh 11451, Kingdom of Saudi Arabia

Sara Al-Musharaf
Division of Metabolic and Vascular Health, University of Warwick, CV47AL, Coventry, UK

Soundararajan Krishnaswamy and Kaiser Wani
Prince Mutaib Chair for Biomarkers of Osteoporosis, Department of Biochemistry, College of Science, King Saud University, Riyadh 11451, Saudi Arabia

Naji J. Aljohani
Obesity, Endocrine and Metabolism Center, King Fahad Medical City, Faculty of Medicine, King Saud bin Abdulaziz University for Health Sciences, Riyadh 11525, Saudi Arabia

A. Afrah Alharbi, Buthaynah A. Alraqebah and Nasser M. Al-Daghri
Prince Mutaib Chair for Biomarkers of Osteoporosis, Department of Biochemistry, College of Science, King Saud University, Riyadh 11451, Saudi Arabia
Obesity, Endocrine and Metabolism Center, King Fahad Medical City, Faculty of Medicine, King Saud bin Abdulaziz University for Health Sciences, Riyadh 11525, Saudi Arabia

Amal Al-Serehi
Maternal-Fetal Medicine Department, King Fahad Medical City, Riyadh 59406, Saudi Arabia

Aisha Mansoor Ali
Diabetes Care Center, King Salman Bin Abdulaziz Hospital, Riyadh, Saudi Arabia

Eman Sheshah
Obstetrics and Gynaecology Department, King Salman Bin Abdulaziz Hospital, Riyadh 11564, Saudi Arabia

Mona A. Fouda and Naemah M. Alshingetti
Department of Medicine, Endocrinology Division, College of Medicine, King Saud University, Riyadh 11461, Saudi Arabia

Iqbah Z. Turkistani and Gawaher Al-Saeed
Department of Obstetrics and Gynecology, College of Medicine, King Saud University, Riyadh 11461, Saudi Arabia

Jens H. Stupin, Joachim W. Dudenhausen and Wolfgang Henrich
Clinic of Obstetrics, Charité - Universitätsmedizin Berlin, corporate member of Freie Universität Berlin, Humboldt-Universität zu Berlin, and Berlin Institute of Health, Campus Virchow-Klinikum, Berlin, Germany

Raffael Ott, Kerstin Melchior, Rebecca C. Rancourt, Karen Schellong, Thomas Ziska and Andreas Plagemann
Clinic of Obstetrics, Charité - Universitätsmedizin Berlin, corporate member of Freie Universität Berlin, Humboldt-Universität zu Berlin, and Berlin Institute of Health, Campus Virchow-Klinikum, Berlin, Germany
Division of 'Experimental Obstetrics, Charité - Universitätsmedizin Berlin, corporate member of Freie Universität Berlin, Humboldt-Universität zu Berlin, and Berlin Institute of Health, Campus Virchow-Klinikum, Berlin, Germany

Andrea Loui and Elisabeth Eilers
Department of Neonatology, Charité - Universitätsmedizin Berlin, corporate member of Freie Universität Berlin, Humboldt-Universität zu Berlin, and Berlin Institute of Health, Campus Virchow-Klinikum, Berlin, Germany

Hugo Ingar, Walter Castillo and Rina Zumaeta
Instituto Nacional Materno Perinatal de Lima, Lima, Perú

Percy Pacora
Departamentos de Medicina y Ginecología y Obstetricia, Universidad Nacional Mayor de San Marcos, Lima, Perú

Gloria T. Larrabure-Torrealva and Pedro A. Mascaro
Instituto Nacional Materno Perinatal de Lima, Lima, Perú
Departamentos de Medicina y Ginecología y Obstetricia, Universidad Nacional Mayor de San Marcos, Lima, Perú

Stephanie Martinez, Miguel Angel Luque-Fernandez, Bizu Gelaye and Michelle A. Williams
Department of Epidemiology, Harvard T.H. Chan School of Public Health, 677 Huntington Avenue, Kresge 505F, Boston, MA 02115, USA

Mirtha Grande and Vicky Motta
Asociación Civil Proyectos en Salud, A.C. PROESA, Lima, Perú

Sixto E. Sanchez
Asociación Civil Proyectos en Salud, A.C. PROESA, Lima, Perú
Facultad de Medicina, Universidad Particular San Martin de Porres, Lima, Peru

Hee Joong Lee
Department of Obstetrics & Gynecology, College of Medicine, The Catholic University of Korea, Seoul, Republic of Korea

Errol Norwitz
Department of Obstetrics & Gynecology, Tufts University School of Medicine, Boston, MA, USA

Banghyun Lee
Department of Obstetrics and Gynecology, Hallym University Kangdong Sacred Heart Hospital, 150, Seongan-ro, Gangdong-gu, Seoul, Republic of Korea

Xiyan He, Xueping Yang, Nan Guo and Yan Mao
Department of Obstetrics, Gansu Provincial Hospital, Lanzhou, China

Xiaotong Sun
The First Clinical Medical College, Lanzhou University, Lanzhou, China
Department of Obstetrics, Gansu Provincial Hospital, Lanzhou, China

Tao Qu and Xianghong Xu
Department of Biotherapy Center, Gansu Provincial Hospital, Lanzhou, China

Xiaodong Sun
Department of Endocrinology, Affiliated Hospital of Weifang Medical University, Weifang, China

Xuehong Zhang
The First Clinical Medical College, Lanzhou University, Lanzhou, China
The Reproductive Medicine Special Hospital of the First Hospital of Lanzhou University, Lanzhou, China
Key Laboratory for Reproductive Medicine and Embryo of Gansu, Lanzhou, China

Weihua Wang
Houston Fertility Laboratory, Houston, TX, USA

Natarajan Padmapriya, Shirong Cai and Iris Shen Zhe
Department of Obstetrics & Gynaecology, Yong Loo Lin School of Medicine, National University of Singapore, Singapore, Singapore

Jonathan Y. Bernard
Singapore Institute for Clinical Sciences, Agency for Science and Technology Research (A*STAR), Singapore, Singapore

Yap-Seng Chong
Department of Obstetrics & Gynaecology, Yong Loo Lin School of Medicine, National University of Singapore, Singapore, Singapore
Singapore Institute for Clinical Sciences, Agency for Science and Technology Research (A*STAR), Singapore, Singapore

Shen Liang
Biostatistics Unit, Yong Loo Lin School of Medicine, National University of Singapore, Singapore, Singapore

See Ling Loy
KK Women's and Children's Hospital, Singapore, Singapore

Kenneth Kwek and Jerry Kok Yen Chan
KK Women's and Children's Hospital, Singapore, Singapore
Duke-National University of Singapore, Singapore, Singapore

Keith M. Godfrey
Medical Research Council Lifecourse Epidemiology Unit, Southampton, UK
NIHR Southampton Biomedical Research Centre, University of Southampton, Southampton, UK

Peter D. Gluckman
Singapore Institute for Clinical Sciences, Agency for Science and Technology Research (A*STAR), Singapore, Singapore
Liggins Institute, University of Auckland, Auckland, New Zealand

Seang Mei Saw
Saw Swee Hock School of Public Health, National University of Singapore, Singapore, Singapore

Falk Müller-Riemenschneider
Saw Swee Hock School of Public Health, National University of Singapore, Singapore, Singapore
Institute for Social Medicine, Epidemiology and Health Economics, Charite University Medical Centre, Berlin, Germany

Ib C. Bygbjerg and Thilde Rheinländer
Department of Public Health, University of Copenhagen, Oester Farimagsgade 5, 1014 Copenhagen, Denmark

Karoline Kragelund Nielsen
Department of Public Health, University of Copenhagen, Oester Farimagsgade 5, 1014 Copenhagen, Denmark
Steno Diabetes Center Copenhagen, Niels Steensens Vej 6, 2820 Gentofte, Denmark

Anil Kapur
World Diabetes Foundation, Brogaardsvej 70, 2820 Gentofte, Denmark

Peter Damm
Center for Pregnant Women with Diabetes, Department of Obstetrics, Rigshospitalet, The Institute of Clinical Medicine, Faculty of Health and Medical Sciences, University of Copenhagen, Blegdamsvej 9, 2100 Copenhagen, Denmark

Veerasamy Seshiah
Dr. Seshiah Diabetes Research Institute and Dr. Balaji Diabetes Care Centre, 729 Poonamallee High Road, Aminjikarai, Chennai, Tamil Nadu 600029, India

A. Jenna Beckham
Department of Obstetrics and Gynecology, University of North Carolina School of Medicine, Chapel Hill, NC, USA

La-Shell Johnson
Partnerships for Women's Endocrine and Reproductive Health (PoWER), University of North Carolina School of Medicine, Chapel Hill, NC, USA

Wanda K. Nicholson
Department of Obstetrics and Gynecology, University of North Carolina School of Medicine, Chapel Hill, NC, USA
Partnerships for Women's Endocrine and Reproductive Health (PoWER), University of North Carolina School of Medicine, Chapel Hill, NC, USA
Diabetes and Obesity Core, Center for Women's Health Research, University of North Carolina School of Medicine, Chapel Hill, NC, USA
The Diabetes Center, University of North Carolina School of Medicine, Chapel Hill, USA
Cecil G. Sheps Center for Health Services Research, University of North Carolina School of Medicine, Chapel Hill, NC, USA

Deborah Tate
Department of Nutrition, University of North Carolin School of Medicine, Chapel Hill, USA
Department of Health Behavior, University of North Carolina Gillings Global School of Public Health, Chapel Hill, USA
Program on Obesity Treatment, University of North Carolina Gillings Global School of Public Health, Chapel Hill, NC, USA

Karen Hatley and Molly Diamond
Department of Nutrition, University of North Carolin School of Medicine, Chapel Hill, USA
Program on Obesity Treatment, University of North Carolina Gillings Global School of Public Health, Chapel Hill, NC, USA

Sherri L. Green
Cecil G. Sheps Center for Health Services Research, University of North Carolina School of Medicine, Chapel Hill, NC, USA

Bettina Utz and Vincent De Brouwere
Public Health Department, Institute of Tropical Medicine (ITM), Nationalestraat 155, 2000 Antwerp, Belgium

Mikel Donazar-Ezcurra
Department of Preventive Medicine and Public Health, University of Navarra, C/Irunlarrea1, 31008 Pamplona, Navarra, Spain

Cristina López-del Burgo
Department of Preventive Medicine and Public Health, University of Navarra, C/Irunlarrea1, 31008 Pamplona, Navarra, Spain
IDISNA, Navarra's Health Research Institute, Pamplona, Navarra, Spain
Institute for Culture and Society, University of Navarra, Pamplona, Navarra, Spain

Maira Bes-Rastrollo
Department of Preventive Medicine and Public Health, University of Navarra, C/Irunlarrea1, 31008 Pamplona, Navarra, Spain
IDISNA, Navarra's Health Research Institute, Pamplona, Navarra, Spain
CIBERobn, Instituto de Salud Carlos III, Madrid, Spain

Sonak D. Pastakia
Department of Pharmacy Practice, Purdue Kenya Partnership, Eldoret 30100, Kenya

Benson Njuguna and Beryl Ajwang' Onyango
Department of Pharmacy, Moi Teaching and Referral Hospital, Eldoret 30100, Kenya

Sierra Washington
Department of Reproductive Medicine, University of California, San Diego, CA 92103, USA

Astrid Christoffersen-Deb
Department of Obstetrics & Gyneacology, University of Toronto, Toronto, ON M5G 1E2, Canada

Wycliffe K Kosgei
Division of Reproductive Health, Moi Teaching and Referral Hospital, Eldoret 30100, Kenya

Ponnusamy Saravanan
Department of Diabetes, Endocrinology & Metabolism, Warwick Medical School, University of Warwick, Coventry CV4 7AL, UK
Diabetes and Endocrine Centre, George Eliot Hospital, Nuneaton CV107DJ, UK

Andreas Beyerlein
Institute of Diabetes Research, Helmholtz Zentrum München, Neuherberg, Germany
Forschergruppe Diabetes der Technischen Universität München, Munich, Germany

Daniela Koller
Department of Health Services Management, Munich School of Management, Ludwig-Maximilians-Universität München, Munich, Germany

Werner Maier
German Center for Diabetes Research (DZD), Partner, Neuherberg, Germany
Institute of Health Economics and Health Care Management, Helmholtz Zentrum München, Neuherberg, Germany

Anette-Gabriele Ziegler
Institute of Diabetes Research, Helmholtz Zentrum München, Neuherberg, Germany
Forschergruppe Diabetes der Technischen Universität München, Munich, Germany
Forschergruppe Diabetes e.V. am Helmholtz Zentrum München, Munich, Germany
German Center for Diabetes Research (DZD), Partner, Neuherberg, Germany

Nicholas Lack
German Bavarian Quality Assurance Institute for Medical Care, Munich, Germany

Shimin Hu, Xin Huang and Hongzhuan Tan
Department of Epidemiology and Health Statistics, School of Public Health of Central South University, Changsha, Hunan 410007, PR China

Qian Liu
Department of Epidemiology and Health Statistics, School of Public Health of Central South University, Changsha, Hunan 410007, PR China
Criminal Investigation Division, Changsha Public Security Bureau, Hunan 410004, China

Shanshan Han
Australian Research Centre for Health of Women and Babies (ARCH), Robinson Research Institute, School of Medicine, Discipline of Obstetrics and Gynaecology, The University of Adelaide, 72 King William Road, North Adelaide 5006, South Australia, Australia

Philippa F. Middleton
Australian Research Centre for Health of Women and Babies (ARCH), Robinson Research Institute, School of Medicine, Discipline of Obstetrics and Gynaecology, The University of Adelaide, 72 King William Road, North Adelaide 5006, South Australia, Australia
Women's and Children's Health Research Institute, 72 King William Road, North Adelaide 5006, South Australia, Australia

Thach S. Tran
Garvan Institute of Medical Research, 384 Victoria Street,Darlinghurst 2010, NSW, Australia

Caroline A. Crowther
Australian Research Centre for Health of Women and Babies (ARCH), Robinson Research Institute, School of Medicine, Discipline of Obstetrics and Gynaecology, The University of Adelaide, 72 King William Road, North Adelaide 5006, South Australia, Australia
Liggins Institute, The University of Auckland, Victoria Street West, West Auckland 1142, Auckland, New Zealand

Katrien Benhalima, Karolien Robyns and Chantal Mathieu
Department of Endocrinology, UZ Gasthuisberg, KU Leuven, Herestraat 49, 3000 Leuven, Belgium

Frank Nobels, Paul Van Crombrugge and Natascha Deprez
Department of Endocrinology, OLV ziekenhuis Aalst-Asse-Ninove, Moorselbaan 164, 9300 Aalst, Belgium

Bruno Seynhave
Department of Obstetrics and Gynecology, OLV ziekenhuis Aalst-Asse-Ninove, Moorselbaan 164, 9300 Aalst, Belgium

Roland Devlieger and Johan Verhaeghe
Department of Obstetrics and Gynecology, UZ Gasthuisberg, KU Leuven, Herestraat 49, 3000 Leuven, Belgium

Mary Carolan-Olah
Nursing and Midwifery, College of Health and Biomedicine, Victoria University, St Alban's Campus, Melbourne 8001, Australia

Cheryl Steele and Gillian Krenzin
Western Health, Diabetes Education Service, Western Hospital, Gordon St., Footscray, VIC 3011, Australia

Index

CPSIA information can be obtained
at www.ICGtesting.com
Printed in the USA
LVHW062015100122
708212LV00002B/259